THE ENCYCLOPEDIA OF

BLINDNESS AND VISION IMPAIRMENT

Second Edition

THE ENCYCLOPEDIA OF

BLINDNESS AND VISION IMPAIRMENT

Second Edition

Jill Sardegna; Susan Shelly;
Allan Richard Rutzen, M.D.;
Scott M. Steidl, M.D., D.M.A.

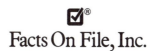
Facts On File, Inc.

Facts On File, Inc.
132 West 31st Street
New York NY 10001

Library of Congress Cataloging-in-Publication Data

The encyclopedia of blindness and vision impairment / Jill Sardegna . . . [et al.].—2nd ed.
p. cm. — (The Facts on File library of health and living)
First ed. cataloged under the m.e.: Sardegna, Jill according to AACR2.
Includes bibliographical references and index.
ISBN 0-8160-4280-2 (hardcover : alk. paper)
1. Blindness—Dictionaries. 2. Blind, Apparatus for the—Dictionaries.
3. Vision disorders—Dictionaries. 4. Visually handicapped—Dictionaries. I. Sardegna, Jill. II. Series.
[DNLM: 1. Vision Disorders—encyclopedias.]
RE91 .S27 2002
362.4′1′03—dc21   2001055653

Facts On File books are available at special discounts when purchased in bulk quantities for businesses, associations, institutions, or sales promotions. Please call our Special Sales Department in New York at (212) 967-8800 or (800) 322-8755.

You can find Facts On File on the World Wide Web at http://www.factsonfile.com

Text and cover design by Cathy Rincon

Printed in the United States of America

VB FOF 10 9 8 7 6 5 4 3 2 1

This book is printed on acid-free paper.

For
Emily and Jack
and
Mary and Julius

To Ann,
For the flowers in my life

CONTENTS

PREFACE TO THE FIRST EDITION

The Encyclopedia of Blindness and Vision Impairment is the first A-to-Z compendium on the subject of blindness and its inherent issues and topics. In more than 500 entries, the volume encompasses all aspects of blindness, including health issues, surgery and medications, social issues, myths and misconceptions, economic issues, education, adaptive aids, and organizations.

The encyclopedia can be of use to both the professional and lay person. For the lay person, we have tried to cover the issue with a minimum of technical jargon while accurately presenting the facts. Though not intended as a diagnostic tool, the text provides basic information to enable the user to make informed decisions with the help of his physician.

For the professional we have been thorough and avoided the simplistic, providing a handy guide covering aspects of vision impairment that may fall outside the particular individual's expertise.

We understand that a volume of this limited size may not meet every need of all who use it. Because of the concise format, we may have failed to include entries needed by some individuals or given other entries limited treatment. The book,

however, will prove useful as a basic guide and can serve as a reference to other sources of information. This volume includes a brief list of references at the end of each main article and a substantial bibliography.

In an effort to maximize limited space, we have occasionally attempted to save words by using the phrase "the blind" rather than more ideal alternatives such as "blind individuals" or "people who are blind." In a similar manner, the pronoun "he" appears in place of "he or she."

We have taken care to avoid significant errors of fact or interpretation. We accept, however, that in a volume of this scope and length, minor errors may have inadvertently been included. Changing statistics and daily medical breakthroughs may render the described current treatments and techniques outdated. We intend to remain current in the field and update the information in future editions.

—Jill Sardegna
San Jose, California

—T. Otis Paul, M.D.
San Francisco, California

PREFACE TO THE SECOND EDITION

Sight is one of human beings' most precious and yet most taken-for-granted gifts. Most of us routinely go about our daily business, relying on our sight to get around, complete our work, recognize friends and family, read, and generally make our lives easier and more enjoyable. Too often, only when we develop problems with our eyes or eyesight do we appreciate what a miracle the sense of sight is—or was.

The Encyclopedia of Blindness and Vision Impairment, Second Edition, is an A–Z compendium on the subject of blindness and issues and topics that relate to blindness. It addresses topics as far-ranging as the mechanics of the eye to traditional biases and prejudices against blind people. It seeks to help readers achieve a better understanding of how the eyes work and of the problems that can occur with the eyes and with vision. It also addresses laws affecting blind or visually impaired individuals, procedures and medicines used to treat vision problems, and diseases and disorders that can affect the eyes and their sight.

The encyclopedia is designed to be a functional tool for a consumer or patient looking for information relating to the eyes, as well as for the professional who is looking for information outside of his or her area of expertise. While the book is not intended to be used as a diagnostic tool, it should be useful in providing readers with information that can be used to make informed decisions in conjunction with their doctors.

A great deal has changed regarding blindness and vision problems since the publication of the previous edition more than 10 years ago. This new edition features many new entries, as well as many that have been significantly revised and updated. Among the new topics covered are increasingly common technologies and treatments such as keratotomy, LASIK surgery, and progressive addition lenses; newly recognized potential causes of vision damage, such as automobile air bags and shaken baby syndrome; and new options for the blind, such as Braille music, the Employment Assistance Referral Network, and guide horses. Also included are such recent milestones as the World Blind Sailing Championship and the Mount Everest expedition of Eric Weihenmayer, who became the first blind person to climb the legendary peak.

More than 100 entries have been updated to reflect new developments and information, particularly medical breakthroughs and current research, improvements and advances in existing devices and technology to aid the blind and vision-impaired, and changes to laws and government programs. Eleven appendixes have been completely redone to provide accurate information about various schools, organizations, associations, and publications of interest to the blind and vision impaired. All information included in this book is as current as possible. However, with rapidly occurring medical advances and constantly changing statistics, some of the information may be outdated, and minor errors may have inadvertently been included in this work.

—Susan Shelly
Shillington, Pennsylvania

—Allan Rutzen, M.D., and Scott Steidl, M.D.
University of Maryland School of Medicine

ACKNOWLEDGMENTS

Professional people working with all aspects of blindness and vision impairment generously gave of their time and talents to advise, counsel and inform us. We would like to acknowledge their contributions and offer our appreciation to Roger R. Cackler, County of Santa Clara Social Services, Dr. Peter D'Alena, Richard E. Dietl, The President's Committee on Employment of People with Disabilities, Juliet Esterly, Council of Rehabilitation Specialists, Dr. Deborah Gilden, Smith-Kettlewell Institute of Visual Sciences, Jessie A. Goehner, National Industries for the Blind, Joseph J. Hennessey, Western Blind Rehabilitation Center, E.K. Hudson, National Association for Parents of the Visually Impaired, Michelle Laboda, American Academy of Ophthalmology, Diane Lipton and Pam Stenberg, Disability Rights, Education, and Defense Fund, Joe Jackson, Media Access Office, Michael Larsen and Elizabeth Pomada, Sally Mangold, California State University, San Francisco, Marc Mauer, National Federation of the Blind, George McNally, United Cerebral Palsy, Michaelann R. Meehan, RP Foundation Fighting Blindness, Tom Moore, Eye Bank Association of America, Mary Ellen Mulholland and Dr. Sandra Timmerman, American Foundation for the Blind, Dr. Harry Murphy and Neil Scott, California State University, Northridge, Diane B. Piastro, Carol Ranalli, James C. Riley, California State Department of Rehabilitation, Arnay Rosenblat, National Multiple Sclerosis Society, Victoria Sheffield, Helen Keller International, Sandy Smith and Kenneth Stuckey, Perkins School for the Blind, Michael A. Thoennes, Foundation for the Junior Blind, Todd Turiff, National Society to Prevent Blindness, Heidi Williams, Vivian Younger, our friends at ABLEDATA, M.C. Migel Memorial Library and Information Center and National Rehabilitation Information Center. Our special thanks to our editors, Nicholas Bakalar and Kate Kelly.

Thanks also to Allan Rutzen, M.D., F.A.C.S., and Scott Steidl, M.D., of the University of Maryland School of Medicine; the Wyomissing Optometric Center in Wyomissing, Pennsylvania; and to Bert Holtje and Gene Brissie of James Peter Associates.

ENTRIES A–Z

abacus The abacus is used to teach mathematics skills to blind and visually impaired students. The Cranmer abacus is an adaptive device that has a backing behind the beads to prevent accidental movement or sliding.

It is used to add, subtract, multiply, and divide whole numbers and decimals. Calculations can be done faster on a talking computer or a calculator, but the Cranmer abacus is considered to be faster and easier to use than a BRAILLE WRITER, TAYLOR SLATE, or PEGBOARD. Schools for blind students offer courses in the use of the Cranmer abacus.

ABLEDATA A database that lists and describes products for people with disabilities. It is funded by the National Institute on Disability and Rehabilitation Research of the U.S. Department of Education.

As the nation's largest information source on disability-related products, it contains over 17,000 commercially available products for use in personal care, transportation, communication, independent living, and recreation. Each product entry lists the generic name, brand name, manufacturer, availability, cost, and product description. Products are listed from over 2,000 companies. The database is updated continuously.

Individuals may request a custom search of ABLEDATA by telephone or written request. Searches of eight or fewer pages are free of charge. Single copies of fact sheets containing detailed information about specific products are available free of charge. An ABLEDATA thesaurus is available for a fee and includes the listing of categories and product names.

Individuals may access the database for independent searching on the Internet at www.abledata. com.

Contact:

ABLEDATA
8401 Colesville Road, Suite 200
Silver Spring, MD 20910
800-227-0216 (ph)
301-608-8958 (fax)

Access-Able Travel Source An online service that provides access information about travel to disabled persons, including those who are blind or visually impaired. Access-Able provides information about cruise lines, various hotels and destinations, and tips for travelers with special needs. It also has links to other travel and disability sites, information about travel magazines and travel agents, and real-life travel stories from disabled people who have used Access-Able.

Contact:

Access-Able Travel Source
www.access-able.com

accessibility The ability to enter and navigate through a building or environment and to use all its facilities or services. To ensure integration of disabled persons into all aspects of society, Congress has issued laws and regulations that prohibit those who accept federal funds from discriminating against disabled persons by limiting accessibility.

Federal accessibility standards are outlined by the American National Standards Institute (ANSI) in the document "The American National Standard Specifications for Making Buildings and Facilities Accessible to, and Usable by, the Physically Handicapped." Compliance with the standards is monitored by the Architectural and Transportation Barriers Compliance Board, an organization within the Department of Health, Education and Welfare.

Although ANSI works with architects, public officials, organizations that serve the disabled, and disabled individuals, the federal requirements may not be the complete solution to accessibility. The standards represent only minimum levels of accessibility and do not encourage efforts to exceed these levels. Federal regulations do not solve problems that result from the conflicting needs of two or more types of disabilities; for example, street crossing curb cuts that serve wheelchair users may be hazardous for visually impaired persons.

Accessibility requirements for visually impaired persons may be inadequate as well. The standards are generally misunderstood and underdeveloped because blind people and those working professionally in services for the visually impaired have been unable to reach a consensus on accessibility needs. Excellent methods of orientation and mobility have been developed to enable visually impaired persons to successfully compensate for their sight loss. As a result, the visually impaired segment of the disabled community may lack the urgency felt by other members who cannot compensate for physical barriers.

Groups representing blind and visually impaired persons are in place and working to improve accessibility. The World Wide Web Consortium is in the process of finalizing accessibility guidelines to assure that all people have equal access to the Internet. These efforts are a collaboration of industry, disability, and research organizations, as well as various governments from around the world.

For more information about federal accessibility standards and ANSI, contact:

American National Standards Institute
1819 L Street, NW, Suite 600
Washington, DC 20036
212-642-4900
www.ansi.org

accommodation   The adjustment the lens of the eye makes in order to focus on close or distant objects. Our ability for accommodation begins to diminish at around age 10, but the decline is not normally noticed until about age 40. Accommodation also refers to the method of bringing an object closer to the eye in order to see it better. This method, also known as the approach system, is used by people with low vision.

Act to Promote the Education of the Blind
Passed by Congress in 1879, this act mandates that the AMERICAN PRINTING HOUSE FOR THE BLIND, a nonprofit agency, produce and distribute specially designed and adapted educational materials to blind students in public schools in America.

Such materials are necessary so that blind students have equal access to public education, and include textbooks in Braille and large type, tangible teaching devices, educational tests, and special instructional aids, tools, and materials adapted for students who are legally blind. The American Printing House for the Blind received federal funding to produce and distribute materials.

activities of daily living   See DAILY LIVING SKILLS.

acyclovir   Acyclovir, also known as ACV or Zovirax, is an ANTIVIRAL DRUG used to treat ocular herpes. The drug suppresses the enzyme thymidine kinase, which is vital to the virus. Acyclovir is distinctive in that, unlike other antiviral medications, it attacks the viral cells only and disregards normal cells.

Acyclovir is available in pill, cream, injection, or ointment form. It is commonly used to treat HERPES SIMPLEX type 1 and type 2 of the skin, mouth, eyes, brain, genitals and lungs and in newborn infants. It has also been proven effective against the HERPES ZOSTER virus associated with shingles and chicken pox. There are no significant side effects associated with this drug.

Acyclovir is not a cure. The drug can attack the virus only when it is active. It inhibits the virus from reproducing, but the virus retreats to the ganglion and remains latent. The virus may become reactive at any time, because the drug is ineffective against herpes during periods of latency.

Acyclovir is available through prescription only. Cream or ointment forms of this drug should never be placed in the eye directly.

adaptive aids   Adaptive aids (or daily-living aids, independent-living aids) are devices and tools that have been adapted or invented to enable visually impaired persons to perform sight-related tasks independently. Often, an unadapted tool or utensil is marked with raised dots, braille, or large print to become an adaptive aid. Other aids are equipped with voice simulators.

Adaptive aids may require prescription by an OPHTHALMOLOGIST or low-vision specialist and may require special training for use. Adaptive aids are available through adaptive-aids catalogs or are constructed or adapted by the users themselves.

Health aids are instruments that can be used by visually impaired persons to monitor their health or administer medicine. Devices for monitoring temperature, blood pressure, pulse, and glucose are marked in braille or announce the measurement in a synthesized voice. Pill splitters divide pills into even halves, and guides are available for measuring liquid medications. Diabetes-related devices measure insulin to preset levels and serve as needle guides. Many syringes are marked in large print.

Household aids include cooking devices, such as a liquid level indicator (which hooks over the lip of a cup and beeps or vibrates as the liquid nears the top of the cup), one-cup beverage makers (which heat liquids for soup, coffee, etc.), electromagnetic stoves (which heat food without flames or heating elements), elbow-length oven mitts, and knife slicing guides.

Other aids for the home include self-threading needles, sewing-machine magnifiers, magnetic padlocks (which require no combination and open with a magnetic sensor), raised large-print telephone dials, one-button automatic telephone-dialing systems, and brailled clothing tags.

Magnification aids, or MAGNIFIERS, include hand-held devices such as a bar magnifier, which enlarges one line of print, and hand-held aspheric magnifiers, which magnifies three to 10 times the normal size. Magnifiers may lie on the page as a sheet magnifier, may be held by stands at a precise distance from the page or object, or may be attached to spectacles and swung down into place when needed. Magnifiers may be telescopic and enable the user to see street signs or other distant objects.

Electronic magnifiers or visual aids include CLOSED-CIRCUIT TELEVISION (CCTV), which employs a camera and a zoom lens to magnify a page of print

60 times normal size. Portable models are available and constantly improving.

NONOPTICAL or *environmental aids* improve vision but do not use lens magnification. These factors improve the environment rather than the device or object of regard. They include illumination, light transmission, reflection control, and contrast.

Illumination is improved through use of brighter or dimmer room lighting, as needed according to the cause of disability. Light transmission is improved through lenses, filters, and absorptive lenses, which reduce glare and highlight contrast.

Reflection is controlled by visors, sideshields, specially treated lenses, and typoscopes. Contrast is enhanced by using highly contrasting colors near one another, such as black ink on white paper or fluorescent strips on stair risers.

TALKING AIDS, or *auditory aids*, allow the user to access information by the sense of hearing. They are devices that play or read the text, message, measurement, or degree according to a preset interval of time or on activation of the voice.

Tape recorders are used to play and/or record communications and recorded materials such as TALKING BOOKS. Some models are available with stop/start foot pedals to allow for typing while listening. Many tape recorders and players contain variable speed adjustments to reduce the time spent listening.

Speech compressors are machines that control the speed of the audio of a tape by deleting portions of the pauses between words or by shortening vowel sounds. The material is rerecorded in the shorter version, and the sound of the speech is not affected.

Accelerated speech is text that is recorded at normal speed but reproduced and played at an accelerated speed. Highly accelerated speech may produce a distortion in the sound of the voice, although some models contain pitch-controlling options.

Talking books and other recorded texts are available through talking-book programs or the Library of Congress. Books on cassette tape are also available through commercial publishers.

Synthetic speech is the computerized production of sounds into words and is used in the voice output of reading machines and computers. The Kurzweil

Reading Machine is a talking device that uses a computer-controlled camera to scan lines of print. A voice synthesizer "reads" the print to the user.

Talking adaptive aids are tools that supply a voice reading of the information normally gained by sight. Such aids include the talking scale, clock, watch, timer, blood-pressure monitor, thermometer, blood-glucose monitoring kit, talking wallet (which identifies bills of $1–$10 denominations), label makers, calculators, and computer-speech output.

Tools and instruments include rulers, yardsticks, and tape measures with raised tactual readings or braille markings, saw guides with raised markings at specific degree points, drill guides and squares, calipers, and micrometers with raised-dot markings. Light probes and metal or voltage detectors locate light or flame, metal objects, or live electrical current and sound an audible signal to alert the user.

TRAVEL AIDS allow the user to move in an environment safely and independently. These include canes, folding or rigid, and electronic travel aids that are prescribed by an optometrist or ophthalmologist and include the laser cane, the Pathsounder, the Sonic Guide, and the Mowat Sensor, all of which require specialized training to use.

Electronic travel aids send out light beams or ultrasound waves that come into contact with objects in the path. When the beam or waves hit an object, the device responds by vibrating or emitting a sound.

ORIENTATION AIDS familiarize a visually impaired traveler to the layout of a particular building or site. Orientation aids include tactile maps, three-dimensional maps that include raised lines and are read with the fingertips, models, three-dimensional scale representations of the site, and verbal recordings of site descriptions or travel routes.

Watches, clocks, and timers are available in a variety of forms. Watch covers are designed to open so the user can feel the hands in relation to the raised dots at each hour. Time pieces may be tactually marked with dots at each hour or at set intervals on the dial. Many feature large print or bold, high-contrast numbers. Some designs announce the time audibly at the touch of a button, and others automatically announce the time at set intervals.

Writing and communication aids enable users to perform writing and reading tasks independently.

Braille books, magazines, musical materials, and maps are available to those who read braille. Large-print materials employ larger lettering for use by those with partial vision. Written materials are recorded on tape or gramophone and are available to visually impaired persons.

A script-writing guide is a template with an opening that corresponds to one line of space on a lined page. The device can be lowered one line at a time as the writer progresses down the page. Many designs allow adaptations for drawing vertical lines and for use on nonstandard-size paper.

Bold-line paper is lined writing paper with heavy, dark lines in place of standard light blue lines. The bold lines (often used with a thick-tipped felt pen) may be all that is necessary to allow persons with low vision to write independently.

Templates or stencils are available in myriad forms for tasks that range from envelope addressing to check writing. They are made from plastic or metal and have openings or windows that correspond to the type of document. Many templates can be made to order to suit the user's needs or documents. A signature guide is a template that has one opening to place on the signature line.

A RAISED-LINE DRAWING KIT involves a penlike stylus for forming letters or drawings on special plastic paper or mylar covering a drawing board. Drawn lines are visible and can be tactually traced. A similar device, a dot inverter, involves embossed dots that can be used to make simple maps or figures.

THERMOFORM is a system that uses an oven to heat plastic sheets. The heated sheets can be embossed into dots or shapes including braille letters or maps. The thermoform sheets can be used to duplicate braille pages from a master sheet.

Label makers include designs that make adhesive-backed or magnetic labels in large print, braille, raised-line letters, or "talking" labels.

Three-D markers allow writing three-dimensional letters or figures that can be felt with the fingertips. The ink may be brightly colored and may be used on cloth, plastic, and metal.

Braille writers or braillers are used to type braille. A slate and a stylus are portable writing devices for printing braille.

The OPTACON is a reading device used by those who read braille. The user sweeps a line of print with a small camera held in one hand. The other hand rests on a console that receives the print and converts it to a series of vibrating pins that simulate print letters.

Standard typewriters or word processors can be used for those with touch typing skills. Computers that print braille or standard print are available with speech output.

Many advances in computer access for visually impaired persons have been made in recent years. Special tools are available that convert documents into text, which can be read by a screen-reading program that synthesizes text as audible speech.

In some cases, regular computers can be converted and made accessible to blind or visually impaired users.

See also COMPUTERS.

advocacy An advocate is one who pleads the case of another. Advocacy among persons with disabilities often centers on working to change legislation, to fill unmet needs or to take advantage of denied opportunities or rights ensured by law. Advocacy measures may involve issues of legislation, medical rights, housing rights, fair compensation, nondiscrimination, employment rights, educational rights, use of public transportation or facilities, and rights of privacy.

The Rehabilitation Act of 1973 established the discretionary creation of advocates or client assistants at the state level. These assistants work as ombudsmen with disabled individuals and service providers to ensure that individuals receive the services they seek. Many states have established specific state protection and advocacy agencies to serve as advocates. Local governmental social service offices may provide additional help in gaining appropriate services and aid.

Professional, consumer, and advocacy organizations and agencies for the blind and visually impaired on the national, state, and local level serve as self-advocates by informing and educating lawmakers, providing services and information to the public, and offering referral services.

Parents of disabled children frequently merge to form advocacy groups. Whether working individually for their own children, or in groups to represent the needs of similarly disabled children, parents are an effective force. For example, during the epidemic of cases of retrolental fibroplasia in the 1940s and 1950s and later in the 1960s following an epidemic of rubella, parents formed advocacy groups that forced schools to provide special education for their visually impaired and multihandicapped children and to include these children into public schools and mainstream classes.

A parents advocacy group active today is the National Organization of Parents of Blind Children, affiliated with the National Federation of the Blind. It can be accessed on the Internet at www.nfb.org/nopbc.

Successful advocacy usually includes phases of preparation, action, and evaluation. During the preparation phase, the advocate identifies the specific need, researches the existing organizations that provide services and aid and identifies which agency or individual is best prepared to fill the need.

In the action phase, the advocate contacts the agency or individual, convinces the individual of the needs of the disabled person and the ability, appropriateness or responsibility of the agency to provide for those needs, works with the individual to target specific methods to meet needs and develops a timetable or plan for fulfilling the needs.

During the evaluation phase, the advocate determines whether the needs have been met according to the agreement and remains in contact with the agency until the needs are met.

age-related maculopathy (ARM) See MACULAR DISEASE.

aging More than 50 percent of all individuals with severe vision impairments are over 65. In addition, a study by Lighthouse International showed that one in six people age 45 or older report some type of visual impairment. More than half of these people describe the impairment as severe. Changes with age occur both in the external and internal portions of the eye. Externally, the globe itself may seem to have sunken into the skull. This is the result of a breakdown or natural degeneration of the retrobulbar fat that supports the globe in the bony socket. Fortunately, the bony socket, called the orbit, is not susceptible to osteoporosis, as are other bones in the body. The orbit does not weaken or become thin and brittle with aging.

The eyelids may lose elasticity and tone causing PTOSIS (drooping eyelid). This may cause a reduction in the area of visual field.

ENTROPION (a turning inward of the eyelid) and ECTROPION (a turning outward of the eyelid) are common complaints associated with aging. Both conditions can be successfully treated with surgery if they produce discomfort or a threat to vision.

The CONJUNCTIVA, or white portion of the eye, becomes slack and more susceptible to chronic inflammations with age. As it slackens, a section may become caught between the lids during blinking. Harmless degenerative plaques may appear on the white of the eye.

ARCUS SENILIS may appear on the margin of the cornea. This harmless white circle bordering the CORNEA is a common occurrence in the elderly. Composed of cholesterol and its derivatives, the presence of arcus senilis does not necessarily indicate an overall raised cholesterol level.

Most aging eyes become presbyopic, a condition in which the hardened lens is unable to bend and focus effectively on objects at close range. PRESBYOPIA usually surfaces near age 45 and affects both nearsighted and farsighted eyes. The condition is treated with reading glasses or bifocals.

The lens often becomes opacified with age. Degrees of OPACIFICATION vary and are not termed CATARACT until a significant opacification develops. The lens may yellow and cause color vision changes and nearsightedness.

The pupil loses its ability to accommodate quickly with changing light. The pupil becomes smaller and reduces the light entering the eye to approximately 30 percent of normal levels.

The VITREOUS of the aging eye may contain opacities that become visible to the individual as floaters, or spots that bounce or float in the field of vision. The vitreous may collapse or detach from the retina. This may cause a more serious condition, RETINAL DETACHMENT, and vision loss.

The arteries and veins of the RETINA become narrower with age, reducing the flow of blood. The aging retina is duller and exhibits a less responsive light reflex. The optic disc may be paler also.

VISUAL ACUITY, or the ability to see small objects under normal lighting and contrast conditions, may suffer with age. The reduction may occur as a result of the smaller pupil and/or the aging, opacified lens. Decreased visual acuity may affect the ability to perform tasks such as reading or driving.

The aging eye requires more light than a younger eye. It is estimated that for every 13 years of life, twice the amount of light is needed to function effectively. This may be due to the smaller pupil and less transparent lens.

CONTRAST sensitivity and spatial perception reductions may occur with age. The ability to detect and recognize contrast is controlled by the neural circuitry of the retina and brain. As neuronal changes occur, contrast sensitivity decreases. Spatial perception depends on contrast detection, so any reduction in contrast perception affects this ability as well.

Adaptation, the ability to be sensitive to changing light levels and adjust to them, is diminished by age. An elderly eye may require more time to recover from glare or a bright light such as a flashbulb or car headlights. This is a result of the smaller, less adaptive pupil and the opacified lens.

Color vision may fade or change with age. The yellowing lens tends to absorb and scatter blue light, rendering blues darker and less intense. The unimpeded red and yellow light is allowed to pass through and cast a warm, reddish glow onto objects.

In addition to visual changes, vision loss occurs as a result of diseases that are associated with aging. The four leading causes of vision loss among elderly individuals are AGE-RELATED MACULOPATHY, cataracts, GLAUCOMA, and DIABETIC RETINOPATHY.

Age-Related Maculopathy (ARM) is a progressive disease in which the macula, or area of sharpest central sight, deteriorates. Central vision and contrast enhancement is lost but peripheral vision often remains intact. Some types of macular disease may be treated with laser therapy, and other advances in the treatment of ARM are occurring rapidly. Doctors and scientists are optimistic about new treatments for ARM, and are working hard to find a cure for this disease.

Cataracts are opacifications or cloudy spots on the lens of the eye. Senile cataracts, those associated with aging, are usually progressive and may exist for several years before requiring surgical removal. Removal of cataracts is highly successful, and entails removal of the lens. The lens is replaced by an artificial intraocular lens or by a contact lens or glasses. The results of cataract removal, although generally successful, vary from person to person.

Glaucoma is an increase in the intraocular pressure. This occurs when the eye produces an overabundance of AQUEOUS FLUID or when the eye fails to drain the fluid adequately. The increase in pressure may damage organs of the eye and result in vision loss. Glaucoma can be treated and controlled with medication or surgery.

Diabetic retinopathy is an eye disease that results from diabetes. The small blood vessels that support and nourish the retina become damaged and weak. These may hemorrhage and cause an accumulation of fluid in the retina that limits or alters vision. New, weaker vessels may proliferate, hemorrhage and form vision-limiting scar tissue. The scar tissue may trigger a retinal detachment, and permanent vision loss may result.

Aging eyes may benefit by changes in the environment and lifestyle of the individual. Increased lighting and color contrast coupled with reduced glare may aid residual vision, increase effectiveness in the performance of tasks, and enhance safety. ADAPTIVE AIDS may improve or enhance remaining vision, aid in the performance of skills and tasks, and increase independence. Biannual eye examinations for those over 40 may uncover an eye disorder at its earliest and most treatable stage.

American Foundation for the Blind. *Aging and Vision.* New York: AFB, 1987.

Carroll, Thomas J. "A Look at Aging," *The New Outlook* (April 1972): pp. 97–103.

Denby, Dorothy. "Aging and Blindness," *Aging and the Human Condition,* New York: Human Services Press, Inc. 1982.

Galloway, N. R. *Common Eye Diseases and their Management.* Berlin: Springer-Verlag, 1985.

American Society on Aging. Visual Disorders and Aging. www.asaging.org/ameritech/V002_visual_disorders. html, 2000.

AIDS Acquired immunodeficiency syndrome, or AIDS, is a disease of the immune system characterized by a deficiency of thymus-derived lymphocytes. These lymphocytes, identified by the phenotypic marker T4, function as helpers to the immune system. The lack of T4 lymphocytes leads to a breakdown in the immune response and allows the body to become host to opportunistic infections and neoplasm (tumor) development. AIDS is caused by a virus called HIV (human immunodeficiency virus). Having HIV is not the same as having AIDS. AIDS is the late stage of HIV infection.

Visual disorders or disturbances affect over 50 percent of AIDS patients. One-third of these patients have cytomegalovirus retinitis, an infection of the retina caused by the cytomegalovirus (CMV). Cytomegalovirus is a member of the herpes virus family and may cause primary, latent, and persistent infections.

Cytomegalovirus retinitis progressively destroys tissue that leads to scar formation, and possible retinal detachments. Symptoms of the condition include blind spots, blurred vision, and loss of peripheral vision, although the infection may be present without any apparent symptoms. The infection progresses rapidly and may cause blindness if left untreated.

Current treatment for cytomegalovirus retinitis involves the use of two ANTIVIRAL DRUGS: ganciclovir and foscarnet. Ganciclovir stops the progression of the disease and may save the residual vision. The drug is contraindicated for use with AZT. The drug is given by daily intravenous infusion, but an oral form has recently been developed and is in testing.

Foscarnet also stops the progression of the infection. It is given intravenously but can be taken in conjunction with AZT. Foscarnet may be less effective in preventing relapses of CMV retinitis after the initial high-dose induction phase of treatment. Foscarnet may have the additional advantage of being effective in combatting HIV activity.

Aid to Families with Dependent Children (AFDC) A federal cash-assistance program for needy children. The program is administered by each state's Department of Social Services.

Eligible children are those who have been deprived of support or care of one or both parents by death, disability, absence, or unemployment. Children may be eligible for the program if they are under age 17. Children 18 years old and enrolled in high school full time may be eligible.

The parent or caretaker is usually included in the grant, and two-parent households may be eligible if both parents are unemployed. Parents must register for work, unless they are exempt from employment.

Children living in foster homes also may qualify for AFDC funds.

Some state AFDC programs, such as that in California, include a homeless assistance (HA) component that grants payments to acquire temporary shelter and/or permanent housing. An AFDC eligible family qualifies for HA funds if the family lacks a permanent nightly residence, has a nightly residence that is a publicly or privately operated shelter for temporary living accommodations, or lives in a public or private place that is not designed for residence, such as a bus station or building lobby.

air bags Protective devices that are installed in many cars. Air bags, also known as inflatable restraint systems, are designed to inflate immediately upon impact, in the course of an automobile accident. They are designed to prevent the driver and front-seat passenger from being thrown against the steering wheel, dashboard, or window or from being thrown from the car.

Although they are credited with saving lives and preventing many injuries, there are risks, including eye injuries, associated with air bags. This is particularly true with regard to children.

An article in the August 2000 issue of *Ophthalmology,* the journal published by the American Academy of Ophthalmology, concluded that air bags can cause serious eye injuries to children and that to avoid such injuries, children should not be permitted to ride in the front seat of an automobile.

Some possible eye injuries that could result from air bag deployment include cataracts, glaucoma, blood in the front chamber of the eye, alkali burn, temporary loss of consciousness and visual acuity, laceration of the eyelid, inflammation of the iris, corneal lesions and abrasions, black eye, and swelling and hemorrhage of blood vessels under the outer surface of the eyeball.

albinism A hereditary condition in which all or part of the body lacks pigment. Albinism may affect the skin, eyes, and hair of the individual. It is thought to be caused by an enzyme deficiency involving the metabolism of melanin during prenatal development.

There are two major types of albinism: oculocutaneous albinism and ocular albinism. Oculocutaneous albinism involves a lack of pigmentation in the eyes, skin, and hair. The condition is subdivided into two groups, tyrosinase-positive or tyrosinase-negative, according to the presence or absence of the enzyme tyrosinase in the hair bulbs. Tyrosinase inhibits the formation of pigment in the body. Tyrosinase-negative individuals have white hair, pink skin, and pale blue eyes, and tyrosinase-positive individuals produce some melanin and vary as to physical condition and coloring.

Ocular albinism involves the lack of, or reduced amount of, pigmentation of the eye. Individuals with ocular albinism may exhibit no lack of pigmentation of the skin and hair.

Those with ocular albinism and tyrosinase-negative oculocutaneous albinism usually experience severe visual disorders. These may include a visual acuity of 20/200 or less, NYSTAGMUS (an involuntary movement or jerking of the eyes), AMBLYOPIA (a condition in which the brain does not receive information from one or both eyes as a result of a failure of the vision development as an infant or child), iris transillumination (the ability of light to pass through the normally pigmented iris), lack of fundus pigmentation, and PHOTOPHOBIA (a sensitivity to light).

Albinism cannot be cured. Symptoms such as loss of visual acuity, nystagmus, amblyopia, and photophobia may be treated with therapy, surgery, corrective lenses, or light-reducing lenses.

alcohol amblyopia A visual condition unique to alcoholics or those who have a history of chronic, severe drinking problems. The disorder involves lost vision, including SCOTOMAS (blind spots) and decreased visual acuity within the central portion of the visual field. The painless, bilateral sight loss gradually worsens. The disorder is caused by the toxic effects of alcohol on the OPTIC NERVE. The toxicity causes optic neuropathy, a condition in which the optic nerve swells.

Alcohol amblyopia may be linked with a thiamine (vitamin B_1) deficiency, a condition that can lead to optic-nerve damage. Alcohol consumption may interfere with the absorption or activation of nutrients and vitamins within the body, including thiamine and zinc.

Alcohol amblyopia may be treated with proper diet and vitamin supplements. The condition is usually reversible but may lead to permanent vision loss if untreated.

Burde, Ronald M., Peter J. Savino and Jonathan D. Trobe, *Clinical Decisions in Neuro-Ophthalmology.* St. Louis: C.V. Mosby Company, 1985.

Havener, William H. *Ocular Pharmacology.* St. Louis: C.V. Mosby Company, 1970.

O'Brien, Robert, and Morris Chafetz. *The Encyclopedia of Alcoholism.* New York: Facts On File Publications, 1982.

Alliance for Eye and Vision Research

The Alliance for Eye and Vision Research is a nonprofit organization founded in 1993 by the Association for Research in Vision and Ophthalmology, the American Academy of Ophthalmology, and the Association of University Professors of Ophthalmology. Its goal is to achieve the best eye care possible for all Americans and to educate the public and Congress about the importance of the research conducted by the National Eye Institute that affects public vision and eye care.

The Alliance is the parent group of the National Alliance for Eye and Vision Research, which is primarily a lobbying organization.

Contact:

Alliance for Eye and Vision Research
426 C Street, NE
Washington, DC 20002
202-544-1880
202-543-2565 (fax)
www.eyeresearch.org

Alva Access Group

Alva Access Group is a Netherlands-based company that specializes in the development and production of Braille displays and software that make computers accessible for those who are blind or visually impaired.

Its primary products, in addition to Braille displays, are a screen magnifying software program called inLARGE and a screen reader software program called outSPOKEN. Its products can be integrated in most computer systems and operate in all commonly used languages and all common Braille tables.

Alva, which was founded in 1984, acquired Berkley Systems, a software development and publishing company that specializes in products for the visually impaired, in 1996.

For the worldwide distribution of its products, ALVA maintains and supports a widespread distribution network.

Contact:

Alva Access Group, Inc.
436 14th Street, Suite 700
Oakland, CA 94612
510-451-2582
510-451-0878 (fax)
www.aagi.com

amaurosis The loss of sight due to disease.

amblyopia Also known as "lazy eye," a condition in which an otherwise healthy eye provides poor vision. This occurs in an infant or child when one eye presents less visual information to the brain than the other eye due to abnormal vision development. The weaker eye's corresponding visual brain cells have impaired function and receive less information from the eye. According to the National Eye Institute, amblyopia occurs in approximately 2 percent to 4 percent of the population and is a major cause of visual impairment in young children. It is frequently unilateral, but can be bilateral.

In normal vision, each eye looks at an object and sends electrical impulses to the brain describing each separate image of that object. The brain's visual cells receive and translate these impulses into one three-dimensional image as "seen" in the brain.

When one eye is crossed (STRABISMUS), causing different images sent to the brain, or when one eye sends more accurate information to the brain, this interferes with the image-making process. The messages of one eye may be suppressed or ignored by the brain. The ignored eye becomes nonfunctional.

The vision cells of the brain that serve the ignored eye become dysfunctional, causing the eye to lose vision and become amblyopic. Children are especially susceptible to amblyopia since visual systems take years to fully develop and can be altered easily in the formative years.

Amblyopia can be caused by any disorder or condition that interrupts normal vision processing. Strabismus, or crossed eyes, is responsible in approximately 50 percent of all cases.

Conditions that block an image from the eye's retina can also induce amblyopia. CATARACTS, ptosis (a drooping eyelid), corneal scarring, or nontransparent sections in other parts of the eye can cause amblyopia in children. These obstructions may cause an eye to send impaired images to the brain. The developing visual system within a child's brain may cease to accept the impaired information, and the corresponding brain cells become amblyopic.

ANISOMETROPIA often causes amblyopia. Anisometropic eyes have unequal refractive powers, requiring a stronger lens prescription in one eye than another. Without corrective lenses, one eye sends less reliable and accurate information to the brain. The brain concentrates on the information from the better eye and ignores that from the weaker eye. Occasionally, minor degrees of anisometropia exhibit no symptoms.

Amblyopia may be caused by hereditary diseases or conditions such as albinism or by the accompanying strabismus caused by hereditary conditions. To treat amblyopia, the original cause such as cataract, strabismus or anisometropia must be diagnosed and corrected. Therapy for the amblyopia itself follows and includes the prescription eyeglasses and/or a patch for the nonamblyopic eye. Once the better eye is patched, the brain is forced to accept information from the amblyopic eye. Visual brain-cell deterioration begins to reverse itself, and the eye becomes functional again. The patch may be worn a portion of the day or all day, and recovery may take up to several months.

Since a young child's brain cells can reverse themselves and regenerate more effectively during the first few years of life, it is important to diagnose and treat amblyopia as early as possible. Children of any age can be screened for amblyopia during an ophthalmologic examination, but it is more effective after six months and most effective at five years of age. Treatment is very successful in children up to age six. After age nine, treatment is much less effective.

TOBACCO or ALCOHOL AMBLYOPIA are conditions in which the excessive use of tobacco or alcohol impairs central vision. The vision is often blurred and is accompanied by numbness or tingling in the hands and fingers. The condition usually rights itself when tobacco or alcohol use is discontinued or drastically reduced.

American Academy of Ophthalmology   The largest association of ophthalmologists in the United States. More than 90 percent of all practicing American ophthalmologists are Academy members, and an additional 5,000 ophthalmologists are international members.

The academy was incorporated in 1979 when the parent organization, the American Academy of Ophthalmology and Otolaryngology, was divided into two separate academies: one for the eye, the other for the ear, nose and throat. In 1981, the American Association of Ophthalmology merged with the academy.

The goal of the academy is to help the public maintain healthy eyes and vision. The primary focus of the Academy is education. The Academy holds a five-day annual meeting offering scientific papers, symposia, instructional courses, multimedia presentations, and exhibits to educate ophthalmologists and other interested parties about new advances in eye care and treatment.

Courses are offered throughout the year, in locations around the country, with hands-on laboratory instruction and updates on important developments in ophthalmology. The academy offers its members educational programs and materials covering practice management, Medicare billing and coding guidelines, and policy and procedures.

The academy develops and produces education and training materials, texts, videotapes, slide-script programs, and a subscription series for practicing ophthalmologists, nonophthalmic physicians, and other medical eye-care practitioners. The academy produces public- and patient-information materials and maintains a public-information program through the news media. Policy and information statements concerning current eye-care topics are developed and disseminated to the public.

The academy's Office of Governmental Relations in Washington, D.C., represents ophthalmologists and their patients in state and federal legislative matters by monitoring and submitting statements on proposed regulations and legislation.

In 1980, the academy established the Foundation of the American Academy of Ophthalmology, a charitable organization that supports and develops public-service programs, preserves ophthalmic historical collections, and fosters innovative programs to promote and enhance optimal public eye care. As a first project, the foundation developed the Museum of Ophthalmology, a historical collection that traces the development and growth of ophthalmology.

The foundation sponsors the National Eye Care Project, a program to aid disadvantaged elderly persons. The program provides eye care and services to maintain and protect the eyes and vision of elderly people who cannot afford to pay for ophthalmologic care.

Contact:

The American Academy of Ophthalmology
P.O. Box 7424
San Francisco, CA 94120-7424
415-561-8500 (ph)
415-561-8575 (fax)
www.eyenet.org

American Association of the Deaf-Blind

(AADB) The American Association of the Deaf-Blind, Inc. (AADB), formerly the American League for Deaf-Blind, was founded in 1937. It is a nonprofit organization dedicated to the advancement of economic, educational and social welfare of deaf-blind persons. Membership consists of deaf-blind individuals, their families and friends, professionals working within the health-care field, and interested individuals.

The organization maintains service programs, represents the deaf-blind community during public-policy matters, refers individuals to services, and compiles statistics.

AADB holds an annual convention. AADB members meet with parents and community agencies to provide training in methods of communication and discussion of needs for deaf-blind persons.

AADB maintains a library of information concerning deaf-blindness and publishes the *Deaf-Blind American*, a quarterly journal.

Contact:

American Association of the Deaf-Blind
814 Thayer Avenue
Silver Spring, MD 20910
800-735-2258 (ph)
301-588-8705 (fax)
301-588-6545 (tty)
www.tr.wov.edu/dblink/aadbz.htm

American Council of the Blind

(ACB) A nonprofit organization that serves as a national clearinghouse for information on blindness and organizations and institutions that serve the blind.

The organization works to improve conditions and services concerning those with visual impairments. It provides advisory assistance on issues concerning disability-related legislation, affirmative action, civil rights, education of disabled persons, increased participation in vending facility programs, improvement of Social Security and other federal benefits, reading and library services, low-vision technology, and eye research.

The ACB provides professional support in cases of class action and public interest litigation. It offers group health insurance and supports public education concerning the needs and abilities of the visually impaired. The organization awards Floyd Qualls Memorial postsecondary scholarships each year to visually impaired students.

The ACB publishes the bimonthly *The Braille Forum* and holds an annual convention. It also operates ACB Radio, a webcasting service with three Internet radio stations. It can be accessed at www.Live365.com.

Contact:

American Council of the Blind
1155 15th Street NW, Suite 720
Washington, DC 20005
800-424-8666 (ph)
202-467-5085 (fax)
http://acb.org

American Foundation for the Blind   (AFB)   A national, nonprofit organization, founded in 1921, dedicated to providing direct service and programs, referral services and improvement of the standards of service for blind and visually impaired people. AFB works in conjunction with public schools and universities, senior centers, businesses, and more than 1,000 specialized agencies. Headquartered in New York City, AFB has regional centers in Washington, D.C., New York, San Francisco, Chicago, Dallas, and Atlanta.

AFB provides national consultation services to schools, agencies, and organizations of and for blind people on topics concerning visual impairment, including education, orientation and mobility, low vision, early childhood, employment and aging. It offers regional consultation services for technical assistance, staff training, regional fundraising, public education, and public-relations program development.

AFB serves as a clearinghouse for information about blindness and visual impairment. It publishes and distributes books, pamphlets, periodicals and audio/visual materials. It maintains a public education program that utilizes publications, personal presentations, exhibits, and media releases.

AFB houses the National Technology Center (NTC), a research and development facility that explores, develops and evaluates technological devices for visually impaired people and consults with manufacturers in the development of new devices. The NTC maintains a database of consumer information about products, training programs, funding resources, and evaluation reports.

AFB also houses the M.C. Migel Memorial Library and Information Center. The 37,000-volume collection of printed materials is one of the largest collections on blindness and the largest circulating library on blindness in the United States.

Much of the library's collection is accessible to blind and visually impaired people via on-site computerized reading devices. The library holds the Helen Keller archives, a collection of letters, photographs and memorabilia given to AFB by Helen Keller, who worked for the AFB for more than 40 years, and her teacher, Anne Sullivan Macy.

AFB records and manufactures over 500 titles of talking books each year for the Library of Congress. It conducts research, surveys the needs of visually impaired people and studies the current services provided by agencies. It consults with Congress and governmental agencies on legislative issues. It manufactures and sells publications, and products for visually impaired people.

AFB publishes *The Journal of Visual Impairment and Blindness, AFB News, Long Cane News* and *AFB Directory of Services for Blind and Visually Impaired Persons in the United States.* AFB began publishing *Access World* in January 2000. Printed six times a year, the publication provides the latest information on adaptive technology and visual impairments. AFB sponsors the annual Helen Keller Seminar and the annual Josephine L. Taylor Leadership Institute for professionals in the field.

Contact:

American Foundation for the Blind
11 Penn Plaza, Suite 300
New York, NY 10001
212-502-7661 (ph)
212-502-7777 (fax)
www.afb.org

American Printing House for the Blind   (APH)   Founded in 1858, the American Printing House for the Blind (APH) is the oldest American nonprofit organization for the blind. It is the largest independent publishing house of materials for the visually impaired in the world.

The APH publishes books and magazines in BRAILLE, large print, tape, and flexible disc. It provides writing tools and recording equipment, vocational materials, educational aids, and computer products to visually impaired adults and students.

The educational aids and materials are used to teach math, science, reading, and social studies to students of all ages. Other aids aim to improve LOW

VISION or sensory, motor, and conceptual skills. Tools include braille writing equipment, study and school supplies, recording and playback machines, and specialized lamps. APH also provides hardware and software materials for use with microcomputers, such as speech-synthesizing devices and enlarged screen images.

APH maintains a Department of Educational Research to conduct studies about blindness. Through this research, new materials and product manufacturing methods are developed. APH also provides a national data base of materials for the visually impaired called *Louis,* in honor of Louis Braille. The comprehensive database contains more than 135,000 listings for large type, Braille, recorded, computer disk, and tactile graphic publications. It is fully speech accessible.

The American Printing House maintains a library of 3,500 volumes and publishes the magazine *APH Slate.* It holds an annual convention in Louisville, Kentucky.

Contact:

American Printing House for the Blind
P.O. Box 6085, 1839 Frankfort Avenue
Louisville, KY 40206
800-223-1893 (ph)
502-899-2274 (fax)
http://aph.org

American National Standards Institute The American National Standards Institute (ANSI) was founded in 1918 to administer and coordinate a voluntary standardization system among the American private sector. It is a private, nonprofit organization that is supported by many different organizations from both the private and public sectors.

ANSI is important to blind and visually impaired people because it works with architects, public officials, and organizations to establish standards aimed at creating accessibility for all disabled persons. Although ANSI does not develop standards, it facilitates their development by encouraging consensus concerning the standards among various groups.

ANSI has more than 1,000 company, organization, government agency, institutional, and inter-

national members. It is headquartered in Washington, D.C., and has offices in New York City.

Contact (Washington):

American National Standards Institute
1819 L Street, NW, 6th Floor
Washington, D.C., 20036
202-293-8020 (ph)
202-293-9287 (fax)

Contact (New York):

American National Standards Institute
11 West 42 Street, 13th Floor
New York, NY 10036
212-642-4900 (ph)
212-398-0023 (fax)
www.ansi.org

American Thermoform Corporation (ATC) A company that produces Brailon materials, Braille text duplicators, Braille printers, computer Braille paper, Braille translation software, thermoform machines, and graphic machines.

Brailon is the trade name for the paper used in a thermoform duplicator. Each plastic sheet is placed atop a page of Brailled paper and inserted into a thermoform machine. The machine heats the Brailon sheet and creates a duplicate of the Brailled sheet. The company introduced Dot & Print in June 2000. A Braille and print printer, the machine allows someone to produce Braille and print on the same piece of paper, utilizing one printer. It also prints Braille only or print only.

Contact:

American Thermoform Corporation
1758 Brackett Street,
La Verne, CA 91750
800-331-3676 (ph)
909-593-8001 (fax)
www.atcbrleqp.com

Americans With Disabilities Act (ADA) An act passed by Congress on July 26, 1990, that "prohibits discrimination on the basis of disability in employment, programs and services provided by state and local government, goods and services provided by private companies, and in commercial facilities."

The act was intended to make all areas—including the workplace, recreational facilities, restaurants, places of worship, schools, and so forth —accessible to those with any kind of disability, including blindness or vision disorders. It is aimed at giving disabled people the same rights, access, and opportunities in areas such as employment, health care, child care, and participation in everyday civic life. As a result, elevators and automated teller machines must include Braille instructions, and public documents and financial statements must be available in alternative formats, such as Braille, large print, and audiotape. Curbs must be cut out at the corner to allow wheelchair access, and wheelchair ramps must be included in buildings covered under the act. TTY terminals are required in public buildings for people who are deaf or have speech disabilities. There are many regulations contained within the act.

Recently, the ADA has been extended to apply to cyberspace. In 1996, the U.S. Department of Justice, which oversees the ADA, stated that the act applies to Internet access. Any entity that is included under the ADA is required to "provide effective communication, regardless of whether they generally communicate through print media, audio media, or computerized media such as the Internet." The act also requires that covered entities that use the Internet for communications regarding their programs, goods, or services must be prepared to offer those communications through accessible means.

A disabled person who feels that his or her rights are being violated because of a covered entity's noncompliance with the ADA is entitled to file a complaint with the U.S. Department of Justice.

More information about the ADA in general, compliance with the act, or how to file a complaint is available by calling a toll-free ADA information line. The line is maintained by the U.S. Department of Justice. The number is 1-800-514-0301.

ametropia   A vision problem caused by the eye's inability to focus properly. Ametropia occurs when the CORNEA and the LENS of the eye cannot effectively focus light, and the resulting image, onto the RETINA. This focusing impairment is also called REFRACTIVE ERROR.

Refractive errors such as HYPEROPIA (farsightedness), MYOPIA (nearsightedness), ASTIGMATISM (distorted image) or PRESBYOPIA (aging eyes) result in blurred vision. Ametropia can be diagnosed in a routine ophthalmologic examination and is usually corrected with eyeglasses or contact lenses.

Amsler grid   A specialized testing device, invented by Professor Marc Amsler and used to detect disorders and SCOTOMA (blind spots) in the central field of vision. It is routinely used to screen patients for AGE-RELATED MACULOPATHY during the ophthalmologic exam.

The Amsler grid is a black-on-white grid of 400 squares. It is composed of 20 horizontal squares by 20 vertical squares. A black dot is in the center of the grid where the two central horizontal and vertical lines intersect.

With one eye covered, the patient is asked to look at the center dot. The patient is asked whether the center dot is visible, all the sides are visible, the entire grid is visible, any lines are wavy or bent, there are any blurs, color differentiations or distortions within the grid. If any lines appear wavy, if some of the lines disappear, or if all four corners are not visible, scotomas or age-related maculopathy may be present.

aneurysm   A diseased or weakened section of a blood vessel that fills with blood and dilates. Aneurysms may occur within blood vessels throughout the body.

Aneurysms within the blood vessels of the brain may be the result of ARTERIOSCLEROSIS. They may rupture and bleed into the cerebral fluid, a condition called a subarachnoid hemorrhage. A subarachnoid hemorrhage may cause increased pressure within the brain and decreased blood supply, resulting in a STROKE. Paralysis of the limbs, sudden changes in the field of vision, speech and memory disorders and thinking or reasoning problems may follow.

Aneurysms of the eye's RETINA may occur as a result of another disease or disorder such as DIABETIC RETINOPATHY. In this disease, the retinal vessels are weakened by diabetes. They tend to bulge and leak, hemorrhaging into the retina and causing vision loss. As the disease progresses, neovascularization occurs producing weakened blood vessels that rupture, hemorrhage and may cause RETINAL DETACHMENT and scar tissue resulting in permanent vision loss.

aniridia   Aniridia (or irideremia) is the absence of the IRIS within the eye. It is a congenital or acquired condition. Congenital aniridia is a genetically determined condition. In many cases, a vestigial portion of the iris root or margin is present. The congenital condition is usually bilateral and often seen in conjunction with congenital CATARACT. GLAUCOMA tends to develop in early adolescence in approximately 25 percent of congenital aniridia cases, due to the abnormal angle of the anterior chamber and blockage by the iris root.

Individuals with congenital aniridia are photophobic and may experience AMBLYOPIA (loss of vision in one eye due to disuse) and NYSTAGMUS (involuntary jerking of the eyes). Associated retinal abnormalities or malformations may exist. The condition, which develops at about the 12th week of pregnancy, is very rare, affecting 1 in 500,000 to 1 in a million children.

Acquired aniridia occurs as a result of trauma or injury. The iris is dislodged or torn from the CILIARY BODY. It contracts into a small pellet and moves to the outlet of the anterior chamber, where it may form a blockage and cause secondary glaucoma.

The glaucoma of both types of aniridia is treated with medications or with surgical procedures such as goniotomy or trabeculotomy if the medication proves ineffective. The prognosis for the vision of those with aniridia is generally poor.

anisocoria   A condition in which the pupils differ in size. Average-size pupils range from three to four millimeters.

All pupils are small at birth. Differences in size become more apparent as the individual grows and achieves maximum pupil size by adolescence. The pupil may become smaller with advancing age.

Approximately 17 percent of the population have minor amounts of anisocoria, but only 4 percent have pronounced cases. The difference in size

may vary from minute measurements to noticeable degrees. The size difference may be variable during the course of a day.

On the average, women tend to have larger pupils than men have, and blue or less pigmented irises are larger than brown, more pigmented irises. Myopic (nearsighted) individuals usually have larger pupils than those with HYPEROPIA (farsightedness).

Anisocoria may be congenital or acquired, as from ingestion of oral contraceptives. The condition may be a first indication of pupillary defects but may also exist in the absence of ocular disorder. One or both anisocoric pupils that fail to properly react to light may indicate neurological problems.

anisometropia   A common condition in which the eyes have unequal refractive power or unequal ability to focus and see. The degree of anisometropia can be determined during an ophthalmologic examination. Anisometropia is corrected by prescribing a stronger prescriptive lens for one eye than the other to equalize the eyes' refractive powers. Contact lenses often can greatly reduce the effects of anisometropia.

Without correction, anisometropia can cause AMBLYOPIA in children. The weaker anisometropic eye sends less reliable information to the brain than does the stronger eye. The visual cells of the brain ignore the information of this eye, become dysfunctional and cause the eye, however healthy, to become amblyopic.

anterior chamber   A section of the eye between the CORNEA and the LENS. The chamber is filled with a clear liquid called AQUEOUS FLUID.

The cornea and the lens of the eye lack blood vessels, which deliver nutrients and carry away waste. The aqueous fluid, produced by the CILIARY BODY, provides these services as it circulates within the anterior chamber. The aqueous fluid leaves the chamber through the Schlemm's canal, a channel where the IRIS and the cornea meet. If the channel becomes blocked, fluid may build up in the eye and cause a rise in intraocular pressure, a condition known as GLAUCOMA.

antibiotics DRUGS that fight infections caused by bacterial microorganisms. They are commonly prescribed for those who have a bacterial eye infection or who undergo eye surgery. Antibiotics are often taken prior to surgery to avoid the possibility of infection.

Antibiotics may be topical (applied outside the body) or systemic (taken internally). Antibiotics prescribed to treat eye disorders may be in ointment, eye-drop, or pill form.

Antibiotics are classified as one of two types, bacteriocidal or bacteriostatic. Bacteriocidal antibiotics, such as penicillin, ampicillin, and amoxicillin, disrupt the natural cell formation of microorganisms to eliminate them. Bacteriostatic antibiotics, such as tetracycline, doxycycline, and erythromycin, hinder reproductive chemical processes to eradicate the unwanted microorganisms.

When an infection is suspected in the eye, a culture may be taken from the conjunctival sac. A wide-spectrum antibiotic may be prescribed until the cause of the infection is isolated. Once the cause is determined, both systemic and topical antibiotics may be required.

antiviral drugs DRUGS that fight viruses that infect the body. Viruses that affect the eye usually result in inflammation or infection. These infections may lead to serious, vision-limiting conditions such as KERATITIS (corneal inflammation) or IRITIS (inflammation of the IRIS).

Since HERPES SIMPLEX is a major cause of viral infection in the eye, several antiviral drugs have been developed for the purpose of treating this condition. Drugs most often prescribed include IDOXURIDINE, TRIFLURIDINE, ACYCLOVIR, and ARA-A.

Idoxuridine and trifluridine were the first drugs to be developed to treat the inflammation of the CORNEA (or keratitis), associated with ocular herpes. They are also known by the names Herplex, Stoxil, Dendrid, TFT, F3T, and Viroptic. These drugs are antimetabolite agents that affect the metabolic system of the body. Highly toxic, they cannot differentiate between healthy human cells and viral cells in the body. They may destroy the healthy cells in the process of ridding the body of unwanted viral cells. Because of their toxicity, these drugs are not taken intravenously or internally. They are available in ointment or drop form only.

A new group of drugs, including acyclovir and ARA-A, has since been developed that attack only the viral cells and leave the body's healthy cells intact. These drugs, also known by the names ACV, Zovirax, vidarabine, Vira-A, and adenine arabinoside, are less toxic and can be prescribed in drop, ointment, injection, or pill form.

None of these drugs is a cure for the herpes simplex virus. They can treat the virus only when it is active in the body. The drugs discourage the virus from generating new cells, and the virus then retreats into the ganglion of the body where it remains latent. The drugs are ineffective against the virus during periods of latency. The drugs cannot stop the virus from becoming active, which could occur at any time.

Antibiotics may also be used to treat viruses. TRACHOMA, a leading cause of blindness in the world, is often successfully treated with tetracycline hydrochloride ointment.

aphakia Aphakia refers to an eye without a LENS. After CATARACT surgery, during which the lens of the eye is removed, the eye is aphakic. A monocular aphake is a person without the lens from one eye. A bilateral aphake is a person missing both lenses.

Without the lens, the eye is unable to accommodate or adjust to focus on an object. Commonly, elderly cataract surgery patients experience limited accommodation before surgery and therefore surgery-induced aphakia minimally affects their vision. People with aphakia are at a greater risk for some types of retinal detachment than those who are not aphakic.

Aphakia also distorts the size of objects, makes images appear larger, and may bend or curve straight lines. Distance judgment problems may result. Changes in color-perception may also occur. Colors may appear brighter, pinker, or bluer.

Aphakia can be corrected with glasses, contact lenses, or intraocular lenses, also called IOLs.

appetite suppressants Systematic use of appetite suppressants, including amphetamines, dextroamphetamines, methamphetamines, and phenmetrazine compounds, can affect the eyes, causing such side effects as pupil dilation and impaired vision. These drugs also can cause difficulty with accommodation and convergence, which can make reading difficult. Persistent use of these drugs also can lead to closed-angle glaucoma in some people.

aqueous fluid The aqueous fluid (or aqueous humor) is the clear liquid that fills the ANTERIOR CHAMBER of the eye, located between the CORNEA and the LENS. The cornea and lens must be transparent to function and, therefore contain no blood vessels. The aqueous fluid functions as blood vessels by delivering the nutrients and antibodies and carrying away the waste normally.

The clear, thin fluid is produced by the CILIARY BODY at a rate of approximately two cubic millimeters (about one drop) per minute. The nutrients and antibodies are pumped from blood vessels within the ciliary body and mix with the aqueous.

The aqueous flows from the ciliary body, behind the IRIS, across the lens, through the PUPIL into the anterior chamber, and along the back surface of the cornea. It circulates in the anterior chamber, bringing nutrients and carrying away waste from the avascular cornea and lens.

The aqueous fluid drains from the eye at the base of the cornea, an outflow channel called the Schlemm's canal. The aqueous fluid is strained of waste and collected in the canal. It then flows to small veins in the sclera and joins the body's blood stream.

When the draining channels become blocked or if the eye overproduces aqueous, the fluid may build up. Intraocular pressure builds within the eye, damaging the nerve endings of the RETINA. This condition is known as GLAUCOMA.

ARA-A An ANTIVIRAL DRUG prescribed in the treatment of ocular herpes. Available in ointment and pill form, it is also known by the names vidarabine, Vira-A and adenine arabinoside. Unlike IDU or TFT, drugs that attack healthy as well as infected cells, ARA-A is less toxic and attacks only viral cells.

ARA-A is used to treat HERPES SIMPLEX types 1 and 2 of the eyes, including herpes KERATITIS, a condition involving the cornea. It is also effective in the treatment of herpetic encephalitis, a brain infection.

ARA-A is not a cure for herpes keratitis or herpetic encephalitis. It can only destroy viral cells when the virus is active. During periods of herpetic latency, the drug is ineffective.

architectural barriers See ACCESSIBILITY.

Architectural Barriers Act The Architectural Barriers Act of 1968 requires buildings designed, constructed, or altered with federal funds to be accessible to physically disabled persons. The Act was amended to include access to public buildings and government-leased buildings for public use or where disabled individuals might be employed. Later legislation required government agencies to perform continuous surveys to ensure compliance with the Act.

The Rehabilitation Act of 1973 founded the Architectural and Transportation Barriers Compliance Board, which ensures compliance with the Act. The board reports to Congress and the president each year. Complaints about facilities that do not comply with the act must be submitted in writing to:

The Access Board, Office of Compliance and
  Enforcement
1331 P Street, NW, Suite 100
Washington, D.C. 20004-111

(See ACCESSIBILITY.)

U.S. Department of Education. *Summary of Existing Legislation Affecting Persons with Disabilities.* Washington, D.C.: USDE, 1988.

arcus senilis Arcus senilis is a grey or white ring or arc that appears on the edge of the IRIS, or colored part of the eye, where it borders the SCLERA, or white part of the eye. The ring is actually located on the margin of the CORNEA, the clear, protective covering of the eye.

The condition is caused by aging and is most often noticed in dark-eyed people. Arcus senilis is a harmless condition that does not affect vision and is not a sign of another eye disorder. Arcus senilis also is known as a cornea ring.

argon laser The argon is a LASER often used to treat DIABETIC RETINOPATHY, a leading cause of blindness in the United States. A complication of diabetes, diabetic retinopathy occurs as a result of damage to retinal blood vessels that leak or hemorrhage. The retinal tissue loses oxygen normally brought by the vessels and develops new vessels (neovascularization) that tend to be weak and bleed. Continuous leaking and the formation of retinal scars may lead to blindness.

If neovascularization has occurred, unhealthy, oxygen-deprived tissue is treated with the laser. The directed energy of the laser causes scarring and prohibits the tissue from forming new, weak vessels.

The argon laser, which was invented in 1964 by William Bridges, a scientist at Hughes Aircraft, may be used to treat subretinal neovascularization, a disorder caused by AGE-RELATED MACULOPATHY (ARM), a major cause of blindness associated with aging. ARM produces scarring of the macula, the region of the RETINA that allows for sharpest vision. Subretinal neovascularization is caused by a break in the pigment epithelium, a layer below the retina. A collection of blood vessels below the retina bleeds into the retina through the break and causes scarring.

During argon laser treatment, burns are placed around the neovascularization areas to cauterize the bleeding. However, the bluegreen light of the argon laser is absorbed by the pigment of the inner retina, above the deeper affected layers. This may cause damage to the inner retina.

The red krypton laser is often substituted for the argon on this procedure since it is absorbed only in the melanin pigment of the deepest layers of the retina where the neovascularization occurs. Treatment with the krypton laser is preferred since it allows the inner, unaffected retinal layers to remain untouched while treating only the deep, affected layers.

Laser therapy called laser trabeculoplasty may be an alternative to surgery in the treatment of GLAUCOMA, a disease in which the intraocular fluid fails to properly drain from the eye, accumulates and causes elevated intraocular pressure. If untreated, glaucoma causes a loss of peripheral vision and eventual blindness.

When medication fails to lower the intraocular pressure, laser trabeculoplasty with the argon may be used to open the drainage area located where the cornea meets the IRIS. A series of burns are placed in the drainage area, which causes scarring and openings within the meshwork of drainage channels. The fluid drains more easily from the eye, and intraocular pressure is reduced.

Berland, Theodore, and Richard A. Perritt. *Living With Your Eye Operation.* New York: St. Martin's Press, 1974.

Eden, John. *The Eye Book.* New York: Penguin Books, 1978.

Krames Communications. *The Retina Book.* Daly City, Calif.: KC, 1987.

Reynolds, James D., "Lasers in Ophthalmology." *Health-Net Library.* Columbus: CompuServe, 1989.

Shulman, Jules. *Cataracts.* New York: Simon and Schuster, 1984.

arterial occlusion A blockage of the arteries of the RETINA. When this occurs, blood is prevented from reaching the retina, and vision is threatened. Arterial occlusions may be caused by carotid artery stenosis, retinal artery emboli, retinal artery occlusion and temporal (also called giant cell) arteritis.

Arterial occlusion occurs most frequently in people between the ages of 50 and 80.

Carotid artery stenosis occurs when one of the carotid arteries, which lie on each side of the neck and supply blood to the brain, becomes narrowed with arteriosclerotic plaque. The blood flow to the brain and the eye is decreased, and a TIA, transient ischemic attack, or ministroke may occur.

TIAs are warning signals of more serious impending strokes and include the symptoms of tingling in the face or limbs, difficulty speaking, headache, dizziness, vision disturbances, inability to swallow, mental confusion, and loss of memory.

During a carotid artery stenosis or TIA, vision may be suddenly lost in one eye. The loss is usually painless and generally lasts for a short period of time. Temporary loss of vision of this type may be accepted as a symptom or warning sign of a TIA.

Individuals with any symptom or combination of symptoms of a TIA should be examined by a physician immediately. Treatment for carotid stenosis may include anticoagulants or a surgical procedure called carotid endarterectomy, which removes arteriosclerotic plaque from the carotid artery.

Retinal artery emboli are small particles of blood clots that enter the blood's circulation and become wedged in a retinal artery. These emboli may cause obstructions that result in vision loss.

The loss of vision is usually swift and painless. If treatment is not begun within minutes, vision may be permanently lost. Results from current treatments to restore vision are often disappointing. Therapy should include treatment of the underlying cause such as arteriosclerosis, hypertension, and heart disease.

Retinal artery occlusion is a blockage of the retinal artery that does not involve emboli. This is most common in hypertension patients as a result of ARTERIOSCLEROSIS. The sight loss is usually sudden, painless and permanent. Treatment is directed to the underlying hypertension and arteriosclerosis.

Temporal or giant-cell arteritis is a chronic condition that involves inflammation of all the body's arteries. The inflammation causes the artery walls to thicken, which may block the flow of blood to vital organs, including the eyes. Symptoms include dizziness, headache, weight loss, scalp tenderness, jaw pain, depression, low-grade fever, and vision loss. Vision loss may be sudden and permanent.

The disease may be diagnosed with a blood test that reveals the presence of giant cells and a biopsy. The disease is treated with corticosteroids. Vision in one eye may be lost before the diagnosis is made but careful monitoring and treatment of the unaffected eye may prevent further loss of vision.

Temporal arteritis may last from two to three months and is rarely seen in patients under 50 years of age. Approximately 25 percent of cases result in permanent blindness.

(See HYPERTENSIVE RETINOPATHY, STROKE and VENOUS OCCLUSION.)

American Heart Association. *1989 Stroke Facts.* Dallas: AHA, 1988.

Galloway, N. R. *Common Eye Diseases and Their Management.* Berlin: Springer-Verlag, 1985.

Gurwood, Andrew S., Alan G. Kabat, and Joseph W. Sowka. "Handbook of Ocular Disease Management." *Review of Optometry Online,* Jobson Publishing, 2002.

Reynolds, James D. "Ocular Artery and Vein Occlusion." *HealthNet Library,* Columbus: CompuServe, 1989.

arteriosclerosis   A condition in which the arteries become narrow and blocked, also known as hardening of the arteries. The condition is a leading cause of stroke and is associated with heart disease and other disorders. Arteriosclerosis produces fatty material, called plaque, that accumulates and lines the artery walls. The arteries become smaller in diameter, then clogged. This results in decreased blood circulation or cessation of the blood flow. As the body's organs receive less blood and oxygen, they may fail to function properly. When the blood flow is blocked, blood fails to reach the brain, and a STROKE results.

Arteriosclerosis is a factor in the formation of blood clots. Platelets, blood-clotting cells in the blood, tend to adhere to the arteriosclerotic plaque and further block the arteries. When the clot of platelets is jarred loose from the artery, it is termed an embolism. The embolism can travel through the blood stream, become wedged into a smaller blood vessel and cause a stroke.

Arteriosclerosis may also cause heart attacks, heart failure, heart disease, angina, kidney damage, poor circulation, and vision loss. It is associated with aging and high blood pressure, or hypertension, and is linked to obesity, improper diet, smoking, stress, and lack of exercise.

Arteriosclerosis may affect the eyes as the blood vessels of the RETINA become constricted. A normal RETINA, the light-sensitive layer in the back of the eye, gathers light information about an object and encodes it into electrical impulses. The impulses travel along the optic nerve to the brain where they are translated into an image. A retina impaired by arteriosclerosis cannot function adequately, and vision may be blurred or lost.

Retinal arteriosclerosis, when coupled with hypertension, is a condition called HYPERTENSIVE RETINOPATHY. Although the condition alone is rarely vision-threatening, it may lead to other eye diseases such as AGE-RELATED MACULOPATHY.

Age-related MACULOPATHY (ARM) is a condition in which the macula, the center of the retina and point of clearest vision, deteriorates. As the macula degenerates, central vision is lost. ARM may be caused by heredity, chronic sun exposure, or arteriosclerosis. It is a progressive disease without a cure but that can sometimes be treated with photocoagulation or laser treatments.

Arteriosclerosis is often present without symptoms. The condition may be detected during a medical or ophthalmologic examination. It is treated with medication for high blood pressure or anticoagulants that increase blood circulation and discourage the accumulation of plaque. Patients are often urged to make changes in diet and exercise and to reduce smoking and stress.

arteritis   See ARTERIAL OCCLUSION.

Artic Technologies   A company founded in 1984 to develop products using speech synthesis, such as custom computers and braille notetakers, to be used by the blind. Artic updates its products frequently to take advantage, and keep abreast, of changing technology.

Contact:

Artic Technologies
55 Park Street
Troy, MI, 48083
248-588-7370 (ph)
248-588-2650 (fax)
www.artictech.com

artificial tears   Artificial tears are used to treat dry eye, a condition brought about by allergy, keratoconjunctivitis (corneal and conjunctival inflammation), extreme vitamin-A deficiency, TRACHOMA, chemical burns, and disorders and diseases, such as BELL'S PALSY. Many artificial tears are available without prescription.

These drugs are known by the generic names hydroxyethylcellulose, hydroxyproplycellulose, hydroxypropl methylcellulose, methylcellulose, polyvinyl alcohol, and other polymeric solutions. Numerous trade names include Clerz, Lacrisert, Isopto Alkaline, Muro Tears, Methopto, Methulose, Aqua Tears, Liquifilm Tears, aqua-FLOW, Refresh, Adapettes, Comfort Drops, Moisture Eyes, and Hypo Tears.

Henkind, Paul, Martin Mayers and Arthur Berger, eds. *Physicians' Desk Reference for Ophthalmology 1987.* Oradell, N.J.: Medical Economics Company Inc., 1987.

artificial vision system   A system that uses technology to produce images that can be detected and recognized by blind people. Developed by Dr. William H. Dobelle, the device is battery operated and weighs about 10 pounds. It works through a miniature digital video camera and an ultrasonic distance sensor, which are built into a pair of sunglasses. The sensor connects through a cable to a small computer, which the blind person wears around his or her waist.

The computer processes the video and distance signals, then uses computer-imaging technology to transmit the image to the person wearing the device. Once the image has been transmitted, the computer triggers a second computer, which sends pulses to 68 platinum electrodes that have been surgically implanted onto the part of the brain that controls vision. The second computer is screwed into the wearer's skull bone, with its shaft protruding through the skin.

When the electrodes are stimulated, they generate a display of phosphenes, which are bursts of light caused by pressure on the eyeball. Phosphenes appear as black-and-white images, and the wearer of the device possibly can learn to recognize patterns and distinguish images. Reportedly, one blind man who received the artificial vision system made such progress that he was able to recognize different character sets commonly used in visual acuity tests. The system also has an electronic interface that is a radio frequency. It can replace the camera and allows patients to watch television and use a computer.

The artificial vision system, also called a visual prosthesis, is still in the testing stages, but is expected to be available on a limited commercial basis sometime in 2002. Dobelle, who heads the Dobelle Institute at Columbia Presbyterian Medical Center in New York City, and the Institute Dobelle AG in Zurich, Switzerland, has been working on the vision system for 30 years.

Reuters Health. "Artificial Vision System Gives 'Sight' to the Blind." *Rx.com Magazine,* January 18, 2000.

A-scan An A-scan is a test that uses ultrasonic waves to determine the length of the eye. An A-scan is performed prior to CATARACT surgery to pre-determine the power of an intraocular lens implant or to ascertain whether an implant is necessary.

The average eye is approximately 24 millimeters from the CORNEA to the RETINA. A shorter eye is usually farsighted, or hyperopic. A longer eye is usually nearsighted, or myopic. A shorter eye needs a stronger lens to focus properly. A longer eye needs a weaker lens to focus. An extremely long eye may not require an implant.

The information from this painless test is analyzed by a computer along with the results of KERATOMETRY. The computer evaluates the information and determines the power of the needed implant.

Association for Education and Rehabilitation of the Blind and Visually Impaired (AER) An organization founded in 1984 as a consolidation of the Association for Education of the Visually Handicapped (AEVH) and the American Association of Workers for the Blind (AAWB). The goal of the organization is to promote the advancement of education and rehabilitation of blind and visually impaired persons.

It is a private nonprofit organization of 41 state groups and 7 regional groups. The organization has over 6,000 members internationally.

The membership includes anyone interested in the education, vocational rehabilitation, guidance, or occupational placement of visually impaired persons. The membership encompasses educators, administrators, ophthalmologists, social workers, professionals in the field of rehabilitation, parents, agencies, organizations, and schools.

AER works with universities and colleges to provide workshops and conferences and extend opportunities for the visually impaired. It maintains certification programs, presents awards, offers job-exchange services, and provides public information services.

AER holds a biennial convention and issues two publications, *AER Report,* a bimonthly newsletter,

Re:View, a quarterly journal, and "Job Exchange," a monthly listing of available jobs within the field.
  Contact:

Association for the Education of the Blind and
  Visually Impaired
4600 Duke Street, Suite 430
Alexandria, Virginia 22347
703-823-9690 (ph)
703-823-9695 (fax)
www.aerbvi.org

Association of Parents Having a Kid in Contacts (APHAKIC) An on-line group for parents of children with vision problems, especially those who wear contacts or other corrective lenses. The website offers advice, information and support for parents, as well as recommendations for ophthalmologists and other eye specialists.

The group has an on-line newsletter and offers discussion groups and bulletin boards where parents can share questions and concerns. APHAKIC can be accessed on the Internet at http://members.aol.com/aphakic.

astigmatism A common disorder in which the visual image is distorted because the corneal surface is not completely spherical. Light entering the eye at different angles is focused unequally, creating the distortion. An individual with astigmatism may not recognize the distortion because the brain compensates for it and presents a reasonable image.

Symptoms of astigmatism include eye strain and headaches. Cylindrical lenses are prescribed in the form of eyeglasses or contact lenses and may be combined with a prescription for near- or farsightedness. Patients may experience a feeling of being tilted or off balance for the first few days of wearing the cylindrical lenses as the brain learns to read the new, correct image.

Astigmatism levels off after the eye stops growing, but can change with age, due to PRESBYOPIA, changes in the eyelid, and cataract formation.

attitudes Attitudes toward blind persons are formed by and reflect the society in that blind people live. Historically, blind or visually impaired persons have been viewed negatively as either liabilities or wards of the society. Although strides have been made by visually impaired individuals in modern history, they are to some extent still viewed as a separate group—"the blind" rather than as blind individuals.

Society lacks full social, economic and vocational integration of the visually impaired. Therefore, large segments of society have little contact with, or knowledge of, the true abilities and individuality of blind people. This segregation perpetuates "handicapism," a term for stereotyping, prejudice, and discrimination by society against disabled people. Handicapism reinforces negative stereotypes and increases barriers to integration.

Society develops and maintains stereotypes about disabled people through superstitious beliefs, fairy tales, folklore, comic books, literature, religious beliefs, the media, and many charity organizations that serve disabled persons. These serve as information sources when personal experiences are limited.

The most commonly held stereotypes place visually impaired persons (or any disabled person) in one of two roles: either very good and righteous or very bad and evil. The stereotype of the blind person as heroic is common. The individual is considered admirable by "overcoming all obstacles" to achieve modest, everyday goals such as going to school or holding a job. This undermines the feasibility of such goals for most blind people.

The situation is also sometimes exaggerated to portray the blind person who has overcome all odds to achieve ambitious goals by use of compensating powers or abilities. In films and literature, blind persons are falsely attributed with ESP, heightened hearing or touch, or higher IQs as powers that develop through Nature's compensation program to offset the loss of sight.

Films and literature often depict blind persons as righteous and in positions of jeopardy, so that plots of good versus evil can be enacted. This reinforces the stereotype of blind persons as victims of violence, people to be pitied.

The pitiful character is seen as helpless and perpetuates the reasoning that blind people lack independence and must be cared for. This reduces

blind persons to being considered burdens on society. It ignores the fact that blind people can be self-supporting and self-sufficient. According to the stereotype, blind people are considered generally unhappy persons who lead dependent, bitter, unsatisfying lives.

The stereotype of blind persons as evil or sinister also exists. Negative blindness stereotypes stem from our very language. Phrases such as "blind alley," "blind stupor" or "blind fury" reinforce the concept of blindness with darkness, fear, ignorance, and evil.

Historically, blindness was considered a mark of disapproval from the gods or a punishment for sins. In ancient societies, blind children were left in the elements to die. Literature such as the Oedipus legend depicts the hero's self-imposed blindness as a punishment for his sins.

According to another stereotypical attitude, blind people are held to be self-pitying. In response to complaints about discrimination, society often instructs that the individual should "get on with life" or "when life gives you lemons, make lemonade." The individual is considered bitter and angry rather than an activist.

Blind people are generally regarded as physically and recreationally less active than others, although the lack of sight may be their only physical limitation. Blind skydivers, swimmers, bowlers, golfers, and skiers abound but are rarely depicted in the media or noted by society.

The misconception of the blind person as sedentary and homebound is tied to the belief that blindness is a disease rather than a sensory loss. This breeds the fear that, like a disease, blindness can be "caught" or transmitted.

Blind persons using a dog guide are generally accepted as the norm, although a very small percentage of blind persons actually own a dog guide. Society mistakenly holds that the dog knows the directions to the destination, checks the color of the traffic lights, and directs its owner when to cross the street. In reality, the dog is directed by the owner, is color-blind, and is basically used only to avoid obstacles and occasionally protect its owner from danger.

Seldom depicted, but in reality more common, is the concept of the blind person who uses a long cane. Although a person traveling with a cane is generally competent, graceful, and self-assured, the stereotype features a distracted bumbler who inadvertently destroys objects with a wildly swinging cane. This stereotype gives rise to the concept of the blind person as laughable or foolish.

Another stereotypical view is that blind persons are less intelligent than their sighted peers. It is held that since sighted persons require vision to learn and confirm knowledge, the lack of sight disallows learning.

The loss of sight is also linked with the loss of all the senses, particularly hearing. This prompts some people to shout questions at a blind person who has normal hearing.

Blind persons are often believed by society to be nonsexual. Castration and blindness are linked in the Oedipus legend, in the result of blindness from venereal disease and in the superstition that masturbation leads to blindness.

In light of these stereotypes, sighted people may react with conflicting emotions when interacting with blind people. A sighted person may feel fear, anxiety, pity, revulsion, superiority, generosity, shame, helplessness, or suspicion. These attitudes negatively influence hiring practices, legislative priorities, economic opportunities, and social potentialities of disabled persons.

Although many of these stereotypes and attitudes still prevail, there are indications that public attitude toward people with disabilities is starting to change. In 1991, the polling firm Louis Harris & Associates conducted the first poll regarding public attitude toward disabled people. The poll, commissioned by the National Organization on Disability, revealed that movies depicting people who are in some way disabled are making the public more aware of, and empathetic toward, those who are disabled.

Films such as *Rain Man,* in which a main character is autistic, and *Children of a Lesser God,* in which a main character is deaf and played by a deaf actress, were cited as examples of movies that have influenced attitudes. Harris said that people who are exposed to conditions such as blindness, either in actuality or through a film, become more comfortable and familiar with them.

"Clearly, familiarity breeds an empathy, an understanding, a sense of equality," Harris said. "Lack of familiarity breeds concerns, doubts, and outright hostility."

Biklen, Douglas, and Robert Bogdan. "Media Portrayals of Disabled People: A Study in Stereotypes," *Interracial Books for Children Bulletin* vol. 8, nos. 6–7 (1977), pp. 4–9.

Goldberg, Maxwell H., and John R. Swinton. *Blindness Research: The Expanding Frontiers.* University Park: Pennsylvania State University Press, 1969.

Lukoff, Irving, et al. *Attitudes Toward Blind Persons.* New York: American Foundation for the Blind, 1972.

Weinberg, Nancy, and Rosina Santana. "Comic Books: Champions of the Disabled Stereotype." *Rehabilitation Literature* vol. 39, nos. 11–12 (November–December 1978), pp. 327–331.

auditory aids   Auditory aids and devices enable the visually impaired user to access information with the sense of hearing. These include tape recorders and players, speech compressors, accelerated speech, talking books, synthetic speech, and talking aids.

Cassette tape recorders are used to record or play back recorded material. Some models are available with stop/start foot pedals to allow for typing while listening.

Speech compressors are machines that control the speed of the audio of a tape by deleting portions of the pauses between words or by shortening vowel sounds. The material is rerecorded in the shorter version. The sound of the speech is not affected.

Accelerated speech is text that is recorded at normal speed but reproduced and played at an accelerated speed. Highly accelerated speech may produce a distortion in the sound of the voice, although some models contain pitch-controlling options.

Talking books and other recorded texts are recorded by, and available through, talking-book programs or the Library of Congress. Books on cassette tape are also available through commercial publishers.

Synthetic speech is the computerized production of sounds into words and is used in the voice output of reading machines and computers. The

Kurzweil Reading Machine converts print placed onto its scanner into synthetic speech.

Talking aids are tools that provide auditory readings or speech to supply the reading or information normally gained by sight. These include the talking scale, clock, watch, timer, blood-pressure monitor, thermometer, blood-glucose monitoring kit, talking wallet (which identifies bills of $1–$10 denominations), label maker, and calculator.

Bell's palsy   A disorder involving unilateral facial weakness or paralysis. The condition usually has its onset over a two- to five-day period. During that time, the patient may experience a loss of facial sensation, a numbness, drooling, delay in blinking, inability to close the eye, excessive tearing, paralysis of one side of the face, or noticeable drooping of the mouth or face. Half of those with Bell's palsy experience pain behind the ear, but the condition does not cause hearing impairments.

The symptoms of Bell's palsy, named for Sir Charles Bell, the 19th-century physician who first described the disease, may be confused with those of a stroke. Bell's-palsy symptoms, however, usually affect the entire side of the face from forehead to chin, whereas stroke symptoms are usually located below the eye. Bell's-palsy symptoms do not include classic stroke indications, such as weakness in limbs, slurred speech or double vision.

Bell's palsy is caused by a swelling of the facial nerve due to immune disorders or a viral disease. The nerve is constricted, the blood supply is limited and the nerve becomes ischemic, or anemic, due to lack of blood flow. Nerve degeneration may follow.

Individuals who contract Bell's palsy are typically in good health, but a history of DIABETES, SARCOIDOSIS, or LYME DISEASE has been linked to the disorder. It has been associated with influenza, colds, and headaches and may be triggered by such illnesses. Bell's palsy may occur to either sex at any age but is most prevalent after the age of 40.

Bell's palsy poses the greatest threat to the eye's CORNEA, the clear, protective cover of the eye. When the eyelid, which normally protects the cornea, functions incorrectly, the cornea becomes dry and is vulnerable to the elements. Constant exposure may result in KERATITIS (corneal infection), ulceration or injury, causing a loss of vision.

The eye may be treated with occasional applications of ARTIFICIAL TEARS such as methylcellulose solution during the day and a lubricating cream or ointment such as Lacri-Lube S.O.P. at night. The eye may be taped shut or protected with an eyeshield.

Dryness or irritation, increased sensitivity to light or symptoms of infection may develop and require further treatment. A partial TARSORRHAPHY, a surgical procedure in which the upper and lower eyelids are stitched together at the corner, may be performed. The tarsorrhaphy is reversible and may be temporarily effective but may cause corneal breakdown, irritation to the cornea from eyelashes or scars along the lashline.

The treatment of Bell's palsy may include physical therapy, a combination of heat application and facial massage or facial exercises. In severe cases, corticosteroids may be prescribed for 10–14 days.

In 85 percent of cases, recovery begins to occur within 10 days to 3 weeks. The remaining 15 percent of cases may require up to 12 months to recover. The condition tends to recur in 10 percent of cases and usually affects the opposite side of the face. Pregnancy has been linked to recurrences, as has multiple sclerosis.

Dyke, Peter J., Gunter Haase and Mark May. "Diagnosis and Care of Bell's Palsy." *Patient Care* (October 1988): 107–118.
The Bell's Palsy Network Frequently Asked Questions. www.bellspalsy.net, 1997.

bifocals   Bifocals or bifocal lenses contain two prescription lenses put together in one lens. Each contact or eyeglass lens has two focusing abilities, one for seeing near objects and one for seeing distant objects.

Bifocals are usually needed after age 40. They are a common aid in the treatment of PRESBYOPIA, aging eyes. As the eye ages, its LENS loses the ability to focus on close objects.

Prescription of reading glasses alone would solve the problem, but the wearer would have to remove the glasses to see distant objects. The wearer requiring a distance vision correction would have to constantly switch between reading glasses and distance glasses. Bifocals eliminate the necessity of swapping glasses when changing tasks.

Although modern bifocals are essentially the same two pairs of glasses combined into one frame that Benjamin Franklin invented, today's lenses are custom-designed for the wearer. The reading and distance segments of each lens may be small or large and placed high or low in the frame. The lens size and placement are determined by the needs of the wearer. Using an updated method of polishing, bifocals today can be made without a noticeable line. These are called "blended bifocals," and are preferred by many people.

The clerk whose job requires copious amounts of reading and occasional distance viewing will need a large reading segment and a smaller section for distance at the top of the lens. The factory supervisor who manages a long assembly line will need a smaller reading section located low in the lens to avoid obstructing a distance view.

Bifocal wearers must adopt new head movements to use bifocals correctly and safely. The wearer may have to raise his chin when reading something at a level higher than normal or learn to lower his head, rather than just his eyes, when navigating a cluttered path.

binocular indirect ophthalmoscope   See OPH-THALMOSCOPE.

biomicroscope   The biomicroscope (or slit lamp) is an instrument used to examine the eye. It magnifies the ANTERIOR CHAMBER of the eye, including the CORNEA, IRIS and LENS.

A biomicroscope examination is one step in a routine eye exam. It is painless. The patient places his chin on a chin rest centered at the bottom of an open square-shaped frame. A bright light in front of the frame shines a vertical beam of light through the cornea. The light that is reflected back gives an illuminated, magnified cross-section of the front part of the eye.

The biomicroscope examination is used to check for abrasions, erosion or scarring, inflammation, presence of blood vessels, or change of shape in the cornea; inflammation or thinning of the SCLERA, inflammation or irregularities of the iris; and sub-luxated or shifted lens and CATARACTS.

The biomicroscope may also be used to examine the eye during tests such as those to determine intraocular pressure (TONOGRAPHY) or the junction of the cornea and the iris (GONIOSCOPY). It also is used as a tool in some laser treatment procedures.

bioptics   Optical aids that consist of small telescopes fused onto the upper portion of spectacles, on one or both lenses. The bottom portion of the spectacles contains the individual's corrective prescription.

The bioptics involving both eyes enable the low-vision user to view distances when walking or driving or to view closer objects or material if magnification is needed. The bioptics that involve one eye only are used for near and intermediate distance viewing for reading material.

Bioptics are prescribed by an ophthalmologist or low-vision expert and must be properly centered to the eyes of the wearer. Magnification may extend to six times normal size when used for distance viewing. Wide-angle lenses may be incorporated into the device. Thirty states permit driving with the aid of bioptics. Regulations vary from state to state.

blepharitis   Blepharitis is a common condition of the eyelids. The margin of the eyelid becomes swollen and red with inflammation, and a crusty discharge may gather at the base of the lashes. Some lash loss may occur, but in milder cases the lashes grow back. In severe cases, the lash follicles are destroyed and permanent lash loss results.

Causes of blepharitis, sometimes called eyelash dandruff, are unknown. It is often associated with allergies, a disorder in the lipid layer of the tear film or seborrhoea of the scalp. Although blepharitis is a difficult condition to treat, it rarely results in loss of vision.

It is important to keep the eyelid area very clean in order to cut the buildup of secretions. Ophthalmologists may treat the symptoms of blepharitis with ANTIBIOTICS, but since there is no cure, the disorder may become chronic. Chronic blepharitis may involve CONJUNCTIVITIS and inflammation of the CORNEA.

Blinded Veterans Association (BVA) An association founded in 1945 by a group of veterans blinded in World War II. In 1958, the BVA was chartered by an act of Congress to represent all blinded veterans. It is the only service association committed exclusively to meeting the needs of veterans with severe vision impairments. This nonprofit organization has a membership of 6,500, consisting of veterans who have lost their sight while serving in the armed forces and veterans who have since lost their vision in ways unrelated to the armed services.

The BVA maintains two major outreach programs: The Field Service Program and the Outreach Employment Program. Blinded veterans serving as representatives of the Field Service Program provide emotional support, encouragement and assistance to fellow veterans seeking services, rehabilitation training and benefits from local, state, and Veterans Administration agencies. In 1988, the Field Service Program made nearly 1,400 contacts to assist visually impaired veterans.

The Outreach Employment Program assists veterans in finding satisfying employment and developing independence. Blinded veterans serving as representatives of this program aid in all aspects of job placement, ranging from resume writing to acquisition of vocational training. Both programs are available to veterans at no cost.

The BVA also serves as a clearinghouse for information to alert veterans and others to new legislation, rights, benefits and technology. The BVA maintains a public-awareness program regarding the capabilities and productivity of blinded veterans.

The association publishes the journal *BVA Bulletin* and a newsletter, *BVA Update*. The BVA holds an annual convention in August.

Contact:

Blinded Veterans Association
477 H Street, N.W.
Washington, D.C. 20001–2694
800-669-7079
www.bva.org

blindisms Stereotypical mannerisms or behaviors of blind children or infants are commonly called "blindisms." The term is misleading, since the same mannerisms are also stereotypical of children with other disabilities, such as autism.

These stereotypical behaviors include rocking, shaking or turning the head, shaking the hands, mouthing the hands or objects, and eye poking or pressing. The repetitive and unconsciously performed mannerisms are most often found in those who are congenitally blind but may be acquired by those with adventitious blindness.

Some studies indicate that children create these mannerisms of self-stimulation to compensate for the lack of sensory stimulation and activity in their lives. Others cite the lack of opportunity and ability of blind children to imitate the acceptable behaviors of others and to develop a sense of unacceptable behaviors.

Behaviors related to the vision loss may appear to be blindisms. A child may hold the head unnaturally to one side in order to make the best use of residual vision or a reduced visual field or may grimace in an effort to see an image.

Blindisms may lead to social segregation if the mannerisms are considered distracting or unsightly. They may falsely indicate to others the presence of mental retardation, autism, or emotional disorders. Blindisms may become injurious to the individual, since eye rubbing and poking can cause bruising and callous formation.

Blindisms may be prevented by the use of stimulating, physical activity (including the use of motion furniture such as rocking chairs and swings), development of an interest in the environment and frequent opportunities for new experiences.

Established blindisms may be corrected if the child is given a substitute activity for the physical movement. The effort of flapping the hands may be redirected to playing an instrument or fondling a stuffed toy.

Bonfanti, Barbara H. "Effects of Training on Nonverbal and Verbal Behaviors of Congenitally Blind Adults," *Journal of Visual Impairment and Blindness* (January 1979): 1–9.

The Canadian National Institute for the Blind. *The Impact of Vision Loss on the Development of Children from Birth to 12 Years.* www.cnib.ca/pamphlets_publications/vision, 2000.

Cutsworth, T. *The Blind in School and Society.* New York: American Foundation for the Blind Inc., 1951.

Eichel, Valerie J. "A Taxonomy for Mannerisms of Blind Children." *Journal of Visual Impairment and Blindness* (May 1979): 167–177.

Fraiberg, S. *Insights from the Blind.* New York: Basic Books, 1977.

Harper, Florine Watson. "Gestures of the Blind." *Education of the Visually Handicapped* (Spring 1978): 14–20.

Hoshmand, Lisa T. "Blindisms: Some Observations and Propositions." *Education of the Visually Handicapped* (May 1975): 56–59.

Knight, John J. "Mannerisms in the Congenitally Blind Child." *The New Outlook* (November 1972): 297–301.

Miller, Barbara S., and William H. Miller. "Extinguishing 'Blindisms': A Paradigm for Intervention." *Education of the Visually Handicapped* (Spring 1976): 7–14.

Scholl, Geraldine, ed. *Foundations of Education for Blind and Visually Handicapped Children and Youth.* New York: American Foundation for the Blind Inc., 1986.

Warren, D. H. *Blindness and Early Childhood Development.* New York: American Foundation for the Blind Inc., 1984.

blindness   Blindness, or loss of vision, is a condition that is prevalent throughout the world. The World Health Organization estimates that there are between 40 million and 45 million blind people in the world, and an additional 120 million suffering from disabling low vision. In addition, the organization predicts that, unless decisive public health action is taken, the numbers of people who are blind or visually impaired will double by the year 2025.

Worldwide, the most common causes of blindness are CATARACT, TRACHOMA, and GLAUCOMA. These three conditions account for more than 70 percent of the world's blindness. Nine out of 10 of the world's blind people live in developing countries, with nearly 60 percent of all the blind people in the world living in sub-Saharan Africa, China, and India. The World Health Organization estimates that up to 80 percent of global blindness is preventable through nutritional, therapeutic, and sanitation-improvement programs. Other common causes of blindness worldwide are Vitamin A deficiency, ONCHOCERCIASIS, LEPROSY, DIABETIC RETINOPATHY, MACULAR DISEASE, RETINITIS PIGMENTOSA, eye injuries, and congenital or hereditary disorders.

In the United States, there are about 1 million people who are legally blind, and another 2.3 million who are visually impaired, according to Prevent Blindness America, formerly known as the National Society to Prevent Blindness. The most common causes of blindness in the United States are age-related glaucoma, macular degeneration, diabetic retinopathy, and hereditary disorders such as retinitis pigmentosa and Stargardt's disease.

The terms *blind* and *blindness* are defined in a variety of ways according to the user. Rehabilitation experts, doctors and ophthalmologists, educators and leaders in the field determine and define the terms according to their own preferences and viewpoints.

Over the past 150 years, blindness has been described using various terms including medically blind, legally blind, partially blind, partially seeing, low vision, functionally blind, braille blind, vocationally blind, economically blind, visually defective, visually impaired, visually handicapped and visually disabled.

Medical diagnostic guidelines define blindness as no light perception (NLP), or light perception and projection, or central acuity up to hand movements plus a large field loss. *Hand movement* and *hand motion* are terms used to describe someone who cannot see the separate fingers but who can discern some movement when the hand is waved. Light perception, or LP, describes the person who can perceive only light or its absence. NLP or no light perception refers to one who is unable to discern any light.

The American Foundation for the Blind recommends that the term *blind* be reserved for those individuals with no usable sight at all, and that the terms *visually impaired, low vision* or *partially sighted* be used to describe persons with some usable vision, regardless of how little.

Legal blindness is the term used by the Internal Revenue Service and other governmental agencies to determine whether an individual is eligible for federal or state benefits. The classification for legal blindness is determined by measuring visual acuity (how much detail one sees at a specific distance) and visual field (the area of vision).

A person is classified as legally blind if the visual acuity of the better eye, with correction, is 20/200 or less. This involves a loss of central vision.

One may also be described as legally blind if the visual field of the better eye, even with 20/20 vision, is limited to 20 degrees or less. An individual with loss in the visual field may experience peripheral or central vision loss.

Loss in the peripheral, or side, vision may result in tunnel vision. Loss in the central, or straight-ahead, vision may result in difficulty in seeing an object in the center or direct line of sight. Because the classification involves measurement of the better eye only, people who are blind in one eye are not considered legally blind.

Legally blind people should not necessarily be considered totally blind. The term includes a wide range of visual abilities, since two individuals with 20/200 visual acuity or 20 degree visual fields may have vastly different vision levels. Over 75 percent of legally blind individuals have some remaining vision. These people are often able to utilize their remaining vision to work, read, travel and continue their daily routine by using adaptive devices or by developing accommodating body or head movements.

Partially seeing is a term that replaced *partially blind*. It is defined as a central visual acuity of between 20/60 and 20/200 in the better eye with correction. *Low vision* is defined as between 20/50 and 20/200 in the better eye with correction.

Functionally blind refers to the ability of the individual to function or perform daily tasks. Certain diagnoses relate to specific functional guidelines. For instance, NLP requires braille for reading and long canes or dog guides for independent traveling. "Braille blind" refers to a person's inability to read large print even with optical aids and, therefore, the person's need for braille.

Vocationally blind and *economically blind* are terms little used today. Each refers to an inability of blind people to earn a living, an outdated notion. *Visually defective* is a negative, archaic term.

Visually impaired is a term that describes a recognizable defect or malfunctioning of the eye. Impairments are diagnosed and defined by a medical doctor. Visual impairments range from total blindness to low vision.

The term *visually impaired* is also used frequently to describe those persons who have sight loss in one or both eyes but are not legally blind. These include individuals who cannot read newsprint with prescriptive lenses (severely impaired) or who are monocularly blind or who have otherwise unclassified visual impairments.

Handicapped refers to individuals who are disadvantaged in the performance of tasks due to expectations or attitudes about their impairment. The term *visually handicapped* is commonly used almost interchangeably with *visually impaired*. When applied to children, *visually handicapped* notes the requirement for special education provisions due to sight loss.

Visually disabled applies to the actual effect the impairment has on the functioning of the individual. It is the limitation or restriction caused by the lack of sight. Disabilities are not necessarily handicaps.

Terms such as congenital blindness, adventitious blindness, cortical blindness, hysterical blindness, and snow blindness are well defined and accepted. Each refers to the cause of vision loss.

Congenitally blind refers to an individual blind at birth or during the first five years of life. A congenitally blind child may not have visual memory.

Adventitiously blind refers to an individual who becomes blind after five years of age. This individual will probably have some visual memory and can use visualization.

Cortical blindness occurs as a result of lesions on both occipital lobes where the visual cortex is located. The lobes control the visual field of each eye. Lesions on both lobes causes bilateral loss of vision with normally reactive pupils. A lesion on one occipital lobe may result in hemianopsia, loss of half the field of vision, but does not affect the central vision acuity.

Cortical blindness is most common in aging eyes affected by vascular disease. There may be a history of cerebrovascular incidents and loss of cerebral function. Cortical blindness may be a temporary condition that follows a cerebrovascular embolism or circulatory occlusion caused by a stroke, myocardial infarction, or heart surgery.

Hysterical blindness is a condition of blindness caused by the need to physically resolve an emotional upset or shock. The condition is usually bilateral and often occurs suddenly. Often the blindness is not total and is restricted to a particular field. Additional symptoms include lack of regard for the loss of sight, ability to travel within surroundings, and normal blink response. An eye examination reveals that the pupils react normally and the fundus (back of the eye) appears normal, discounting damage to the optic nerve, cortical blindness, chiasmal lesions, or other ocular disease. The condition is usually diagnosed in light of information gathered through the eye examination and study of the patient's psychological history. Treatment of hysterical blindness may include reassurance that the condition will right itself, evidence of ability to see, and placebo medicine therapy. The patient may recover from the hysterical blindness only to replace it with another physical illness. Psychiatric counseling is often recommended to address the underlying emotional problem.

Snow blindness is the term for an eye injury caused by intense light reflected off snow. The bright light in prolonged exposure produces an ultraviolet burn on the cornea of the eye. Symptoms of snow blindness are bilateral and include extreme pain, a feeling of sand in the eyes, and severe sensitivity to light. The symptoms are usually delayed two to nine hours after exposure.

The burn heals itself within two to three days. Antibiotic or steroid drops may be prescribed to ease discomfort and discourage infection. Snow blindness can be prevented by wearing protective goggles or glasses. (See TERMINOLOGY, VISION IMPAIRMENT, WORLD BLINDNESS.)

American Foundation for the Blind. *Low Vision Questions and Answers.* New York: AFB, 1987.
Barraga, Natalie C. *Visual Handicaps and Learning.* Belmont, Calif.: Wadsworth Publishing Company Inc., 1976.
ERIC Clearinghouse on Handicapped and Gifted Children. *ERIC Digest: Visual Impairments.* Reston, Va.: ERIC, 1982.
Foundation for the Junior Blind. *California Services for Persons with Visual Impairments.* Los Angeles: FJB, 1987.
Galloway, N. R. *Common Eye Diseases and Their Management.* Berlin: Springer-Verlag, 1985.
Kelley, Jerry D., ed. *Recreational Programming for Visually Impaired Children and Youth.* New York: American Foundation for the Blind, 1981.
National Association for Visually Handicapped. *Problems of the Partially Sighted.* New York: NAVH, 1980.
National Information Center for Handicapped Children and Youth. *General Information about Handicaps and People with Handicaps.* Washington, D.C.: NICHCY, 1982.
Prevent Blindness America. *Facts and Figures,* www.preventblindness.org, 1998–2000.
Scholl, Geraldine T. *Foundations of Education for Blind and Visually Handicapped Children and Youth,* New York: American Foundation for the Blind, 1986.
World Health Organization. Blindness and Visual Disability. www.who.int, 1998.

blind spot The blind spot is a point of blindness or blocked vision found in normal PERIPHERAL VISION. This spot is caused by the OPTIC DISC. The optic disc is the spot on the RETINA where the OPTIC NERVE meets the eye.

The retina is the light-sensitive layer of the back of the eye. It contains cells called RODS AND CONES, which receive light and provide information about the viewed object. The retina encodes this information into electrical impulses. The impulses are sent to the brain via the optic nerve, a cord of nerve fibers that connects the brain to the eye and supplies blood to the retina. The brain translates the impulses into an image. The optic nerve is joined to the retina at the optic disc. The optic disc is devoid of photosensitive rods or cones and is unable to collect information about an object. As a result, the disc is "blind."

Since the blind spot is small and located within the peripheral (side) field of vision, it does not interfere with normal vision. The optic disc may be observed during an ophthalmologic exam or by moving an object into the field of the blind spot.

This is easily accomplished by marking a piece of white paper with an *X*. Approximately two inches to the right of the *X*, mark a dark circle. Close the left eye and look directly and steadily at the *X*. Move the paper forward or back until the circle disappears. This circle lies in the sphere of the optic disc.

The blind spot does not affect normal vision. Constant eye movements deflect attention from the blind area and the brain compensates for its lack by completing any incomplete lines and filling in any gaps.

books for the blind   See NATIONAL LIBRARY SERVICE FOR THE BLIND AND PHYSICALLY HANDICAPPED.

braille   A tactile language made up of a system of raised dots. The reader of braille feels the dots to recognize the letter. Braille makes reading, writing, note taking, and communicating possible for visually impaired, blind, and deaf-blind users.

Braille was invented in 1824 by LOUIS BRAILLE, a blind French student. He based his system on a method of raised dots and dashes called night writing or Sonography. Sonography was developed by Charles Barbier de la Serre to enable soldiers to read messages passed during night maneuvers. Braille and Barbier met to discuss possible alterations to the system. When Barbier insisted that the method remain unaltered, Braille developed a new system that involved raised dots in a fresh configuration.

Although the braille system was met with enthusiasm by blind users, the system was not first accepted officially by educators until 30 years later, in 1854. This may have been caused by resistance to change from the proven methods of instruction, a lack of willingness on the part of sighted instructors to learn a new method, or the simultaneous development and promotion of other new language systems for the blind.

The braille system is based on a cell, a configuration of dots forming two columns of three dots each. Each letter of the alphabet and each punctuation mark is made up of one or more of the possible six dots that make up a cell. Sixty-three combinations or patterns are possible.

In addition to the alphabet, there are 189 contractions and short forms or abbreviations for words that are formed in the cells. These same braille cells are also assigned different meanings to write music, foreign languages, numbers, and science terms.

Different forms or grades of braille are available. Grade 1 braille is the form developed by Louis Braille and utilizes one character per each letter of the alphabet. It contains no contractions. Grade 2

braille was developed in England and contains over 200 contractions and short forms for common words. In 1932, Grade 2 or Standard English Braille was officially adopted as the braille of choice for English-speaking nations. Grade 3 braille is an expansion of Grade 2. It extends the list of contractions and deletes vowels. Grade 3 is used most often for ease in writing rapidly or for taking notes.

Braille is embossed onto thick paper or plastic sheets by a braille press, braille writer or brailler, braille computer printer, or manual slate and stylus. Because braille requires a large amount of space, the braille edition of a book or magazine is several times longer than the print edition.

Braille is read with the finger tips of the index finger and/or middle finger or ring finger of one or both hands. An average reading speed of a reader using one hand is approximately 104 words per minute. Ambidextrous readers may increase the rate to 200 or more words per minute.

Braille is not used by all visually impaired or blind people. Some visually impaired persons have sufficient remaining vision to read with the use of an optical aid such as a magnifier. Others with less useful residual vision may opt to forgo learning braille due to physical problems such as diabetic neuropathy (decreased sensitivity in the fingers due to diabetes) or because of advanced age.

The wide availability of recorded books, other reading materials and synthetic speech output for computers may have had an effect on the willingness of visually impaired persons to learn braille. However, braille reading is accepted as a necessary skill for learning the basic literacy skills of reading, grammar, and diction.

Braille, Louis   Louis Braille is the inventor of braille, a language of raised dots read by the fingers and used by visually impaired persons.

Braille was born in 1809 in Coupvray, France, the son of a harness maker. At the age of three, he injured his eye while playing with his father's leather-working tools. The initial injury became infected, spread to both eyes and left him completely blind.

He was sent to the Royal Institution for Blind Youth in Paris when he was 10. The students in the school were taught orally through lessons repeated to them by their instructors or through books printed in embossed letters in a system developed by the founder of the school, Valentin Haüy. Later, the school adopted Sonography, an adaptation of a system of night writing developed by an army captain, Charles Barbier de la Serre. The night-writing system was used to write messages and maneuver instructions that could be read in the dark by the fingertips.

Sonography employed a complicated system of raised dots and dashes that spelled words phonetically. It was based on a 12-dot cell for each letter that used considerable space on a page. Braille began to experiment with the writing system, making changes and improvements. Braille met with Barbier, who rejected the changes and insisted that the system remain as introduced.

Over the next three years, Braille worked continuously to develop his own language of dots. In 1824, at the age of 15, his work was complete. He had developed a reading and writing system of dot patterns or characters based on a six-dot cell. Each character represented one letter of the alphabet or one numeral. He went on to adapt systems that could be used for musical notation and a method for drawing letters using a slate and stylus, called Raphigraphy.

Although the Braille method was immediately adopted by pupils at the school, it was officially rejected. This may have been for reasons of fear on the part of sighted teachers, hesitancy to revamp current teaching methods, and reluctance to make obsolete teaching tools that had been difficult and expensive to purchase.

It was not until 1843, at the inauguration of the new building of the Institution for Blind Youth, where an exhibition of the system was given, that braille gained official recognition. In 1854, at the insistence of the students and blind teachers, braille was adopted as a teaching method by the school. Acceptance for the system spread throughout Europe. It was first taught in America in about 1859 or 1860 at the St. Louis School for the Blind. Today, braille is universally used as a language of reading and writing for the blind and visually impaired.

Louis Braille did not live to see the acceptance of his writing system. He died in 1852 of tuberculosis. A century later, in 1952, his remains were moved from his native Coupvray for reburial in the Pantheon, the highest honor that can be bestowed on a French citizen. (See BRAILLE.)

American Foundation for the Blind. *A Different Way of Seeing.* New York: AFB, 1984.
American Foundation for the Blind. *Louis Braille.* New York: AFB, 1987.
American Foundation for the Blind. *Understanding Braille.* New York: AFB, 1970.
Davidson, Margaret. *Louis Braille,* New York: Hastings House Publishers, 1971.
Kugelmass, J. Alvin. *Louis Braille.* New York: Julian Messner, 1951.

braille music   Music printed in braille traditionally was produced manually by a limited number of people who specialized in the service. Musicians often were frustrated by having to wait weeks, sometimes months, to have their music transcribed.

In 1997, a company called Dancing Dots Braille Music Technology introduced a braille music translator program that allows music to be produced locally by sighted copyists. The service is based on a software program called GOODFEEL. With this program, braille music can be produced by people with no special training. Braille scores are produced from the same computer music files that are used to print staff notation.

The technology was spearheaded by Bill McCann, president and founder of Dancing Dots, who is also a blind musician and programmer. The company also offers other music-related products for visually impaired people.

Contact:

Dancing Dots Braille Music Technology
1754 Quarry Lane
P.O. Box 927
Valley Forge, PA 19482-0927
610-783-6692 (ph)
610-783-6732 (fax)
info@dancingdots.com
www.dancingdots.com

braille writer   A braille writer, or brailler, is a machine used to write braille. Similar to the function of a typewriter, braillewriters come in manual or electric forms. They are more practical for large writing tasks than a slate and a stylus, which is the equivalent of paper and a pen for a sighted person. The first brailler, the Hall Braillewriter, was introduced in 1892 by Frank H. Hall, superintendent of the Illinois School for the Blind.

Braille writers have six keys and a space bar. Each key corresponds to a dot of the six dot braille cell. To form a braille letter, the user simultaneously pushes the keys corresponding to the needed dot combination. The dots are pressed onto lightweight manila tag paper. Users can attain writing speeds of up to 60 words per minute.

Braille writers vary in size by maker but generally are approximately 15″ × 9″ × 5″ and weigh 10 pounds. Current braille writers include the Perkins Brailler, the Lavender Braillewriter, and the Hall Braillewriter.

Brailon   The trade name for the paper used in a thermoform duplicator. Each plastic sheet is placed atop a page of brailled paper or tactual paper and inserted into the thermoform machine. The machine heats the Brailon plastic sheet and creates a duplicate of the tactual sheet.

Brailon is used to make duplicates of braille books and other tactual materials such as tactile maps. The Brailon exchange is the agreement of many educational agencies or organizations for the blind to provide a braille copy of a book in exchange for an equal number of Brailon sheets. (See THERMOFORM.)

B-scan   A test performed prior to cataract surgery to view the RETINA. The retina is usually examined with a binocular indirect OPHTHALMOSCOPE, but in some cases, the cataract is dense enough to obstruct the view of the retina. In these instances, a painless, ultrasonic B-scan affords a picture of the hidden retina.

The health of the retina must be determined before cataract surgery to rule out the possibility of a detached retina. Without this knowledge, the surgery could successfully remove the cataract, only to reveal a non-functioning eye.

Business Enterprise Program   (BEP)   A federally supported program administered by each individ-

ual State Department of Rehabilitation. The program was established by the Randolph-Sheppard Act in 1936 and amended in 1974. The program provides employment opportunities to qualified blind persons, licenses blind vendors, and establishes vending facilities in federal, state, county, and some private buildings.

Vending facilities may sell newspapers, periodicals, confections, tobacco products, foods, beverages. and other articles or services. The articles or services may be dispensed automatically or manually and are prepared on the premises. The facility may also be a cafeteria, snack bar, or a dry/wet facility.

To qualify for the BEP training program, an applicant must be a citizen of the United States, legally blind, emotionally and physically qualified to operate a vending facility as verified by medical and vocational evaluation, have independent living skills, and have a reasonable expectation to succeed in the program.

An applicant entering the BEP program must complete a training program. Those who have had prior management experience in food service may be eligible to demonstrate their skills by completing two months on-the-job training with another vendor and passing the final exam covering all the training program material with a grade of 85 percent or better.

The standard training program is seven months long and consists of pretraining evaluation, basic training, and on-the-job practical experience. All trainees must pass a comprehensive final exam.

Those who complete the program are certified as eligible for licensing as a BEP vendor. As locations become available, students are notified and can apply for a specific location. Applicants are interviewed by a selection panel of business people who decides which vendor is to be assigned. Selection is based on prior work experience, education, training, experience, and performance on the oral interview. Vendors are considered trainees until the first year of vending has been completed.

The income from vending machines that compete with BEP vendors may be accrued to a maximum and paid to the vendor. The income may be used to establish a fund for sick leave, vacation, or retirement benefits.

cancer Cancer of the eyes is relatively rare. According to the American Cancer Society, ocular cancer is responsible for approximately 2,500 new cases of cancer each year and for approximately 400 deaths from cancer each year as compared with lung and breast cancers, which are responsible, respectively, for 144,000 and 115,000 new cases of cancer each year.

Cancer of the eyes usually develops into tumors. The tumors may be found in the eyeball, the orbit, or the eyelids. Because ocular tumors are often hidden deep in the eye and therefore resist biopsy, it is often difficult to differentiate a malignant tumor from a nonmalignant or benign tumor.

Cancerous or malignant tumors differ from benign tumors in several ways. The cancerous cells are different from their surrounding tissue, often grow quickly and uncontrollably, rarely stop growing, and tend to spread or metastasize to other parts of the body. Malignant tumors threaten life as well as vision.

The three most common types of malignant tumors are malignant melanoma, retinoblastoma, and metastatic tumors. Each is a serious disorder that benefits from early and appropriate treatment.

MALIGNANT MELANOMA is the most common of all tumors that originate in the eye. This type of tumor grows from melanin-laden cells in the eye's CHOROID, IRIS, or CILIARY BODY. It generally affects one eye only and may develop spontaneously or from a mole within the eye. It is usually slow to grow and metastasize. The onset may be at any age and is more common among whites than blacks. They occur more often in people who have skin melanoma.

Symptoms of malignant melanoma include redness, inflammation, loss of vision, and GLAUCOMA. Pupil distortion may be present in melanoma of the iris. Little is known about the cause and progression of these tumors.

Malignant melanomas are generally treated by enucleation, or removal of the entire eye. An uncertain diagnosis may lead to a period of observation augmented by chemotherapy or radiation treatments. Melanomas of the iris are extremely slow-growing and are often treated during observation. Approximately 60 percent of those diagnosed and treated for malignant melanomas are alive five years after treatment.

RETINOBLASTOMA is the most common type of malignant intraocular (inner eye) tumor in children. It occurs in one out of every 12–20,000 children. This tumor develops in the eye's retina. Retinoblastomas may be hereditary or may develop sporadically. The less common hereditary type is usually present at birth and has its onset near one year of age. In both types, the condition is almost always expressed by age five. It is often bilateral (affects both eyes).

Although hereditary retinoblastomas are present in family histories, any occurrence of bilateral retinoblastoma should be considered hereditary and capable of being passed to further generations. Infants of hereditary families should be screened regularly for tumors.

Sporadic tumors are not hereditary. They are generally unilateral (affecting one eye only) and appear at approximately two years of age.

The first symptoms of retinoblastoma include redness, pain, and inflammation. As the tumor grows, the eyes may cross and the pupil may change from black to white or gray, a condition called leukokoria. The light color is the hue of the tumor visible through the hole of the pupil.

Retinoblastoma is treated by enucleation, radiation, or cryotherapy (freezing treatments). In bilateral cases, the more affected eye may be removed and the other eye may receive chemotherapy or radiation treatments. If left unchecked, the tumor could grow and spread up the optic nerve to the brain.

The cause of retinoblastoma is due to the absence of both retinoblastoma genes on the 13th chromosome. Although it has the one of the highest rates of spontaneous regression among all tumors, little is known about the cause of regression. The cure rate for retinoblastoma ranges from 85 percent to 90 percent.

Metastatic tumors are malignant tumors that originate in other parts of the body and spread to the eyes. Among those that can metastasize to the eyes are tumors of the lung, breast, kidney, and prostate. These secondary tumors are bilateral approximately 25 percent of the time.

Symptoms of metastatic tumors may include redness, pain, vision loss, or glaucoma. Often, symptoms of the ocular tumor may present themselves before those of the primary tumor. Because metastatic tumors look much like primary ocular tumors, diagnosis can be problematic.

Once a metastatic tumor has been diagnosed, the primary tumor can be appropriately treated. Depending on the size and growth rate of the ocular tumor, treatment may include surgery, chemotherapy, or radiation treatments.

Malignant tumors of the eyelids include the basal-cell carcinoma and the squamous-cell carcinoma. The more common basal-cell carcinoma, the result of sun damage to the skin, first appears as a slight bump on the eyelid. It develops into a saucer-like shape with a raised edge.

Since the tumor is on the eyelid, it is easy to remove and submit to biopsy. If left untreated, the tumor may spread to the underlying bone. Advanced basal-cell carcinomas are treated with radiation therapy.

Squamous-cell carcinomas appear in observation much like basal-cell carcinomas but can be identified through biopsy. This type of tumor tends to spread to the lymph nodes of the upper or lower eyelid and may metastasize to other parts of the body.

Rhabdomyosarcoma is a highly malignant tumor of the orbit. It is a rare tumor that develops in children. The tumor spreads rapidly but can be detected by a biopsy taken through the eyelid. Treatment may include radiation or chemotherapy. Cure rates for rhabdomyosarcoma range from 30 percent to 40 percent.

Carroll Center for the Blind The Carroll Center for the Blind Inc. is a rehabilitation center founded in 1936 by Reverend Thomas J. Carroll.

The center offers a residential rehabilitation program, primarily for newly blinded adults aged 16 and older. The average age of clients in this program is 44. The program specializes in mobility, homemaking, self-care, sensory development, braille, handwriting, record keeping, tape recording, communications, shop, low-vision devices, diabetic care, and individual and group counseling. The program lasts approximately 16 weeks.

The Carroll Center operates computer assessment and training programs for those seeking vocational careers, special educators, high school students, and rehabilitation instructors. Residential options are available for these programs.

The Orientation and Mobility Travel Skills service provides the visually impaired with community instructors who teach clients skills in orientation and mobility and provide low-vision services in their own homes. The Outdoor Enrichment Program allows visually impaired persons to participate in recreational activities year-round. Activities include skiing, ice-skating, hiking, canoeing, sailing, and bicycling. The program matches a sighted guide to each participant.

The center coordinates more than 200 volunteers who serve as drivers, readers, clerical workers, rehabilitation aides, and recreation assistants. It serves as a public information and education source, presents programs on blindness and the curriculum of the center to interested organizations or groups, maintains a 1,000-volume library, and operates an information and referral program.

The Carroll Center publishes a biennial newsletter. It publishes a review of aids for visually impaired consumers and directs a braille menu program to produce copies of menus in braille for restaurants throughout Massachusetts. The center holds a semiannual convention in the spring and fall.

Contact:

Carroll Center for the Blind
770 Centre Street
Newton, MA 02158
617-969-6200 or 1-800-852-3131
617-969-6204 (fax)
www.carroll.org

cataract Cataract is a leading cause of blindness in the United States and the world. The National Eye Institute reports that more than half of Americans age 65 or older have a cataract, and, according to Prevent Blindness America, cataracts are responsible for one out of every seven cases of blindness in people 45 years and over.

A cataract is a clouding of the crystalline LENS of the eye, which results in dim or blurred vision. Cataracts may also cause glare or halos in the presence of bright lights or a change in color vision.

One or both eyes may be affected. The individual may have opaque visual areas mixed with clear areas within the same eye. The progressive clouding of the lens is usually slow and may take years to progress to the point where surgery must be performed.

Most cataracts are the natural result of aging. These are termed senile cataracts. Little is known about their cause, although heredity, environment, nutrition and general health may be contributing factors.

Secondary cataracts may be caused by birth defects (congenital cataracts), eye injuries, exposure to ultraviolet or infrared light, medications such as cortisone steroids, or diseases such as Down's syndrome, rubella, MARFAN'S SYNDROME, allergic dermatitis, myotonic dystrophy, and diabetes. Diabetics have an increased risk of cataracts and diabetes is present in approximately 10 percent–15 percent of cataract patients.

Once a cataract is diagnosed, it is monitored by a physician. Corrective lenses may be prescribed to correct the patient's changing vision. Surgery to remove the cataract is performed only when the decreased vision begins to seriously interfere with the patient's ability to function.

With over 500,000 operations performed each year, cataract removal is the most common surgery performed in the United States. There are two main types of cataract surgery: phacoemulsification and extracapsular. During phacoemulsification, which is the most common method of cataract removal, a small incision is made on the side of the cornea, and a tiny probe is inserted into the eye. The probe produces ultrasound waves that break up the cloudy center of the lens. The lens can then be removed using suction. In extracapsular surgery, a slightly longer incision is made on the side of the cornea, and the surgeon removes the hard center of the lens. The remainder of the lens is then removed using suction.

Once the cloudy lens has been removed, it is usually replaced with a clear artificial lens called an intraocular lens (IOL). The IOL becomes a permanent part of the eye and does not require any additional care or attention. The person wearing the IOL does not feel or see it. In some cases, patients cannot have an IOL, due to problems that occur during surgery or as the result of another eye problem. In these cases, a soft contact lens or glasses may be used instead.

Prior to surgery, several tests may be performed to determine the power of an intraocular lens implant or the necessity of an implant. The tests may include keratometry, A-scan, B-scan, and an endothelial cell count.

KERATOMETRY is a test to determine the curvature of the CORNEA. A keratometer is used to measure the curvature in order to prescribe the IOL. A nearsighted eye has a more pronounced curve and requires a weaker degree of lens implant than does a farsighted eye. A very nearsighted eye may require such a weak lens as to make an implant unnecessary.

An A-SCAN uses ultrasound to measure the length of the eye. A nearsighted eye is longer than the normal length of approximately one inch. The more long or nearsighted the eye, the weaker the implant lens required. The results of the keratometry and the A-scan are analyzed by a computer to determine the power of the needed implant.

A B-SCAN uses ultrasound to supply a clear picture of a RETINA obscured by a particularly dense cataract. The B-scan can alert the OPHTHALMOLOGIST to a detached retina, which may nullify the effects of successful cataract surgery.

An endothelial cell count is performed to determine the number of healthy endothelial cells remaining in the CORNEA. The endothelial cells line the cornea and protect it from leakage of AQUEOUS FLUID, which could damage vision. The cells are destroyed with aging and as a side effect of surgery. A minimum number of cells, approximately 1,000, is needed to achieve satisfactory results from the surgery. The cells are photographed by an endothelial cell camera, and the resulting photograph is analyzed for cell quantity.

Cataract surgery is performed with either a local or general anesthetic and is usually done on an outpatient basis. The process may take up to an hour with additional time to induce anesthesia. The patient can continue a normal daily routine, with a few exceptions, such as driving.

Postsurgery treatment includes the prescription of glasses for those with the implant and either aphakic spectacles (cataract glasses) or contact lenses plus glasses for those without an intraocular lens implant. It also may include steroid or cortisone eye drops such as Pred-Forte, Inflamase, Ecopred, or Decadron to control inflammation. Antibiotic drops may be prescribed to fight infection, and medication may be used to treat elevated pressure within the eye. Some people experience blurred vision following cataract surgery. This is because the eye from which the cataract has been removed needs time to adjust so that it can focus properly with the other eye. Patients with IOLs may notice changes in colors. Colors may appear to be very bright or have a blue tinge. Exposure to bright sunlight might cause everything to have a reddish tinge for a short period of time. These color sensitivities are not uncommon and should disappear within a few months.

If part of the natural lens remains in the eye, as sometimes occurs, it can become cloudy in time and result in blurred vision. This can occur months or years after the cataract surgery and is called an after-cataract. After-cataracts are usually treated with a YAG laser, which is a type of infrared laser that creates shocks that destroy membranes within the eye. This procedure is called a YAG laser capsulotomy. Normally it is painless and done on an outpatient basis.

Cataracts are one of the leading causes of WORLD BLINDNESS, and are common to all parts of the world. Lack of trained personnel and facilities limits the number of cataract surgeries performed in the third world. World health and governmental agencies operate limited mobile clinics or surgery units to address the needs of those with cataracts in developing countries.

Bath, Patricia E. "Blindness Prevention Through Programs of Community Ophthalmology in Developing Countries." In *Ophthalmology.* Vol. 2. Edited by K. Shimizu and J. Oosterhuis. Amsterdam: Excerpta Medica, 1979.

Freese, Arthur S. *Cataracts and Their Treatment,* Public Affairs Pamphlet #545. New York: Public Affairs Pamphlets, 1977.

Galloway, N. R. *Common Eye Diseases and Their Management.* Berlin: Springer-Verlag, 1985.

Helen Keller International. *Facts About Helen Keller International.* New York: HKI, 1988.

Kelman, Charles D. *Cataracts: What You Must Know About Them.* New York: Crown Publishing Inc., 1982.

Leflar, Robert B., and Helen Lillie. *Cataracts.* Washington, D.C.: Public Citizen's Health Research Group, 1981.

National Eye Institute. Information for Patients-Cataract. www.neinih.gov, 2000.

Phillips, Calbert I. *Basic Clinical Ophthalmology.* London: Pitman Publishers Limited, 1984.

Prevent Blindness America, Frequently Asked Questions about Cataracts. www.preventblindness.org, 1998–2000.

Reynolds, James D. *Cataracts.* HealthNet Reference Library. Columbus: CompuServe, 1989.

Shulman, Julius. *Cataracts.* New York: Simon and Schuster, 1984.

Center for the Partially Sighted   (CPS)   A comprehensive visual rehabilitation service center founded in 1978 for those with visual impairments but who are not totally blind.

The center offers professional assistance to partially sighted persons in the areas of low-vision examinations, training in the use of loaned and prescribed low-vision aids, professional psychological counseling, support groups, diabetic education groups, transportation services, independent-living skills, orientation and mobility training, and referral to community resources. The center supplies an ongoing follow-up program to assess changing needs. Patients retain contact with the center through telephone calls or home visits.

CPS maintains an internship program to educate and train interns in the field of low vision and serves as a clearinghouse for information about the partially sighted. It disperses information to the public concerning low vision, low-vision examinations and aids, the location of low-vision services elsewhere in North America, orientation and mobility, and other related topics.

Contact:

Center for the Partially Sighted
12301 Wilshire Boulevard, Suite 600
Los Angeles, CA 90025
310-458-3501 (ph)
310-458-8179 (fax)
www.low-vision.org

central vision Central vision is the "straight-ahead" vision in the visual field. Central vision is controlled by the MACULA, a tiny section of the RETINA. Although the macula occupies only 1 percent of the retina, it is responsible for distinguishing all detail in vision.

The retina is the light-sensitive layer between the choroid and the vitreous gel. It contains RODS AND CONES that receive light information about an object in view. The rods react to faint light, movement, and shape, and are responsible for peripheral or side vision. The cones distinguish color and detail but require high levels of light to function. They are responsible for central vision.

The retina encodes the information from the rods and cones into electrical impulses. The impulses are sent via the OPTIC NERVE to the brain, where they are translated into an image.

The cones of the retina are concentrated into a central section called the macula. Within the macula is an indentation called the FOVEA. The fovea contains the greatest concentration of cones and is the site of sharpest vision. Light is focused by the cornea and the LENS onto the macula, and specifically onto the fovea. When the macula or fovea are damaged, central vision is affected.

MACULAR DISEASE is a common problem affecting central vision. It may be caused by an injury, heredity, other diseases such as arteriosclerosis, or aging.

Age-related maculopathy (ARM) is the most common form of this disease. It is a progressive disease in which the macula deteriorates, and central vision is lost. ARM may in some cases be treated with laser therapy, but there is no cure for the disease. It is seldom responsible for total blindness, since some peripheral vision usually remains intact.

ARTERIOSCLEROSIS, or hardening of the arteries, may cause macular degeneration. In this condition, the arteries become clogged and smaller in diameter. Blood circulation slows, and the body's organs are denied oxygen. In some cases, the retinal blood vessels become clogged and the macula degenerates.

AMBLYOPIA of disuse, or lazy eye, is a condition that affects central vision. It is a condition of childhood in which one eye is misaligned to the other. The eyes are unable to focus together and double vision occurs. The vision of the misaligned eye is suppressed by the brain, which accepts only information from the aligned eye. In effect, the unused eye ceases to develop and becomes "blind" or amblyopic. In the treatment of amblyopia, the aligned eye is usually patched to encourage the amblyopic eye to function. The central vision of the amblyopic eye is affected, but it usually retains some peripheral vision.

TOBACCO AMBLYOPIA is a condition in which the excessive use of tobacco impairs central vision. The condition usually rights itself when tobacco use is discontinued or drastically reduced.

The cones responsible for central vision need light to function and to survive. Eyes denied light for long periods may lose central vision. A complete lack of vitamin A in the diet may also result in cone or retinal dysfunction and cause blindness.

cerebral palsy (CP) Cerebral palsy (CP) is not a disease, but rather a group of conditions caused by damage to the motor area of the brain before, during or directly following birth. The condition affects about 500,000 persons in the United States and is the most prevalent lifelong disability in the country.

Over one-third of those with CP are teenagers or young adults. Each year, approximately 5,000 babies are born with CP and an additional 1,500 acquire CP before the age of five.

The condition usually involves nerve and muscle dysfunction and may exhibit such characteristics as difficulty in walking; loss of muscle coordination or manual dexterity; spasms; seizures; tremors; hearing, speech, or vision impairments; learning disabilities; mental retardation; and psychological or behavioral problems.

There are five types of cerebral palsy: spastic, athetoid, rigid, ataxia, and tremor. Spastic CP, the most common type, involves the trait of tense, contracted muscles. Athetoid CP entails uncontrollable, constant movement of the head, limbs, and body. Rigid CP is characterized by contracted muscles that resist movement.

Ataxia encompasses coordination and balance problems. Tremor CP is the most rare and is similar to the athetoid type since it involves uncontrollable tremors or trembling of the limbs that hinders balance and coordination. Most individuals with CP are affected by more than one type of CP, a condition termed "mixed type."

Brain damage that results in CP can be caused by acute or chronic anoxia or oxygen deprivation, a result of premature separation of the placenta from the uterine wall, improper birth position, prolonged or abrupt labor, complications during labor, or obstruction by the umbilical cord.

Other congenital causes may include maternal viral infections such as rubella (German measles), Rh and A-B-O blood-type incompatibilities, poor health, excessive smoking or alcohol consumption by the mother, premature birth and untreated jaundice of the newborn causing kernicterus, a disease that involves damage to the nervous system and is also caused by Rh-factor incompatibility.

Acquired CP is a more rare occurrence and results from an injury to the head due to trauma or infection. Cerebral palsy is not hereditary. It is not a progressive condition and is not communicable. Each case of CP is unique. The amount of damage to the brain, the site of damage and the degree to which the nervous system is involved produce varying symptoms.

Vision may be affected if the damage affects the portion of the brain that controls the eyes or the parts of the eyes that process or transmit information such as the retina or optic nerve. Corrective lenses or surgery may be necessary to improve or correct vision.

Early detection and treatment of CP are essential in achieving the best possible management of the condition. Symptoms of CP in infants may include irritability, difficulties in feeding or sucking, and abnormally delayed development of muscle control or coordination. Less noticeable symptoms may be detectable by a pediatrician during a medical examination.

Cerebral palsy currently cannot be cured, but management or treatment may reduce the limitations it imposes. Treatment may include physical, occupational, speech, language, hearing, or behavioral therapy. Neurological or orthopedic surgery may increase control over muscles. Braces may strengthen and support the body and correct deformities. Medications may reduce rigidity and ease nerve-damage problems.

Congenital cerebral palsy can often be prevented. Pregnant women can maintain good nutrition, avoid alcohol, smoking, and unnecessary X rays or medications, and control diabetes and anemia. Routine tests for Rh incompatibility in the mother and immunization with Rhogam within 72 hours after delivery can eliminate problems in future pregnancies.

Infants with blood incompatibility may receive a blood transfusion. Premature infants and those at high risk can be monitored closely in neonatal intensive care units. Infants and young children can of course be protected from trauma.

There is much help available for those suffering from cerebral palsy and for their families. The United Cerebral Palsy Association, founded in 1949 as a voluntary organization, has more than 150 state and regional affiliates. The agency, through its affiliates, serves more than 30,000 children and adults with cerebral palsy and other disabilities every day. It offers assistive technology training, community living, referrals, employment assistance, advocacy, early intervention programs, therapy, and so forth.

To find out more about the organization that serves your area.

Contact:

United Cerebral Palsy Association
1660 L Street, NW, Suite 700
Washington, DC 20036-5602
800-872-5827 (ph)
202-973-7197 (TTY)
202-776-0414 (fax)
www.ucpa.org
Listings of local affiliates are available from the website.

Mann, Richard C. *Diagnosis: Cerebral Palsy.* Oklahoma City: United Cerebral Palsy of Oklahoma, 1986.
United Cerebral Palsy Association. *What Is Cerebral Palsy?* New York: UCPA, 1978.
UCP Net. Cerebral Palsy-Facts and Figures, www.ucp.org, 2001.

chalazion   An inflammation of the eyelid gland. It is caused by a blockage of the meibomian gland duct.

A chalazion appears as a bump or swelling on either the top or bottom eyelid. It is painless and may develop slowly over many weeks. Treatment of chalazion may include warm compresses and sulfonamide eye drops.

Once the chalazion has grown large enough to press on the eyeball, it may cause damage to vision by producing an astigmatism. In such cases, surgery to remove the chalazion may be required. The eye is patched after surgery, and antibiotic eye drops are often prescribed.

Chalazions may become chronic. Prevention may be achieved through strict hygiene and the application of warm compresses at the first sign of inflammation. If they do reoccur, it could be an indication of a more serious condition and should be checked.

Child Abuse Prevention and Treatment Act   The Child Abuse Prevention and Treatment Act, first enacted in 1974, was amended in 1984 to mandate proper medical treatment of infants born with physical or mental disabilities. The amendments were in response to reports to Congress that appropriate medical treatment was withheld from disabled infants.

The law orders the administration of medical treatment to disabled infants except in the cases of irreversible and chronic coma or if the treatment would only extend the dying process. The law directs state child protection agencies to respond to reports of treatment denial. The act was amended again in 1996 to provide for a community-based family-resource and support-grants program. The program includes temporary childcare for children with disabilities and a crisis nursery program for children who are thought to be at risk.

U.S. Department of Education. *Summary of Existing Legislation Affecting Persons with Disabilities.* Washington, D.C.: USDE, 1988.

Child Nutrition Act   As amended, the Child Nutrition Act of 1966 establishes federal-assistance funds to initiate and manage school-meal programs. The Act outlines programs that supplement and expand those described in the National School Lunch Act. Daytime and residential schools and child-care programs that serve disabled children are eligible to participate in the School Milk, School Breakfast, and Nutrition Education and Training Programs.

The School Milk Program was designed to encourage school children to consume milk. The program funds grants to states to provide free milk to eligible children. Eligible nonprofit schools, child-care centers, and camps are reimbursed for the milk served. Schools and centers are eligible, provided they are not recipients of National School Lunch Act or Child Nutrition Act program funds.

The School Breakfast Program provides breakfasts served at school to eligible children. Eligible nonprofit public or private schools, including those for disabled children, are reimbursed for the breakfasts.

The Nutrition Education and Training Program provides grants to states for training on nutrition and management to instructors and food-service personnel and instructional nutrition programs in school classrooms. (See NATIONAL SCHOOL LUNCH ACT.)

U.S. Department of Education. *Summary of Existing Legislation Affecting Persons with Disabilities.* Washington, D.C.: USDE, 1988.

children   See DEVELOPMENT OF BLIND CHILDREN.

chlamydia A type of sexually transmitted disease that can cause conjunctivitis, both in adults and babies, who are affected at birth. Caused by a bacterium, chlamydia is the leading sexually transmitted disease in the United States. About 4 million new cases occur each year.

Early symptoms include abnormal genital discharge or pain when urinating, but symptoms can be very mild and may not even be noticed. As the disease progresses, it can cause eye infection and proctitis and urethral infection in men.

Newborns affected while in the birth canal may develop conjunctivitis or pneumonia. Typically, symptoms of eye problems will occur within the first 10 days of life. The eye infection can be treated with antibiotics in both newborns and adults. Many doctors advise that all pregnant women be tested for chlamydial infection because of the risk it presents to newborns.

chorioretinitis A secondary condition caused by CHOROIDITIS, a swelling of the CHOROID (also called posterior UVEITIS). Chorioretinitis occurs when the inflammation of the choroid spreads to the underlying RETINA.

The choroid is the pigmented tissue layer between the retina and the SCLERA (white part of the eye). It is the posterior section of the uveal tract, a vascularized tissue layer that supplies blood to the eye and that includes the IRIS and CILIARY BODY in the anterior section.

The retina is the light sensitive layer at the back of the eye. The retina receives light information from the RODS AND CONES located there. It converts the information into electrical impulses that it sends to the brain. The brain transforms the impulses into an image.

Symptoms of choroiditis include redness of the eye, light sensitivity, and lost or blurred vision. The symptoms of choroiditis may not be noticeable to the patient if they are located in the areas of peripheral vision.

Choroiditis may occur spontaneously. It may also be linked to viruses, injuries, TOXOPLASMOSIS, arthritis, tuberculosis, VENEREAL DISEASE, parasites, and SARCOIDOSIS.

Because of the close proximity of the choroid and the retina, the inflammation of choroiditis

often spreads to the overlying retina, resulting in chorioretinitis. When this occurs the vision becomes acutely blurred. If the inflammation involves the macular region of the retina, permanent central-vision loss could occur.

Chorioretinitis may be treated with systemic (given orally) or local corticosteroids.

choroid The choroid is the dark, middle tissue layer between the RETINA and the SCLERA, or white part of the eye. It is the back portion of the uveal tract, a vascularized tissue layer that supplies blood to the eye. Blood circulates through the choroid layer to nourish and support the eye.

The UVEA or uveal tract contains the pigmented portions of the eye. These consist of the IRIS, the CILIARY BODY, and the choroid. When uveitis, or inflammation of the uvea occurs, the choroid may be involved.

Inflammation of the choroid is called CHOROIDITIS or posterior UVEITIS. Symptoms of choroiditis may include pain, redness of the eye, and light sensitivity. However, choroiditis is often present without symptoms, and since it may be present only in the peripheral field, it may persist unnoticed. The inflammation may spread to the retina and the VITREOUS, in which case, the vision becomes blurred.

Choroiditis may be caused by parasites (as it is in TOXOPLASMOSIS), viruses, or other diseases such as tuberculosis or syphilis. Choroiditis and posterior uveitis are usually treated with steroid pills, drops, or ointments.

choroiditis Choroiditis is an inflammation of the CHOROID, the vascular layer between the RETINA and the SCLERA. It is a type of UVEITIS, an inflammation of the uveal tract, and is sometimes referred to as arthritis of the eye.

The uveal tract is composed of the IRIS, the CILIARY BODY, and the choroid. The iris is the colored part of the eye that controls the pupil and enables it to open and shut to control the amount of light entering the eye. The ciliary body produces aqueous fluid and moves the lens to focus properly by changing its shape. The choroid, which supplies blood to the eye, is a vascular layer between the retina and the sclera.

Uveitis is categorized as either anterior or posterior. When the iris and ciliary body are involved, the condition is termed anterior uveitis. When the choroid is involved, it is termed posterior uveitis, or choroiditis.

Choroiditis is usually less painful than anterior uveitis. It may be accompanied by redness of the eye, light sensitivity, and lost or blurred vision. The symptoms of choroiditis that occur in the areas of peripheral vision may not be noticeable to the patient.

Choroiditis may occur spontaneously. It may also be linked to viruses, injuries, TOXOPLASMOSIS, arthritis, tuberculosis, VENEREAL DISEASE, parasites, and SARCOIDOSIS. If choroiditis is not treated, it may spread to the retina, a condition called CHORIORE-TINITIS, and to the VITREOUS. Once in the retina, it may affect the MACULA, and result in a loss of central vision.

Choroiditis is treated with steroid pills or drops. Immunosuppressive medications may be prescribed in severe cases. It tends to reoccur.

ciliary body   The ciliary body is the group of ciliary muscles that are attached to the ZONULE, a group of fibers that hold the LENS in place. The ciliary muscles change the shape of the lens when focusing, and they open and shut the PUPIL.

The ciliary muscles contract to bulge the lens forward and focus on a near object. The muscles expand to flatten the lens and focus on a distant object.

The ciliary body also produces the aqueous fluid of the eye. The aqueous fluid flows through the anterior chamber of the eye where it nourishes the lens and CORNEA and carries away waste. Changes in the ciliary body may affect the production and flow of the aqueous fluid, which can result in an increase in intraocular pressure and glaucoma.

Iritis, an inflammation of the IRIS, can cause inflammation of the ciliary body, known as CYCLI-TIS. This results in pain, redness, light sensitivity, and constricted pupil. Iritis and cyclitis are usually treated with steroid pills, eyedrops, or ointments.

Civil Rights Commission Act   The Civil Rights Commission is a council that investigates claims of discrimination and violations of civil rights. The Commission also conducts fact-finding examinations and provides the public with information from its clearinghouse. The Civil Rights Commission influences public opinion but has no authority to enforce the law against violators.

The Civil Rights Commission Act was amended in 1978 to include provisions that prohibit discrimination on the basis of disability. This allowed the Commission to investigate violations of disabled persons' rights.

U.S. Department of Education. *Summary of Existing Legislation Affecting Persons with Disabilities.* Washington, D.C.: USDE, 1988.

Civil Service Reform Act   The Civil Service Reform Act of 1978 authorized widespread changes in federal employment practices. Among other reforms, the Act allowed agency directors to hire assistants for visually impaired or hearing-impaired employees to enable them to do their jobs effectively. These assistants included reading aides for visually impaired employees and interpreters for hearing-impaired employees.

U.S. Department of Education. *Summary of Existing Legislation Affecting Persons with Disabilities.* Washington, D.C.: USDE, 1988.

closed-circuit television   (CCTV)   A low-vision aid that electronically magnifies a distant object or printed material. It is widely used by visually impaired persons in schools, libraries, offices, and homes.

The CCTV consists of a video camera with a zoom lens and a monitor. The camera focuses on print material or distant objects such as a blackboard and electronically transmits the enlarged image to a video monitor. The user employs hand or foot controls to scan the material and focus on a specific sentence, phrase or word. The user may choose to see the print as black letters on a white background or white letters on a black background.

The CCTV can magnify objects or print from 1 to 60 times normal size without distortion. Since it operates on electronic image intensification rather than optical projection, the image contrast and the illumination light source are better than a projection magnifier.

Closed-circuit televisions are offered in models that allow the user to type or use a personal computer. Portable models are available for use away from home or office.

coloboma   A cleft or notch in the IRIS, RETINA, and/or CHOROID due to incomplete formation or closure of the optic cup during gestation. The cleft produces a section of missing iris, retina, and/or choroid that may extend from the optic disc to the periphery of the FUNDUS.

Coloboma most often appears as a keyhole-shaped pupil. The condition may be bilateral, but usually one eye is more acutely affected than the other. If the iris is minimally affected, vision interference may be insignificant. However, if the retina (particularly the macular area) and choroid are involved, vision loss could be serious.

Coloboma is a birth defect that is inherited in a dominant pattern. It sometimes is accompanied by other developmental flaws. There is currently no treatment to correct coloboma.

color blindness   Difficulty in recognizing or distinguishing one color from another. It may be one of two types, hereditary or acquired. The hereditary variety is the most common. It is present at birth in 1 out of 12 men and 1 out of 200 women. It is a genetic defect that affects both eyes and does not change in severity over a lifetime.

The RETINA contains photoreceptor cells called RODS AND CONES. They change light energy into information about the object in view. The retina changes the information into electrical energy that is sent to the brain and translated into an image.

Each cone contains visual pigments that are sensitive to one of the three primary-color light wavelengths. One group of cones recognizes green, one red and one blue. By blending these three colors, the eye is able to distinguish all the colors of the spectrum. This is known as normal trichromatic color vision.

Color blindness occurs when one group of cones does not recognize its color properly. This may be caused by a lack of visual pigment, called an anopia, or by faulty visual pigment, known as an anomaly. Individuals lacking visual pigment are termed dichromats; those with faulty pigment are termed anomalous trichromats.

Most people with color blindness see some color. Many see all three primary colors but in the wrong proportions and may require brighter shades to recognize a particular hue. Other individuals may be red or green blind. A person with red blindness sees reds and oranges as shades of gray or black. A person with green blindness sees reds, oranges, and greens as much the same shade and cannot distinguish between them. Blue blindness is extremely rare, as is complete color blindness, a condition usually attributable to other visual problems.

Color blindness may be detected during the routine ophthalmologic examination. A common screening device called the Ishihara Test uses circles of different sizes and hues to form a mosaic picture. The picture shows a two-digit number in a background field of circles. Those with normal color vision are able to see the number formed with colored circles. Those with color blindness cannot detect a number from the background field.

There is no cure or treatment for hereditary color blindness although some experimentation is being done with tinted contact lenses, such as the X-CHROM LENS, and filters. The individual may not be able to see color with the lenses but may be able to distinguish between colors better as a result of wearing them.

Acquired color blindness can occur as a result of aging or disorders such as retinal optical-nerve conditions, TOXIC AMBLYOPIA, MACULAR DISEASE, CATARACT, GLAUCOMA, and DIABETIC RETINOPATHY. The diseased eye is generally the only eye affected, and effective treatment of the illness may result in an improvement in color vision.

Drugs can temporarily alter an individual's color vision. Barbiturates given as sedatives and large doses of vitamin A may affect the yellow or yellow-green vision, and caffeine has been shown to affect and alter all colors. The popular drug Viagra also has been found to cause temporary changes in blue/green colors and increased sensitivity to light in some cases.

Committee for Purchase from People Who Are Blind or Severely Disabled A small federal agency established as a result of the JAVITS-WAGNER-O'DAY (JWOD) Act. The act, amended in 1971 to replace the Wagner-O'Day Act of 1938, established a program in which federal agencies can purchase selected goods and services from workshops for the blind.

Members of the Committee for Purchase from People Who Are Blind or Severely Disabled include senior officials from federal procurement agencies, as well as private citizens representing people who are blind or otherwise disabled. Citizens are appointed to the board by the U.S. president. The committee administers the JWOD program, with the mission of creating employment opportunities for blind people.

Contact:

The Committee for Purchase from People Who
   Are Blind or Severely Disabled
1421 Jefferson Davis Highway
Jefferson Plaza 2, Suite 10800
Arlington, VA 22202-3259
703-603-7740 (ph)
703-603-0655 (fax)
www.jwod.gov

computers Computers and related technology are tools used by visually impaired and blind persons to access and manipulate information. Recent developments and inventions, many of which were designed to meet the needs of those with vision losses, allow for full competitiveness in most educational and employment settings.

Persons with low vision or some usable residual vision may find standard print on a computer screen or printed output too small to read. Enlarged output or magnification and large print adaptations have been developed for these users.

These include magnification lenses or devices placed in front of the standard computer screen that enlarge the text two to three times normal size, software programs that magnify the text up to eight times, hardware and software combinations that result in magnification of up to 16 times and closed circuit television systems that magnify the output up to 60 times normal size. Many magnify-

ing systems and programs involve high resolution, which enhances magnification. Large-print capable printers and multiple fonts and character sizes improve readability of hard-copy output.

The standard keyboard may be adapted for use by blind or visually impaired users through home-key indicators such as raised dots or indentations. Other adaptations feature felt appliques, large print appliques, and larger key replacements for the most frequently used keys.

Blind persons may access computer information through audio output that relates information on the screen via a synthetic voice. The speech synthesizers process the text to speech and produce human-sounding voices. The voices are available in various forms of male, female, or robotic voice; adult or child voice; voice pitch; speed rate; and volume. The voice speaks English words, letters, and numbers, and some versions offer foreign languages, singing and music.

Screen-reading software, activated by the standard keyboard or an auxiliary keyboard, enables the user to locate and identify sections of the screen or specific sentences, words or letters to be read. The program can be directed to read specific sections or positions on the screen, such as columns, and to provide audio output during data entry so that the user can audibly verify the text as it is entered.

Optical character readers and the accompanying software recognize print and translate it into computer recognizable data. Some systems read pages of print with a scanner and send them directly to computer files. The files can then be accessed and read aloud by the voice synthesizer. Other systems read the print and immediately speak the text aloud.

Text may be entered into the computer through a braille keyboard by use of specialized software or hardware. Braille embossers or printers produce embossed braille paper output. Paperless braille systems allow access to material through braille tactile displays. The tactile displays use retractable pins to form braille characters read by the fingertips of the user. Another tactile system, the Optacon II, presents information from the computer screen to the user through a vibrating tactile display that represents printed letters.

Many software programs allow for translation from braille to print and print to braille. This enables blind and visually impaired persons to share computer-produced information with sighted persons. Other programs translate to different grades of braille.

Through modems and related support software, users can access telephone lines to exchange machine-readable information, enter remote data banks and participate in electronic bulletin boards. They can access telephone directories, automatically dial the telephone, and accomplish electronic mailing, banking, and shopping. Similar software includes talking calculators and general file-management systems.

The documentation and manuals for such systems and programs may be available in formats other than standard print. Many companies offer this material in audio cassette, large print, braille, or machine-readable formats.

As computer technology improves overall, we also can expect improvements in technology for the blind and visually impaired. Specific information regarding this topic is found under listings for individual products and in the Appendix.

congenital disorders Congenital disorders are those diseases or conditions that appear at birth. They may be inherited or caused in utero by other means. Several eye conditions and diseases are commonly seen congenitally. Congenital CATARACT may be inherited or acquired in utero due to conditions such as rubella. The cataracts may be present in both eyes and vary in severity.

ALBINISM is an inherited condition that involves reduced or absent pigmentation of the skin, hair, and eyes. Ocular albinism affects only the eyes. The condition often causes NYSTAGMUS, myopic ASTIGMATISM, and PHOTOPHOBIA.

ANIRIDIA, the absence of the IRIS, is a congenital condition. Those with aniridia may develop secondary GLAUCOMA as a result of the blockage of the anterior chamber by the iris root. Aniridia may be inherited or may occur as the result of trauma.

Severe cataracts may be removed shortly following the neonatal period, but often the surgery is postponed until the density of the cataracts threat-ens to interfere with the child's performance at school or home. Patients may develop AMBLYOPIA or RETINAL DETACHMENT following surgery.

COLOBOMA is a congenital condition involving a defect in the closure of the optic cup. The defect may cause a wide area of missing retina and CHOROID, or a segment of missing iris. If a segment of the MACULA is involved, vision may be affected. When both eyes are involved, commonly one eye is less severely affected. Coloboma may be inherited.

Corneal degenerations, such as KERATOCONUS, may be inherited and congenital. The condition may appear in both eyes and results in a progressive thinning of the cornea, which may necessitate a corneal graft.

Inherited MACULAR DYSTROPHIES are usually seen at birth or up to the age of six. The condition is marked by a destruction of the macula, the site of sharpest vision in the retina. Macular degeneration blurs and may eventually destroy central vision, although some peripheral vision may be retained.

Congenital NYSTAGMUS involves involuntary movement of the eyes. It may be an inherited condition or may be caused by congenital cataract, albinism, aniridia, optic atrophy, or another disease or disorder.

OPHTHALMIA NEONATORUM is an infection of the conjunctiva and cornea acquired during birth through organisms in the maternal birth canal. The condition was common during the early part of the century but is now rare due to the instillation of silver nitrate into newborns' eyes.

PTOSIS is a congenital, inherited condition in which one or both of the upper lids droop. This may cause an obstruction to vision and can be corrected surgically.

RETINITIS PIGMENTOSA (RP) is an inherited degenerative disease of the retina. It may be present at birth or surface later in childhood or young adulthood. RP destroys peripheral vision and causes night blindness. When an individual with RP has a hearing loss, the condition may be called USHER'S SYNDROME.

RETINOBLASTOMA is a congenital intraocular malignant tumor of the retina. It is usually present at birth in one or both eyes. The condition is usually inherited but may occur in families with no history of the condition. Enucleation (removal of the eye) may be necessary to save the life of the patient.

STRABISMUS (squint) is a nonalignment of the eyes. The condition may be inherited or may develop after an illness or injury. Strabismus may cause double vision and amblyopia of disuse. Because many babies have strabismuslike conditions at birth that later self-correct, strabismus is often not diagnosed until after six months of age.

conjunctiva The conjunctiva is the transparent mucous membrane that covers the inside of the eyelid and the SCLERA, the protective white part of the eye. Conditions that are commonly associated with the conjunctiva include CONJUNCTIVITIS, hemorrhage, pinguecula, and pterygium.

Conjunctivitis, or "pink eye," is an inflammation of the conjunctiva. It may be caused by allergies, viral infections, bacterial infections, or overexposure to light. Symptoms of conjunctivitis may include redness of the eye, itching, burning, or discharge.

A hemorrhage in the conjunctiva, called a subconjunctival hemorrhage, may occur due to an injury, excessive rubbing, or coughing and sneezing. A hemorrhage shows itself as a bright red mark on the sclera (white of the eye). The hemorrhage looks frightening but rarely has any long-term effect and generally goes away without treatment.

Pinguecula is a small, yellowish, raised mark on the sclera. It is usually associated with age and is a harmless condition.

Pterygium is a patch of raised vascular tissue on the sclera. If the pterygium grows into the cornea, it may block vision.

conjunctivitis Conjunctivitis is a common infection of the CONJUNCTIVA. Conjunctivitis can be caused by large doses of ultraviolet light, as in snow-blindness, by allergies to pollen, medications, food or smoke, or by bacteria or viruses. While all forms of conjunctivitis are commonly referred to as "pink eye," only the viral form is pink eye in the true ophthalmic sense.

Conjunctivitis caused by overexposure to light can cause redness of the SCLERA and a burning sen-

sation. Treatment involves shielding the eye from excessive light and allowing it to heal with time.

Viral conjunctivitis—which is truly pink eye because it does, indeed, cause the eye to become pink, as opposed to bright red or yellowish from discharge—is caused by one of the viruses responsible for the common cold. It is extremely contagious. This form of conjunctivitis usually occurs seven to 10 days after contact with an infected person, and causes the eye to become itchy and watery. Like a cold, this form of conjunctivitis can linger for weeks. It can be treated with antihistamine eye drops and cold compresses on the eye to relieve swelling but, generally, it simply has to run its course. Avoiding viral conjunctivitis is difficult because it is so contagious. It can be spread by a pillowcase, towel, washcloth, article of clothing, tissue, and so forth.

Bacterial conjunctivitis normally is characterized by eyes that are noticeably inflamed, bright red, and discharge a thick yellow mucous. It is easy to contract because bacteria are so easily introduced into the eyes. While the conjunctiva, just like the mouth, normally contains bacteria, those bacteria that cause conjunctivitis are not normally present there. Antibiotic eye drops generally are prescribed to treat bacterial conjunctivitis. In some cases, oral antibiotics may be necessary.

Allergic conjunctivitis, which can be caused by a host of irritants ranging from pollen to rabbit fur, results in the eyes becoming red, itchy, swollen, and teary. Some eye-care products, such as the preservatives used in eye drops, also can cause allergic conjunctivitis. Pollutants and chemicals also can cause allergic conjunctivitis. This condition normally is treated with antihistamines and cold compresses. Over-the-counter pain relievers may be used to relieve discomfort.

Conjunctivitis can produce serious damage and should be treated by a physician.

contact lenses An alternative to eyeglasses, contact lenses are small, thin discs of plastic that rest in place on the cornea. Held in position by the natural moisture of the cornea, contacts have several advantages over glasses. Many people find contacts to be more comfortable and convenient than glasses, and they provide better peripheral vision than glasses do. Because the lens rests directly on the eye, size differences that sometimes occur with glasses are minimized, giving a more natural appearance to what you see.

Contacts have become increasingly popular since 1972, when soft lenses were first introduced, but the idea for them has been around for centuries. In fact, Leonardo da Vinci is credited with having come up with the idea for contact lenses in about 1550. It was a scientist in Switzerland, however, who actually made the first contact lens out of glass in the late 1800s. These glass lenses were not successful because they were very uncomfortable to wear. Plastic lenses, which we still use, were introduced in the 1940s, although many innovations and improvements have been made since then. Contact lenses are made today to correct almost any vision problem, and there are many varieties. Basically, however, they are divided into two major categories: hard and soft.

Hard contacts, the kind that were first introduced in the 1940s, can correct nearsightedness, farsightedness, and astigmatism. Hard lenses were much improved upon during the 1970s, when a gas-permeable model was developed. Gas permeable lenses are hard but allow air to flow through them to the eye. They are more flexible than the earlier hard lenses, and they generally fit better. They are made with computer-controlled lathes and can be ground to correct various vision problems. They also can be made into bifocal lenses. Gas-permeable lenses also can be used to correct corneal problems that cause vision to be distorted.

Soft contacts are available to correct nearsightedness, farsightedness, astigmatism, and presbyopia (the inability to focus at near distances). They are flexible, and they absorb and hold water. Soft contacts are sometimes called hydrogels. Many more people can wear soft lenses today than in the past, due to advances in the way they are made. Soft contacts also can be made into bifocal lenses.

Daily-wear contact lenses are those designed to be placed in the eye in the morning and taken out at the end of the day. Extended-wear contacts are those that can be worn for more than 24 hours. Extended-wear lenses are designed to allow the eye to receive sufficient oxygen, so they can be worn even while the wearer is sleeping. Flexible-

wear lenses can occasionally be worn overnight, but they are not designed to be worn constantly. Disposable extended-wear lenses have been available since the late 1980s and are just what they are called—disposable. They are designed to be placed in the eye, worn for about a week, and then thrown away. Lenses that are disposed of after one day of use were introduced in the mid-1990s.

All contact lenses should be kept very clean in order to avoid the risk of infecting the eyes. There are three basic methods of disinfecting contact lenses: with heat, chemicals, or a peroxide oxidative disinfectants. Heat systems destroy bacteria on the lenses with high temperatures. Lenses are first cleaned and rinsed, then they are placed into a heat unit, during which time bacteria are destroyed. Using heat to kill bacteria is a fairly quick process, and there is no need to use solutions that contain preservatives and chemicals, to which some people are allergic. A downside to heat cleaning is that it can cause coatings to build up on the lenses. Also, heat cleaning is not safe for all types of lenses.

Chemical disinfectants kill bacteria over a period of several hours. They are effective at cleaning and disinfecting lenses, but, as mentioned above, can cause allergic reactions in people with sensitivity.

Peroxide oxidative disinfectants were developed in the early 1980s and are considered to have some advantages over heating or chemical systems. Although the disinfectants are based on a hydrogen peroxide solution, they have built-in neutralizers that break down the peroxide so that it does not remain on the contact lenses. Because of the neutralization, there are no chemical residues. Nor is it necessary to heat the lenses.

Bifocal contact lenses are available in both hard and soft lenses and contain two prescriptions to correct refractive errors. Crescent bifocal lenses are similar to traditional bifocal spectacles in that the prescription for distance is at the top part of the lens and the prescription for close vision is in a crescent segment at the bottom. The lenses are either weighted or truncated (flattened) at the bottom to keep them from rotating out of position.

Concentric bifocal lenses differ in that the close vision prescription is in a ring around the inner circle of distance vision prescription. This design circumvents the problem of rotation.

Toric contact lenses are soft lenses that correct astigmatism. In the past, astigmatism had to be corrected with hard lenses because the soft lenses tended to mold themselves to the irregularities of the cornea. The toric lens provides the correction of the hard lens and the comfort of the soft. Like bifocal lenses, toric lenses require a predictable, nonrotating position in the eye. They are often weighted or truncated to discourage rotation. Toric lenses are typically more expensive than other lenses.

The *X-Chrom lens* is a contact lens for those with red-green color blindness. It is a deep red lens worn in the nondominant eye and intensifies the color of red and green objects. This allows the nondominant eye to feed information to the brain about colors it could previously not determine. The dominant eye continues to relate information about colors that it normally sees. The lens is not a cure for color blindness, but rather an aid in the improvement of color perception.

As compared with glasses, contact lenses have the advantage of providing more natural, distortion-free vision, unaffected by weather (raindrops and snowflakes), steam or glasses' frame obstruction. In the presence of high myopia (extreme near-sightedness), APHAKIA (loss of natural lens due to cataract surgery) or corneal diseases, contacts correct vision better than glasses.

Because the contact lens is a foreign substance in the eye, complications such as tearing, redness, itching, corneal abrasions, or infections can arise.

contrast   Contrast enhancement is a non-optical, or environmental, aid that maximizes residual vision. Contrast is enhanced by using dissimilar colors or brightness levels to make an object more visible. Highly contrasting colors near one another enhance contrast. Complementary colors that can be used together to create improved contrast include reds with greens, blues with oranges, and yellows with violet hues.

Light objects on a dark background or the reverse improve contrast. Light plates on a dark tablecloth improve visibility. Black letters on a white or yellow page are more readable than blue letters. Dark stairs are more easily seen when next to a light wall or when lined with a fluorescent strip.

Other aids can be used to improve contrast. A sheet of yellow or amber acetate can be placed over pale or bluish print to increase visibility. A typoscope, or slit reader, isolates one line of print to reduce the page glare and add contrast.

convergence   The coordinated movement of the eyes to focus together on a near object. Convergence is tested in an eye examination by slowly bringing a light or object close to the bridge of the nose. The patient is instructed to keep the object in focus as long as possible.

As the object moves closer to the nose, the eyes turn inward to a cross-eyed position. Divergence occurs when the object can no longer be seen as one image and the eyes move from the convergent position.

The near point of convergence is the last point at which the object could be seen as one image. This point is measured in millimeters as the distance from the bridge of the nose to the object. A normal near point of convergence is approximately 50 millimeters.

Copyright Act   The Copyright Act of 1976 extended copyright privileges and protection to songwriters, artists and authors and outlined infringement exemptions concerning works directed primarily for deaf and blind audiences.

The act cited four exemptions. Broadcast performances of nondramatic literary works are exempted if they are broadcast without commercial advantage by a governmental body on a noncommercial educational station, radio subcarrier, or cable system and directed primarily at blind and deaf individuals.

A broadcast of a single performance of a dramatic literary work is permissible if the work was published at least 10 years before the performance date and is directed primarily at blind audiences and the broadcast is made without commercial advantage through facilities of a radio subcarrier and one performance only is completed by the same actors or by the same organization.

Ten recorded copies of copyrighted materials may be made by a nonprofit organization for broadcast by radio information service carriers for performances aimed at blind or deaf individuals. Braille copies are permitted of imported nondramatic, English language works not produced in the United States or Canada.

The act directed the Register of Copyrights to develop forms and procedures to obtain clearance to reproduce nondramatic literary works in braille or recorded form. Certificate of copyright registration forms now include a section in which the applicant may grant permission to the Library of Congress to reproduce the copyrighted material in braille and phonorecords and distribute the copyrighted material to blind and physically disabled individuals only. The Copyright Act was amending in 1996, allowing nonprofit organizations to reproduce and distribute braille, recorded, and digital books for the blind without having to negotiate with each publisher.

U.S. Department of Education. *Summary of Existing Legislation Affecting Persons with Disabilities.* Washington, D.C.: USDE, 1988.

Department of Education, Statement by Tuck Tinsley, III, Ed.D, on 1998 Request for the American Printing House for the Blind, 1997.

cornea The cornea is the transparent tissue in the front section of the eye. It is the curved, clear cover over the colored IRIS. The cornea is surrounded by the tough, protective SCLERA, the white portion of the eye.

The cornea is instrumental in refracting the light that enters the eye. Light that falls on an object is reflected to the cornea. The cornea refracts or bends and focuses the light before it passes through the PUPIL to the LENS.

The cornea must remain transparent to preserve vision and therefore contains no blood vessels. The nourishment and waste disposal normally provided by the blood's circulatory system is supplied by the AQUEOUS FLUID, a clear liquid produced by the CILIARY BODY. The aqueous circulates through the anterior chamber of the eye, along the back of the cornea, to bring nutrients and carry away waste.

Although the cornea is devoid of blood vessels, it retains numerous pain receptors, making any injury to the corneal tissue extremely painful. Injuries or disorders of the cornea often result in distorted or blurred vision. Common disorders of the cornea include ARCUS SENILIS, KERATITIS, KERATOCONUS, abrasions, vascularization and, ulceration.

Arcus senilis is a harmless, cloudy ring that appears around the corneal edge. It is associated with aging.

Keratitis is an inflammation of the cornea. The inflammation may be caused by an infection due to an injury or abrasion or by transmission of microorganisms through the blood. Keratitis may result in opaque scars and impaired vision.

Keratoconus is a condition in which the center of the cornea thins and protrudes forward into a cone shape. This condition results in an impairment of normal vision. Keratoconus can be treated surgically with a corneal replacement or transplant.

Corneal abrasions are common and occur when the outer layer of the cornea is breached or scratched. Overwear of contact lenses is a frequent cause. Abrasions may result in pain, excessive tearing, and sensitivity to light.

Vascularization of the cornea occurs when blood vessels penetrate the normally avascular cornea. This may be due to an infection, inflammation, injury, or disease.

Corneal ulceration occurs when the surface is worn down by viral (such as herpes), fungal, or bacterial infections. Ulceration may result in permanent scarring and infiltration to the remainder of the cornea.

Healthy human corneas may be transplanted to replace diseased corneas. Corneal transplantation is the most commonly performed human transplant surgery. Over 90 percent of the corneal grafts transplanted in the United States are successful in restoring sight.

corneal degeneration The term for the breakdown of the cornea. Corneal degenerations are fairly rare disorders that may be caused by genetic or environmental conditions. Most disorders that cause corneal degeneration are inherited. Among these hereditary diseases are the two most common, *keratoconus* and FUCH'S ENDOTHELIAL DYSTROPHY.

Keratoconus is a disorder that may be inherited from a recessive trait. The disorder affects both eyes and is usually seen in children or adolescents. In this condition, the central part of the cornea thins and eventually protrudes forward into a cone shape. Distortion and loss of vision result. It is estimated to affect one of every 2,000 persons in the general population.

Keratoconus is a chronic, progressive disease that develops slowly. It can be corrected in mild forms with spectacles and, more advanced forms, with contact lenses.

Advanced conditions of keratoconus may be corrected with corneal transplants, called KERATO-PLASTY. Keratoplasty to correct keratoconus is a highly successful procedure since the cornea remains relatively free of blood vessels.

Fuch's dystrophy is an uncommon hereditary disorder. It is more common in women than in men, and normally appears only after a person is 50. In this disease, the endothelium layer degenerates and impairs vision. Fuch's dystrophy may cause further complications such as corneal edema, a rise in intraocular pressure. Corneal transplantation may improve or restore vision.

Little is known about the causes and development of corneal degenerations. It is thought that some degenerations may result from irregularities within corneal fibroblasts, the cells that develop into fibrous tissue. The fibroblasts are central to the processes of healing a corneal injury.

In addition, some corneal degenerations may be caused by environmental influences. They may result from corneal infections or inflammations (KERATITIS) or from accidental injuries such as alkali burns.

corneal edema A condition in which the CORNEA becomes overly hydrated. In order to remain transparent, the cornea is normally kept relatively dry through oxygen supplied in tears and the drain of water by the corneal endothelium. Any changes to the dehydration process or an influx of fluid can impede the process and allow fluid to accumulate.

Symptoms of corneal edema included blurred vision or the appearance of halos around lights. Later symptoms include severe pain as corneal nerves are damaged. Since the early symptoms are similar to those of CATARACT, an ocular examination is necessary for proper diagnosis.

Corneal edema may be caused by infection, corneal endothelial dysfunction (FUCH'S ENDOTHELIAL DYSTROPHY), a viral corneal inflammation (KERATITIS), a rise in intraocular pressure (as in GLAUCOMA), postoperative changes, trauma, overwear of contact lenses, and ill-fitting contact lenses.

The condition is treated according to its cause. Edema caused by an infection or a corneal endothelial disorder may be treated with STEROIDS or other medications. Viral KERATITIS may be treated with ANTIVIRAL DRUGS. A rise in intraocular pressure may be controlled by glaucoma medication or surgery. Postoperative conditions and trauma may be treated with medications and properly fitted and worn contact lenses may alleviate the symptoms related to their use.

Corneal edema may become a chronic condition. As the condition progresses and worsens, the corneal nerves become ruptured and exposed, causing extreme pain. Treatment of acute edema may include a TARSORRHAPHY, in which a portion of the lids are stitched together, or a corneal graft.

corneal transplant A corneal transplant, or keratoplasty, is the most common form of human transplant surgery performed today. There are more than 40,000 corneal transplants done each year in the United States. Keratoplasty uses a donor CORNEA to replace a diseased cornea. Although cornea transplants are generally successful in restoring vision, about 10 percent of transplanted corneas are rejected. Most rejections, however, can be prevented if treated early. Signs of rejection include sensitivity to light, redness, persistent discomfort, and changes in vision. Immunosuppressive drugs are available to reduce the possibility of cornea rejection, including an oral vaccine developed especially for that purpose.

Donor transplants come from people who have decided that when they die they want their corneas to be donated to others. The donor transplants are often kept in eye banks that help match appropriate corneas to needed hosts.

Donor transplants are selected according to age, cause of death, condition of the eye, and time between death and transplant surgery. Blood and tissue typing are not required as with kidney or heart transplants but time is a critical factor since the cornea should be transplanted within four days of donation.

Donor corneas are most desirable from individuals between the ages of 25 to 35 and who died from injury or disease. The donor corneas are screened for eye disease and the presence of venereal disease.

An individual becomes a candidate for a corneal transplant when all vision in that eye is lost due to injury, corneal dystrophy diseases such as KERATO-CONUS, chemical burn, or infection. A transplant also may be performed to repair injuries or tears in the cornea, to relieve chronic pain, or to correct a cosmetically unattractive eye.

A normal cornea is avascular, or lacks blood vessels. In order to perform a successful keratoplasty, the transplant must be placed into the eye in a manner that discourages vascularization, or the growth of blood vessels, into the cornea. Vascularization of the transplant may destroy it.

Certain disorders or diseases such as keratoconus, or a bulging cornea, lend themselves best to corneal transplants because of the lack of corneal blood vessels involved with this disorder. Other conditions, such as corneal scars, are less effectively corrected with transplants because of heavy vascularization present in the cornea.

The surgery may replace part or all of the host cornea. A section of donor cornea is measured to the precise needs of the host with an instrument called a trephine. This section is removed from the donor cornea with scissors. A corresponding section of host cornea is measured with the trephine and removed with scissors. The donor cornea is placed into the remaining cavity and sewn into position with small sutures.

The procedure is performed with either local or general anesthesia and may take from an hour to an hour and a half. It is often done on an outpatient basis, but many patients require a day or two of hospitalization.

For several weeks after surgery, the patient is discouraged from bending, lifting, or straining. The patient wears a protective eye patch or shield and is treated with EYE DROPS for several months. The stitches are removed after a period of six months to two years. Ophthalmologists recently began using artificial corneas is certain transplant cases. (See EYE BANK.)

corneal ulcer   Corneal ulcers occur when the cornea is worn down or damaged by injury or exposure and bacterial, viral, or fungal infections. Ulceration may lead to scarring and loss of sight. It is a common cause of blindness around the world.

Injuries or overwear of contact lenses usually result in minor corneal abrasions or scratches. The symptoms are extreme pain with a feeling of a foreign body within the eye. Anaesthetic drops may be administered to examine the eye that is then generally bandaged shut. The eye may be allowed to heal itself or an antibiotic ointment may be prescribed to avoid infection.

Ulcers due to exposure occur in cases of injury, facial palsy (Bell's palsy) or unconsciousness in which the lid does not adequately protect the cornea, allowing bacteria to enter and infection to result. Exposure-related ulcers may be treated with eyepads and/or anesthetic ointments.

Ulcers caused by bacteria are often associated with the staphylococcus or streptococcus bacterias. Other bacterias may infect the eye when the cornea is weakened by disease or additional infections. Bacterial ulcers are usually treated with ANTIBIOTICS or antibiotic-steroids.

Ulcers due to viruses are most often caused by the HERPES SIMPLEX virus. In infants, the virus is passed from the mother to the child as it travels through the birth canal. A rash may appear around the eyelids of the newborn, and the child may develop a fever.

The condition is serious and may result in death, blindness, or damage to other organs of the body. The virus is treated with ANTIVIRAL DRUGS and antibiotics.

The herpes virus may appear in adults after development of another illness. The virus, which had remained latent in the body, is reactivated and settles in the eye. This gives rise to KERATITIS, or inflammation, and the formation of star-shaped, or dendritic, ulcers. As the ulcers heal, they may leave scars that could impair vision.

An antiviral drug such as IDOXURIDINE, TRIFLURIDINE, or ACYCLOVIR along with an antibiotic may be prescribed as treatment. These drugs cannot cure the herpes simplex virus, but they effectively stop the reproduction of viral cells and prevent infection. STEROIDS are not recommended since they impair the body's rejection of the herpes simplex virus.

Fungal-related ulcers are most often caused by yeasts. The condition may require hospitalization and treatment with antibiotics. Healing of these ulcers often results in scarring of the cornea.

Damage to the corneal nerve, a vitamin-A deficiency, or the onset of other diseases or disorders may also trigger corneal ulcers. Any situation in which the cornea is inflamed (corneal keratitis) should be monitored for ulcers.

cortical blindness   Cortical blindness is a rare condition that occurs as a result of lesions on the occipital lobes where the visual cortex is located. The lobes control the visual field of each eye.

A lesion on one occipital lobe may result in HEMIANOPSIA, loss of half the field of vision, but does not affect the central vision acuity. Lesions on both lobes cause bilateral loss of vision with normally reactive pupils. This is known as cortical blindness.

Cortical blindness can be a congenital problem, but is most commonly seen in aging eyes affected by vascular disease. There may be a history of cerebrovascular incidents and loss of cerebral function. Cortical blindness may be a temporary condition that follows a cerebrovascular embolism or circulatory occlusion caused by a stroke, myocardial infarction, or heart surgery.

cortisone   A steroid hormone used in drugs to treat eye disorders. Cortisone may be an ingredient in prescribed EYE DROPS, ointments, or pills. It is often used to combat inflammation and prevent scarring, as in corneal disease.

Cortisone must be used with caution since it increases the eye's susceptibility to infection. Antiviral or antibacterial drugs are often taken at the same time to augment the eye's natural defenses.

Cortisone should be used in the eyes for the prescribed period of time only. Long-term use of cortisone may cause GLAUCOMA or CATARACT.

cortisporin ophthalmic antibiotic   A drug used to treat bacterial eye infections. It may be pre-

scribed in drop or ointment form. Equivalent products include Triple-Gen and triple antibiotic. Side effects from use of this drug may include burning or stinging of the eyes, redness, blurred or reduced vision, and headache. Eye pain, changes in vision, and headache indicate a serious problem that should be checked by a physician.

The drug should not be prescribed for fungal or viral eye infections or those that involve the back sections of the eye. Those with an allergy to hydrocortisone or any other ingredient, as well as those with tuberculosis, should not use this drug. Those with inner-ear problems, myasthenia gravis, or kidney disease should use the drug with caution.

The eye infection should be monitored during the time the drug is taken, even if the drug is used for a short period of time. If the drug is used long-term, the eye should be examined regularly for the development of CATARACT or a secondary infection.

Council for Exceptional Children (CEC)   A professional organization founded in 1922 and dedicated to providing appropriate educational experiences for exceptional children. The organization recognizes the special needs of visually impaired, hearing-impaired, physically disabled, mentally retarded, and mentally gifted children, as well as those with speech, behavioral, or learning disorders or disabilities. The membership includes teachers, educators, administrators, counselors, parents, and others involved in the education of gifted or disabled students.

The organization has four major priorities. It advances and improves access to education for exceptional people; improves professional conditions and establishes professional standards for those working with exceptional children; ensures the quality, support, and development of instruction provided to exceptional persons; and improves communication between members and those involved with exceptional children.

The CEC develops and sponsors workshops and conferences, generates programs in special education technology, offers technical aid to government legislators and educators, and maintains a network to champion educational rights. The organization directs the ERIC Clearinghouse on Handicapped and Gifted Children and maintains a library of 63,000 volumes.

CEC publishes the journals *Exceptional Children* and *TEACHING Exceptional Children*. The organization holds an annual convention.

Contact:

Council for Exceptional Children
1110 North Glebe Road, Suite 300
Arlington, Virginia, 22201-5704
888-232-7733 (ph)
703-264-9446 (TTY)
703-264-9493 (fax)
www.cec.sped.org

cryosurgery Cryosurgery is a procedure that uses very low temperatures to induce adhering scars in tissue. Cryosurgery employs a cryoprobe, a pencil-like probe with a tip that is cooled to a temperature between 30 and 70 degrees below freezing. Cryosurgery is used to repair RETINAL DETACH-MENTS.

A retinal detachment occurs whenever the RETINA is disconnected to the back layers of the eye. The retina normally adheres closely to the pigment epithelium and is supported by the VITREOUS gel. When the retina detaches or separates from the epithelium layer, vision is threatened and surgery is needed to reattach it.

In order to reattach the retina, the CHOROID, which lies just below the epithelium and the retina, must be irritated to form adhering scar tissue. The surgeon may use surgical diathermy, a procedure in which a needle transmitting high-frequency electrical current is touched to the SCLERA. The heat of the electricity is transmitted to the choroid, which is stimulated to form scar tissue.

An alternative method uses cryosurgery. The cryoprobe is touched to points on the sclera, which is unaffected by the procedure. A hypodermic needle is then inserted to drain any fluid that has accumulated under the retina.

The surgeon may then make an indentation in the back of the eye and place a silicone buckle or band around the eye to indent it slightly inward. This pushes the epithelium into contact with the retina. Adhering scar tissue forms in the frozen area and ensures that the retina will remain in

position. The band remains permanently in the eye but is neither seen nor felt.

Berland, Theodore, and Richard A. Perritt. *Living With Your Eye Operation.* New York: St. Martin's Press, 1974.
Eden, John. *The Eye Book.* New York: Penguin Books, 1978.
Krames Communications. *The Retina Book.* Daly City, California: KC, 1987.
Reynolds, James D. "Lasers in Ophthalmology," *HealthNet Library.* Columbus: CompuServe, 1989.

crystalline lens The crystalline or natural LENS is the transparent, elastic lens of the eye located behind the posterior chamber. The lens changes shape to focus light that enters the eye through the PUPIL. The lens is held in place by fibers called ZONULES. The zonules are attached to ciliary muscles, which contract or expand to change the shape of the lens. The lens bulges forward to focus on a near object and flattens to focus on a distant object.

The crystalline lens is subject to common eye disorders. It may become subluxated or develop cataracts. A subluxated lens is one that has shifted out of place due to a birth defect or an injury. The placement of the lens, usually downward from its normal position, determines the degree of affected vision.

Cataracts are a clouding or opaque spot on the surface of the lens that may develop over long periods of time. Most cataracts, termed senile cataracts, are those associated with aging. Cataracts may also be caused by birth defects, injuries, over-exposure to light, medications, diabetes, Down's syndrome, Marfan's syndrome, and other diseases.

Cataracts may be removed surgically. In some procedures, a portion of the crystalline lens is removed, and an artificial, plastic lens is placed in the eye. This intraocular lens, or IOL, replaces and serves as a permanent substitute for the removed section of natural lens.

See also EYE, CATARACT, IOL SURGERY.

cyclitis An inflammation of the CILIARY BODY of the eye. The ciliary body lies behind the IRIS and is attached to ZONULES, which hold the LENS in place. The ciliary body produces AQUEOUS FLUID, which flows into the anterior chamber to nourish the CORNEA and lens and carry away waste matter. It also moves the lens, allowing it to focus properly.

Cyclitis is associated with UVEITIS, an inflammation of the uveal tract that sometimes is referred to as arthritis of the eye. The ciliary body, the iris and the CHOROID make up the uveal tract. When the choroid becomes inflamed, as in CHOROIDITIS, it is termed posterior uveitis. When the iris or ciliary body becomes involved, it is termed anterior uveitis. Since the ciliary body is linked so closely to the iris, the inflammation soon spreads from one to the other. Because of this, cyclitis is often seen in cases of IRITIS, or inflammation of the iris.

The symptoms of cyclitis include extreme pain, contracted pupil, blurred vision, light sensitivity, and redness of the eye. It may develop quickly within a 24-hour period.

Cyclitis may develop spontaneously. It has been linked to other conditions such as arthritis, tuberculosis, VENEREAL DISEASE, SARCOIDOSIS, sinus disorders, viruses, and injuries. An ophthalmologic examination plus X rays of the sinuses, skull, and chest, as well as blood tests may be involved to determine the cause of the condition.

Treatment of this condition usually involves steroid eye drops and cycloplegic eye drops to dilate the pupil. Untreated cyclitis may spread to the choroid, retina, and vitreous, or may result in secondary GLAUCOMA.

cycloplegic drops Cycloplegic, or mydriatic, drops are eye drops that dilate the pupils. Cycloplegics are most often used during the ophthalmologic examination to observe the back of the eye. Most drops reach a maximum effect after 15 minutes and last approximately three hours. Stronger cycloplegics may last for 24 hours and are frequently used in young children or for lengthy examinations.

In diseases in which the LENS and the IRIS have developed adhesions, such as IRITIS, cycloplegics may be used to suspend accommodation, or movement, of the PUPIL. Atropine, a drug commonly administered in such cases, may last up to seven days.

Occasionally, the instillation of cycloplegic drops induces GLAUCOMA. This occurs when the dilated pupil further constricts the space in an unusually narrow anterior chamber. This impedes the flow of AQUEOUS FLUID from the eye, and intraocular pressure rises. Pilocarpine or other meiotics, drugs that constrict the pupil, can reverse the problem.

In rare instances, the patient may have an allergy to an ingredient in the cycloplegic eye drops. This may result in irritation, redness of the eye or dermatitis that should dissipate as the effectiveness of the drug wears off.

cytomegalovirus retinitis See AIDS.

dacryocystitis An inflammation of the tear drainage sac caused by an infection. It usually affects one eye only and may become a chronic disorder. It is most commonly found in adult females.

Dacryocystitis may be caused congenitally, from a blockage or obstruction of the tear duct or from a trauma or injury. The resulting infection is caused most often by bacteria such as *Staphylococcus aureus* and beta-hemolytic *Streptococcus* and by fungi such as *Candida albicans*.

Symptoms may include constant tearing, swelling, discharge and tenderness of the eye. A culture of the discharge may identify the infecting agent. The condition can be difficult to treat because the sac is located deep within the tissues surrounding the eye. Also, the condition can be hard to pinpoint and sometimes remains undetected for long periods, leading to scarring and tearing problems.

Dacryocystitis is usually treated with warm compresses and topical or systemic ANTIBIOTICS. Blocked nasolacrimal ducts of infants may be massaged to encourage dilation. If the duct fails to open, it may require surgical dilation. If the condition produces an abscess, it may be drained.

daily living skills Living skills that allow an individual to complete routine activities or daily tasks. Also called activities of daily living skills, techniques of daily living, or independent-living skills, these skills include personal-grooming skills, clothing labeling and care, eating skills, cooking, home-management skills, money management, communication skills, and child care.

Daily living skills are learned by visually impaired persons through self-discovery, informal teaching by parents or peers, school or teacher instruction, or formal rehabilitation training. The goal of daily living skills instruction is to teach the visually impaired person to independently perform a task in a safe, confident, socially acceptable manner. Each skill is separated into distinct parts in a task analysis. The analysis determines the steps needed to complete the task, the sequence of steps, and the adaptations necessary for completion by a visually impaired individual.

See NONVERBAL COMMUNICATION, REHABILITATION.

Kwitko, Marvin L., and Frank J. Weinstock. *Geriatric Ophthalmology.* New York: Grune and Stratton Inc., 1985.
Scholl, Geraldine. *Foundations of Education for Blind and Visually Handicapped Children and Youth.* New York: American Foundation for the Blind Inc., 1986.

Dancing Dots Braille Music Technology A company founded in 1992 by Bill McCann, a blind musician and programmer, to develop and adapt music technology for the blind. It released its first product, the GOODFEEL Braille music translator in 1997.

The GOODFEEL software automates transcription of Braille music, eliminating the need for a human transcriber. The software allows sighted musicians to prepare braille scores without needing to be braille music specialists, and allows blind musicians to make sound recordings, as well as print and Braille editions of their own compositions.

Dancing Dots also is an authorized distributor for many more assistive technology and music products.

Contact:

Dancing Dots Braille Music Technology
1754 Quarry Lane
P.O. Box 927
Valley Forge, PA 19482-0927

610-783-6692 (ph)
610-783-6732 (fax)
www.dancingdots.com

deaf-blind   Deaf-blind persons are those who
have a severe hearing impairment in addition to a
vision impairment. The combination of severities
varies according to the individual and often results
in some residual hearing or vision. Deaf-blind individuals may retain enough residual hearing or sight
to benefit from hearing aids or prescriptive lenses.

Deaf-blindness may be caused genetically and be
present at birth, may develop over time as a result
of RUBELLA or USHER'S SYNDROME or may be the
result of aging. Usher's syndrome is a leading cause
of deaf-blindness and responsible for approximately 10,000 of the deaf-blind individuals in the
United States.

Deaf-blind infants may exhibit autisticlike tendencies and are often misdiagnosed as retarded or
emotionally ill. Parents of deaf-blind infants and
children are urged to hold their children as much
as possible to provide the information that someone is close by. They are encouraged to talk, sing,
and hum to their children and to hold the children
near their chests to allow them to feel the vibration
of the sounds.

If a child has some residual hearing, he can be
encouraged to make sounds. Parents can expose
the child to as many vibrations as possible, from
the vacuum cleaner to the stereo speaker. Parents
can place their hands on the child's face and bend
to the child's face level while talking to the child.

Children can be stimulated with toys or movement to avoid unwanted mannerisms (see
BLINDISMS). Playing with drums, whistles, or other
vibration instruments may be helpful. If the child
has some residual hearing, the association of
sounds and actions or sounds and people helps to
define the world.

Deaf-blind children can be gently urged to sit
up, crawl, stand, and walk with encouragement
from parents. The child should always have support until he can stand by himself. Self-care activities such as eating, toilet training, and dressing can
begin early and should be consistent and reasonable in practice. Specific movements or signals may
be used to cue activities such as meal or bath time.

Once the child learns that motor movements
can be used to communicate, language development begins. The individual's residual vision and
hearing and fine motor skills will determine which
method of communication is used.

Some individuals who retain enough hearing or
become deaf after learning to speak can use speech.
Those without residual hearing may use fingerspelling, American Sign Language (ASL) or Signed
English, three sign languages that can be used by
deaf and totally blind persons.

In order to communicate with sighted and hearing individuals, the deaf-blind person may use the
alphabet glove, the Braille Alphabet Card, or the
Tellatouch device. The alphabet glove is a thin, cot-
ton glove printed with the letters of the alphabet at
specific spots that are memorized by the wearer.
The user or sighted person spells out words by
touching the letters on the glove.

The Braille Alphabet Card is a pocket-size card
that has both braille and printed letters on it. The
deaf-blind individual must read braille to use the
card. The user or the sighted person spells out the
words by touching the letters on the card.

The Tellatouch is a small, typewriterlike device
that raises braille letters under the deaf-blind readers fingertip as the other communicator types on
the keyboard. The device also includes braillewriter
keys for use by blind persons.

Education for deaf-blind children can begin
through early intervention programs or preschools
for deaf-blind persons. Those children with greater
hearing and less sight may be placed in programs
for visually impaired students. Those with greater
residual vision and little or no hearing may be
placed in programs for the hearing impaired.

Deaf-blind children entering kindergarten are
protected by the Education for All Handicapped
Children Act, which ensures them a free, appropriate, public education in the least restrictive setting,
which includes special education according to each
child's needs. A leading advocacy group for deaf-
blind people is the American Association of the
Deaf-Blind.

Contact:

American Association of the Deaf-Blind
814 Thayer Avenue
Silver Spring, MD 20910

800-735-2258 (ph)
301-588-8705 (fax)
301-588-6545 (TTY)

American Foundation for the Blind. *The Preschool Deaf-Blind Child: Suggestions for Parents.* New York: AFB, 1974.

American Foundation for the Blind. *What to Do When You Meet a Deaf-Blind Person,* New York: AFB, 1985.

Esche, Jeanne, and Carol Griffin. *A Handbook for Parents of Deaf-Blind Children.* Lansing, Michigan: Michigan School for the Blind, 1980.

McInnes, J. M., and J. A. Treffry. *Deaf-Blind Infants and Children.* Toronto: University of Toronto Press, 1982.

Scholl, Geraldine T. *Foundations of Education for Blind and Visually Handicapped Children and Youth.* New York: American Foundation for the Blind, 1986.

Walsh, Sara R., and Robert Holzberg, eds. *Understanding and Educating the Deaf-Blind/Severely and Profoundly Handicapped.* Springfield, Illinois: Charles C. Thomas Publisher, 1981.

Dendrid   See IDOXURIDINE.

Department of Education Organization Act of 1979   In 1979, a law was enacted to create a new Department of Education. This Cabinet-level department was formerly the Office of Education, a component of the Department of Health, Education and Welfare. This agency was renamed the Department of Health and Human Services under the Act.

The Department of Education took responsibility for most of the programs previously operated by the Office of Education, including the Overseas Defense Department schools and additional federal educational services and programs. However, jurisdiction of veterans education, the Head Start Program, child nutrition, and National Science Foundation educational, art and humanities programs was given to other agencies.

The act also established an Office of Special Education and Rehabilitative Services.

The mission of the Office of Special Education and Rehabilitative Services (OSERS) is threefold: Office of Special Education Programs supports programs that assist with educating children with special needs; its Rehabilitation Services Administration provides for rehabilitation of youth and adults with disabilities; and, its National Institute on Disability and Rehabilitation Research supports research to improve the quality of life of people with disabilities. More information about the Department of Education's Office of Special Education and Rehabilitative Services can be found on the Internet at www.ed.gov.

U.S. Department of Education. *Summary of Existing Legislation Affecting Persons with Disabilities.* Washington, D.C.: USDE, 1988.

development of blind children   Visually impaired and blind children develop according to the same patterns and stages that govern the development of sighted children. The effect the loss of vision has on each child depends on the severity, the type of loss, the age at which the loss occurred and the child's overall functioning level.

Each visually impaired child is an individual; therefore, there is no typical visually impaired child. Each develops according to his own timetable and abilities. However, many visually impaired children have certain traits and needs in common.

Blind or visually impaired children may depend more on their parents initially. They rely on their parents to bring the world to them. Parents need to fill the gaps presented by the lack of sight with experiences involving all the senses, including making the best use of any residual vision.

Severe impairments may require the children to be hospitalized and separated at birth from their parents for extended periods. At the end of such time, the children may resist cuddling and not like to be held. The parents and children may respond negatively to the lack of eye contact.

Parents of visually impaired babies and children may need to hold, stroke, and talk to their children more than normal in order to reassure the children that someone is near. Although some visually impaired children react negatively to being held or picked up from the crib, this is not a rejection of affection, but may rather be a reaction to the sudden interruption. Babies who lie quietly in the crib may be concentrating on sounds in the environment and become frightened or confused at a sudden jostling. Parents may substitute voice contact for eye contact by speaking and crooning to the children and imitating sounds the children make.

The lack of vision may also affect the ability of children to distinguish between self and nonself. Sighted children develop the concept by use of vision. They are able to see themselves as separate from their environment and from others by watching others come forward or move away. Parents may encourage their visually impaired children to develop this concept through auditory means by talking to their children as they enter and leave a room.

Up to age four months, visually impaired children and sighted children vary little in their development. At about four months of age, the sighted child may become fascinated with watching his hand, an activity that the visually impaired child may miss. This hand-watching encourages the child to direct his attention to the outside world.

Because of the impairment or lack of sight, visually impaired children may not reach out to explore their world and depend on their parents to bring objects to them. Blind or visually impaired babies may mouth objects for a longer period of time during development (extending into childhood) than their sighted peers. An abundance of tactile sensors in the lips makes this a logical way to gain information in the presence of a sight loss.

Vision provides useful stimulation for motor development, motivating babies to hold their heads up, reach for objects, sit, participate in imitative activity, crawl, and walk. Parents of babies with a sight loss may have to develop creative ways to motivate their children into movement to teach them these actions. Babies without this stimulation may become passive.

As the children grow, they may be encouraged to participate in the same activities and sports as their sighted peers, including group games, jump rope, skating, running and riding a tricycle. Visually impaired or blind children who are physically active tend to show little difference in gross motor skills as compared with their sighted peers and have a better awareness of body image and spatial orientation than blind or visually impaired children who are not physically active.

If visually impaired children lack sufficient opportunities for movement, they may develop stereotypical behaviors, sometimes called "blind-isms." These movements include rocking, head swaying, and poking or rubbing the eyes. Often described as a reaction to a need for stimulation and activity, these behaviors may be curtailed by providing a stimulating environment and ample opportunities for movement, including such activities as climbing and riding a rocking horse.

Fine motor skills such as using a crayon, tying shoes, and playing with blocks or pegs should also be stressed. These skills help children explore the world and prepare them for learning to read and write.

Abstract concepts are more difficult for children with a sight loss, since they are often linked to visual concepts. Concepts such as dirty and clean, in and out, open and shut, up and down, and forward and behind are crucial to the full development of any child. Parents of visually impaired children may have to try methods based on other sensory experiences, in repeated exposures, to teach these concepts to their visually impaired children.

Language and speech development tend to be comparable in sighted and visually impaired children. If children have had a limited amount of gross motor experiences, however, language development may be delayed.

Visually impaired and blind children may repeat or echo what other people say for a longer period of time than their sighted peers. This repeating, called *echolalia*, may be an attempt to practice linking words to the concepts they stand for.

Nonverbal communication develops in sighted children when they smile in response to smiles by others. Later, they imitate and experiment with facial expressions to determine the kinds of reaction they can elicit. Visually impaired children may not participate in this kind of imitative activity, which may limit their development of nonverbal communication. As children grow, they can be instructed verbally as to the kinds of facial expressions and postures that are socially acceptable in order to avoid embarrassment and misunderstandings in social interaction.

During preadolescent and adolescent years, the emphasis of development is placed on educational and social needs. Visually impaired and blind children are entitled by law to a free and equal EDUCA-

TION, including special education programs to fit each child's needs, in the least restrictive environment. Children may go to school in a variety of settings and may begin to use ADAPTIVE AIDS and devices to complete their studies.

Social needs center on feelings of belonging. Group participation in activities such as Girl or Boy Scouts, and school sports and clubs increases feelings of confidence and acceptance by peers. Self-acceptance should be stressed and children should actively participate in determining their own activities and future pursuits.

American Foundation for the Blind. *Is Your Child Blind?* New York: AFB, 1975.

American Foundation for the Blind. *Parenting Preschoolers.* New York: AFB, 1987.

American Foundation for the Blind. *Touch the Baby.* New York: AFB, 1987.

National Association for Visually Handicapped. *Family Guide: Growth and Development of the Partially Seeing Child.* New York: NAVH, 1985.

Warren, David H. *Blindness and Early Childhood Development.* New York: American Foundation for the Blind, 1977.

diabetes   Diabetes or diabetes mellitus (DM) is a name for a group of inherited medical conditions or diseases in which the body is unable adequately to process and store glucose. According to the American Diabetes Center, 15.7 million Americans are afflicted with this serious disease. It is the sixth major cause of death by disease.

Diabetes, specifically DIABETIC RETINOPATHY, is one of the chief causes of blindness in the United States. Approximately 150,000 diabetics in the United States experience a significant degree of vision loss, and 3 percent have a severe vision loss as a result of this condition.

Diabetic retinopathy, a disease of the RETINA, is a complication of a general circulatory problem caused by diabetes. This disorder causes the blood vessels that nourish the retina, a light-sensitive inner lining in the back layer of the eye, to weaken, disintegrate, or become blocked. The vessels may leak fluid, bleed, grow unnaturally, bulge, or stop functioning completely.

According to the National Institute of Health, 12 percent of diabetics have experienced CATARACTS, or opacities of the lens, and an additional 11 percent have been diagnosed with GLAUCOMA, a condition in which intraocular pressure builds within the eye and causes vision loss. These rates are over twice those for the general population.

Those most at risk of developing diabetes include members of families with a history of diabetes, women (by a two-to-one margin over men), obese or overweight people, people over 40, blacks, Hispanics, native Americans, and those from low-income groups.

The disease affects many organ groups and causes complications such as retinopathy (disease of the retina), nephropathy (disease of the kidney), neuropathy (disease of the nerves), arteriosclerosis (hardening of the arteries), and skin disorders.

Carbohydrates are broken down into glucose by the body's digestive juices. When glucose enters the blood stream, the beta cells of the pancreas produce and release insulin, which helps the body tissues absorb the energy-producing glucose.

Diabetes is present when the beta cells fail to react to the elevated glucose level in the blood. As a result, the blood glucose level rises above normal, the liver produces sugar from protein in the body, glucose appears in the urine, and the individual experiences frequent urination, constant thirst, and weight loss. If untreated, the disease can cause dangerous levels of acid in the blood and diabetic coma.

Three main types of diabetes exist. Type I, insulin-dependent diabetes mellitus (IDDM), is characterized by insulin dependency; the presence of HLA, DR3 and DR4 genetic markers; the appearance of circulation antibodies that attack the cells of the pancreas; and a predisposition to acquire ketoacidosis, high levels of ketones, fatty acids, and glucose in the blood.

Type I diabetes is also called juvenile-onset diabetes and occurs in children and adolescents. The onset of the disease often follows an infection or virus. Several viruses including rubella, mumps, Coxsackie B, and Echo viruses are being explored as possible links to a cause.

Type II, noninsulin-dependent diabetes mellitus (NIDDM), occurs generally in middle-aged adults. NIDDM patients secrete insulin, lack HLA genetic markers, are insulin resistant, and are usually overweight.

Since six out of seven Type II patients who develop the disease after age 45 are overweight, studies are being conducted to determine whether inheritance may interact with obesity to trigger the disease.

Type III diabetes is a milder form of the disease. It is non-progressive and has no known cause beyond inheritance. It affects young and old alike.

Treatment for diabetes may include dietary measures, exercise, oral drug treatment, insulin injections, daily monitoring of blood glucose levels in the blood or urine, and regularly scheduled medical examinations. It is extremely important that anyone who has diabetes get regular, thorough eye exams. The severity of many diabetes-related eye problems can be reduced if the problem is detected early.

See also DIABETIC RETINOPATHY.

U.S. Department of Health and Human Services, NIH. *Facts About Insulin-Dependent Diabetes.* NIH Publication No. 80-2098. Washington, D.C.: Government Printing Office, 1980.

National Diabetes Data Group, NIH. *Diabetes in America.* NIH Publication No. 85-1468. Washington, D.C.: Government Printing Office, 1985.

American Diabetes Association, Diabetes Facts and Figures, ADA website, 2000.

diabetic retinopathy   A disease of the RETINA and a leading cause of blindness and vision impairment. Seven percent of all blind persons are impaired as a result of diabetic retinopathy, a figure estimated by the National Society to Prevent Blindness as 33,000. It is responsible for 1 in every 10 new cases of blindness in the United States each year.

Approximately 150,000 diabetics in the United States experience a significant degree of vision loss due to diabetic retinopathy. Three percent have a severe vision loss as a result of this condition.

Diabetic retinopathy is a complication of a general circulatory problem caused by diabetes. The diabetes causes the blood vessels that nourish the retina, a light-sensitive inner lining in the back layer of the eye, to weaken, disintegrate, or become blocked. The vessels may leak fluid, bleed, grow unnaturally, bulge, or stop functioning completely.

The risk of developing retinopathy is determined by the age of the patient at diagnosis, and the dura-

tion of the disease. People with Type I (insulin dependent) juvenile diabetes often take longer to develop the disease than people who are diagnosed as having diabetes as adults, but since the younger individuals have the disease for a longer period of time, they are more likely to develop the disease. However, the disease does not always follow a predictable pattern. It can occur within a few years of diagnosis or it may be the first indication of diabetes.

The disease has three stages: exudative or background, preproliferative, and proliferative retinopathy. Each can be detected through a routine examination with an ophthalmoscope. Small red spots or microaneurysms may be visible in early stages of the disease, called background or exudative retinopathy.

In this case, the damage has occurred in the retina and retinal vessels. The vessels may swell, bulge, or leak fluid that can collect in the retina and alter vision. The retina can remain in this stage for years or indefinitely.

Preproliferative retinopathy occurs typically in young people with uncontrolled diabetic conditions. This stage of retinopathy is marked by increased hemorrhages, expansion of retinal vessels, and soft exudates, exuded material from a retinal infarct (dead tissue area that resulted from a vascular obstruction).

Examination of the disease at later stages shows larger hemorrhages indicating proliferative retinopathy. This more dangerous stage concerns the growth of new, abnormal blood vessels, or neovascularization. The new vessels often bleed into the retina and VITREOUS and cause sudden, severe vision loss. Although it is not entirely clear why these new vessels grow, it is thought that it is in response to blood vessel changes caused by a lack of oxygen to the retina. The retina, in effect, sends a chemical message to the damaged blood vessels, which respond by growing and releasing tiny new vessels into the retina.

The formation of scar tissue from the healed vessels can pull the retina away from its position in the back of the eye as the vitreous tends to shrink and move toward the center of the globe. The retina may become detached or torn causing serious or total blindness.

Diagnosis and treatment of some cases of diabetic retinopathy includes FLUORESCEIN ANGIOGRAPHY. During this procedure fluorescent dye is injected into the arm of the patient. The eye is examined as the dye travels through the body, including the eye, where it points out the damaged retinal vessels. The dye test, other than the injection itself, is painless and has few side effects. The dye may cause a patient's skin to look slightly yellow and cause changes in the color of the urine. These side effects normally last only about 12 hours.

Treatment of the damaged vessels may include photocoagulation or laser therapy. During this treatment, an argon laser is focused on the leaking blood vessels and cauterizes them. Over 1,000 laser burns are placed on the retina, excluding the macular area. The cauterization destroys the tissue, discouraging regrowth of abnormal vessels and allowing the limited blood supply to reach and nourish the MACULA, or area of sharpest sight. The procedure is performed with a local anesthetic and involves little discomfort. Overnight hospitalization is usually not required.

Laser therapy may be administered to those with background retinopathy when damage is severe or when accompanied by MACULAR EDEMA. Laser therapy is almost always prescribed for those with proliferative retinopathy. Laser therapy is not a cure. Vision is often not improved, but the progression of the disease can be stopped and greater loss of vision prevented.

VITRECTOMY is also used to treat severe retinopathy. A specialized instrument is inserted into the vitreous where it breaks down blood deposits and scar tissue. It then removes the matter and the diseased vitreous fluid by suction. Simultaneously, a sterile saline fluid is injected to replace the vitreous fluid. Approximately two thirds of those who undergo vitrectomy gain improved vision.

See PROLIFERATIVE RETINOPATHY.

Galloway, N. R. *Common Eye Diseases and Their Management.* Berlin: Springer-Verlag, 1985.

National Society to Prevent Blindness. *Facts and Figures: Diabetic Retinopathy.* New York: NSPB, 1980.

Rhoade, Stephen J., and Stephen P. Ginsberg. *Ophthalmic Technology.* New York: Raven Press, 1987.

Vaughn, Daniel and Taylor Asbury. *General Ophthalmology.* Los Altos, California: Lange Medical Publications, 1977.

Cassel, Gary H., Michael D. Billig, and Harry G. Randall. *The Eye Book.* Baltimore: Johns Hopkins University Press, 1998.

diopter   A unit of measurement for the power of a lens. It measures the extent light rays will bend as they pass through the lens.

Diopters are written in prescriptions as O.D. or O.S. followed by a plus or minus sign and a number. The O.D. stands for the Latin *oculus dexter,* or right eye. The O.S. stands for *oculus sinister,* or left eye.

Plus signs indicate convex or farsighted lenses. Minus signs stand for concave or nearsighted lenses. A +3.00 prescription calls for a 3 diopter convex lens for a farsighted eye. A -1.5 prescription requires a 1-1/2 diopter concave lens for a near-sighted eye. The stronger the lens is, the higher the number.

Prescriptions to correct astigmatism employ cylindrical lenses that are often incorporated into a convex or concave lens to curve it more in one direction. Astigmatism prescriptions indicate the diopter degree of near- or farsightedness, plus the word "axis" and a number from 1 to 180. The axis number refers to the number of degrees on a protractor and determines to which degree the cylindrical lens must be oriented.

The prescription -3.25–2.00 axis 95, calls for 3-1/4 diopters of nearsightedness with 2 diopters of astigmatism. The axis 95 indicates the degree at which the cylindrical lens must be oriented (95 degrees in this case).

diplopia   The term for double vision. Diplopia is often confused with blurred vision when cited as a patient complaint. Blurred vision is a cloudy or hazy image, but diplopia is the sighting of two separate images at the same time.

Diplopia may be constant or intermittent and binocular or monocular. Monocular diplopia occurs if the double image persists when one eye is closed. This is a common form of diplopia and is often caused by cataract. Binocular diplopia occurs when the diplopia is corrected when one eye is closed.

Diplopia may go unnoticed in adults or children due to poor general vision or suppression of image. Children often accommodate to the double image by suppressing the image of one eye, a condition called AMBLYOPIA. This condition may lead to vision loss.

Diplopia is a serious symptom and requires examination of the eyes. The examination involves testing of the gross eye movements to check the degree of separation of images in various positions. The Hess chart, red-glass test, or the cover-uncover test may be used.

The Hess chart test involves placing a red filter in front of one eye and a green filter in front of the other. The patient looks at a screen of small white dots. The patient is asked to point to specific dots with a pointer. The amount of mislocation is measured.

The red-glass test involves placing a red glass in front of the right eye and a green glass in front of the left. The patient looks at a light 20 feet away and then at a separate light 14 inches away. The patient tells the examiner if separate red and green lights are seen while fixating on the near or far light.

During the cover-uncover test the patient looks at a letter or object at 20 feet. One eye is covered and the other is observed to see whether it moves to fixate on the object. If the eye moves, a disorder is present. The other eye is tested at 20 feet and then both are tested at 14 inches.

Diplopia may be caused by misalignment of the eyes, as in STRABISMUS (or a latent strabismus from childhood), an ocular muscle imbalance; third, fourth or sixth cranial nerve palsy; orbital lesions; muscle lesions; cataracts; nerve lesions; multiple sclerosis; myasthenia gravis; injury to the orbit; thyrotoxicosis, in which extraocular muscles become inflamed; stroke; or intracranial tumor.

Diplopia may often be treated with corrective lenses, surgery or medication therapy of the underlying cause.

Burde, Ronald, Peter J. Savino and Jonathan D. Trobe. *Clinical Decisions in Neuro-Ophthalmology.* St. Louis: C.V. Mosby Company, 1985.

Eden, John. *The Eye Book.* New York: Penguin Books, 1978.

Galloway, N. R. *Common Eye Diseases and their Management.* Berlin: Springer-Verlag, 1985.

Phillips, Calbert I. *Basic Clinical Ophthalmology.* London: Pitman Publishers Limited, 1984.

disability   There is no complete consensus on terms concerning the topic of blindness and vision impairment. Rehabilitation experts, doctors, educators, and other leaders in the field determine and define terminology according to their own preferences and viewpoints. In recent years, those involved in the field of blindness and vision impairment have made efforts to standardize terms such as disability to eliminate confusion or misinterpretation.

A disability may be defined as the way an impairment (a diagnosed defect or malfunctioning of a body part or organ) affects an individual's ability to function. It is the limitation, restriction, or disadvantage due to the malfunction.

See TERMINOLOGY.

disability insurance benefits   See SOCIAL SECURITY BENEFITS.

Disability Rights Education and Defense Fund (DREDF)   A nonprofit advocacy group founded in 1979 by leaders in the disability rights movement. It is the only advocacy organization that represents all disabled persons as a class. The goal of DREDF is to change policies and attitudes that contribute to discrimination of disabled persons and prevent them from fully participating in all aspects of life. The organization addresses laws and policies that will ensure disabled persons integration into schools, jobs, and community life.

Nationally, DREDF advises Congress and other policy makers concerning disability civil rights issues; participates in civil rights coalitions, including those representing women's and disability groups; provides a national network of legislative information for disabled persons and their families; and coordinates and submits to the U.S. Supreme Court "friend of the court" briefs on disability rights issues.

On a local level, DREDF provides legal representation to disabled persons and their families in cases of school placement, respite and child care, and discrimination by employers, landlords, and businesses.

It educates and advises the California state legislature on issues affecting the rights of disabled persons.

DREDF publications include the *Disability Rights Education and Defense Fund News.*

Contact:

Disability Rights Education and Defense Fund,
  Inc. Government Affairs Office
1629 K Street NW, Suite 802
Washington, DC, 20006
202-986-0375 (ph)
202-775-7465 (fax)

DREDF's main office is located at:

2212 Sixth Street
Berkeley, CA 94710
510-644-2555 (voice and TTY)
510-841-8645 (fax)
www.dredf.org

divergence   Divergence is the movement of the eyes from a convergent position. Convergence is the turning-in movement of the eyes to focus on a near object. When the object is too close to the nose to be seen as one image, the eyes diverge, or move from the convergent position.

dog guide laws   All of the 50 states, plus Puerto Rico, have enacted statutes that regulate dog guides. All states guarantee the legal right of a blind person to be accompanied by a trained dog guide on all public transportation and in all public accommodations.

Public transportation is described as all modes of public conveyance and includes airplanes, trains, boats, buses, taxis, and elevators. Public accommodations are anywhere the public is invited. They include city streets, stores, restaurants, hotels, lodging places, resorts, amusement parks, educational institutes, and public buildings. The blind person cannot be charged a fee for the dog guide but is liable for any damage to the premises that the dog might cause.

Violation of the law by a person or organization generally results in a fine or imprisonment. Some states allow dog-guide users who are denied their civil rights to take the offending parties to court.

Although the above minimum statutes apply in all 50 states and Puerto Rico, some dog-guide laws designate specific restrictions while others extend rights. Some states require the dog guide to be in harness or compel the owner to muzzle the dog guide upon request. Others specifically note that dog guides may not occupy a seat or that the blind person must carry and show, on request, the identification card issued by the school that trained the dog. Others allow dog guides to be exempt from licensing regulations or fees.

In Hawaii, dog guides, like all dogs entering the state, must undergo a 120-day quarantine. However, dog guide users may stay with their dogs in special cottages on quarantine grounds. Dog guides are not exempt from the regular quarantine fee.

Some state laws order drivers to use every safeguard to avoid injury or endangerment to a dog-guide user traveling the streets. Drivers must yield the right of way to a crossing user and bring the car to a stop if necessary.

Many states include in the dog-guide law assurances that dog-guide users have the right to equal accommodation in commercial housing. The definition for commercial housing varies greatly from state to state. It may be described as one or more of the following: a self-contained dwelling unit; property offered for rent, lease, or compensation; group homes; residential communities; or public-assisted housing. Many states make specific exceptions for single-family private homes that offer one rental room only. Some stipulate that a fee cannot be charged due to the presence of the dog guide; others allow the landlord to levy a limited security deposit against possible damage incurred by the dog guide.

Some states express the right of dog-guide users to have equal employment opportunity in state employment, public schools, or any employment supported by public funds, so long as the person is qualified to perform the job.

A number of Canadian provinces have enacted dog-guide laws that closely resemble the basic statutes of those in the United States. Dog-guide users must carry a current health record for the dog guide, including proof of rabies vaccination, when crossing the Canadian-American border. Users are advised to include an identification card from the dog-guide training school and a muzzle, because in many provinces muzzling is required.

dog guides Dog guides are specially trained dogs that provide protection, independent travel and companionship to blind persons. Approximately 1 percent of the nation's blind persons use dog guides.

The training of dogs began in Germany during World War I. Dogs used to carry messages onto the battlefield were found to locate wounded soldiers and lead rescuers to their aid. As a result, the Germans began to train these dogs as guides for men blinded during the war. Dorothy Harrison Eustis, an American living in Switzerland, learned of this development and developed a training program for dog guides. Eustis returned to the United States and established the first American dog guide school, The Seeing Eye Inc., in 1929. Although modern dog guide schools vary in the services they offer, many breed and train dogs, train dog guide instructors, instruct blind persons on how to use and care for dog guides, and provide public information.

Both male and female Labradors, golden retrievers, and German shepherds are most often preferred as dog guides, although boxers, Doberman pinschers and collies are also used. New puppies are examined and tested at the school to determine physical health, intelligence, responsibility, and willingness to learn and please. Suitable puppies are sent to live with a foster family. The puppies live with the family for approximately one year in which they learn socialization and, in some cases, obedience skills. The 4-H Clubs and other volunteer puppy-raising organizations often work closely with schools to place new puppies in homes. After a year or longer, the dogs return to the dog-guide school for formal training. They are taught basic obedience skills and are introduced to the leather harness that is worn when traveling.

The dogs learn to lead rather than walk in the heel position, to stop at curbs and stairs, to avoid obstacles, both on the ground and overhead, to ignore distractions and to disobey instructions that put the user in danger. The training may last from three to six months. Roughly half of the dogs trained to be dog guides do not pass the training requirements. They are usually offered to the foster family for adoption or placed in other good homes.

After graduation from training, the dog is matched with a blind person. The student and dog live, eat and train together at the school for four weeks. Training sessions include traveling skills, transportation use in both residential and urban settings, and grooming, rewarding, and disciplining the dog guide.

The blind student learns to direct the dog and to understand the signals felt through the U-shaped handle of the leather harness. Dogs are color blind and therefore cannot distinguish a red traffic light from a green. The blind student must listen to traffic to determine when to cross streets as well as direct the dog guide to the desired destination. Since public interference is the greatest distraction to dog guides, users learn to discourage strangers from speaking to or touching the dog while it is in harness.

Applicants for dog guides generally must be legally blind, over 16 years old, able to travel independently, and physically and psychologically able to care for the dog. Although dog guides are often provided free of charge, some training schools require a fee. Most schools will not disqualify an applicant due to lack of funds.

Dog guides generally live and work for 10 years. Dog guides that become sick or disabled are offered to the blind owner to keep as a pet or are returned to the school and placed in an adoptive home. If the dog dies, the blind person may generally return to the school for a new dog. If the dog's owner dies, it may remain with the family, be placed with a new dog guide user, or be retired at the school.

dominant eye In normal, healthy eyes, one eye is usually in some degree dominant over the other. Eye dominance follows the same principle as right- or left-handedness and often complies with hand dominance.

In normal vision, both eyes focus on an object. Each eye sends a slightly different view of the sighted object to the brain where the two views are processed into one three-dimensional image. The normally dominant eye is the sighting eye that finds and focuses on the object, whereas the nondominant eye focuses just off center, the dominant eye is usually used unconsciously to look through a telescope, into a microscope, or through the sight of a camera. To find the dominant eye, punch a hole in a piece of paper and then, without thinking, quickly look through the hole. The eye used to look through the hole is the dominant eye.

Overdominance of one eye may affect or limit vision. If one eye or its muscles are weakened or impaired by conditions such as MYASTHENIA GRAVIS, MULTIPLE SCLEROSIS, brain tumor, STROKE, or infection, the eyes may become uncoordinated and fail to focus on the same object. When this occurs, DIPLOPIA, or double vision, results.

When one eye turns in (esotropia) or out (exotropia), a condition called STRABISMUS, or crossed-eyes, occurs. The aligned eye becomes the dominant eye over the misaligned eye. Diplopia occurs as a result of strabismus. Strabismus may occur at any age but generally is present in young children. Strabismus may affect over 1.6 million children in the United States.

As the brain receives two images from the misaligned eyes, it relies increasingly on the dominant eye for information about the object viewed. It may begin to suppress the information from the nondominant eye, causing the vision to deteriorate from lack of use of the eye. This condition is known as amblyopia. The suppressed or amblyopic eye may become less functional or lose vision due to lack of light stimulation. Amblyopia usually occurs in young children and affects over 2.5 percent of all children in the United States.

An overdominant eye can often be corrected with surgery to repair or reinforce weakened eye muscles, or with nonsurgical techniques such as glasses, exercise therapy, or patching of the dominant eye. Early diagnosis generally results in the most favorable results.

double vision   See DIPLOPIA.

Down's syndrome   Down's (or Down) syndrome, or mongolism, is a genetic condition produced by a chromosomal abnormality involving an additional 21st chromosome. Down's syndrome is marked by mental retardation, mongoloid facial characteristics, small stature, heart abnormalities, and obesity. Down's syndrome occurs most often in children born to women over 35.

Ocular conditions associated with Down's syndrome include high MYOPIA (nearsightedness), hyperplasia of the iris, STRABISMUS, narrow palpebral (eyelid) fissures, epicanthus (vertical folds of the eyelids), and CATARACT. Cataracts may be slight or serious enough to warrant surgical removal.

dreams   Dreams of the blind have long been a subject of interest to psychologists. Research, however, has been sparse, and few investigations have been launched into the activities and objects in dreams of the visually impaired.

Two early studies, Heermann (1838) and Jastrow (1888), drew four major conclusions that are still widely held today. They discovered that no visual images exist in the dreams of the congenitally blind, nor for those blinded before age five, but that the dreams of those who become blind between five and seven may or may not contain visual imagery and that most optical imagery tends to fade markedly with time.

McCartney (1913) discovered that dreams of the blind contained a high ratio of fearful objects in their dreams when compared with those of sighted subjects. Blank (1958) found that dreams of the blind contained more thought and language than those of sighted subjects, and Von Schumann (1959) related that intellectual activity, dynamic body movement, and falling were characteristic traits of dreams of the visually impaired.

Hall (1966, 1972) proposed that dreams, including those of the blind, must be continuous with waking behavior in that they must reflect actions or conscious thoughts or attitudes. The studies discounted the compensation theory that contends that dreams can embody complete reversals of waking tendencies.

Findings from separate investigations by Kirtley and Cannistraci (1973) and Kirtley and Hall (1975) agreed that the dreams of blind or visually impaired persons differed significantly from those of sighted persons in regard to the activities and objects found in the dreams. The investigators concluded that these differences are caused by the physical limitations and "special reality problems" of the blind that exist in their waking life.

Kirtley and Cannistraci created five categories—mobility, aggressive behavior, friendly interactions, self-perception, and perception of the physical environment—to describe the differences between the dreams of sighted and visually impaired persons. In their dreams, the visually impaired were more restricted in physical movement, and settings tended to be indoors rather than outdoors.

The dreams of the blind were lower in incidence of physical aggression, yet when incidents did occur, they were unusually extreme. There were few incidents of self-aggression. Verbal aggression incidents were much more frequent than those of sighted subjects. The study showed that the dreams of the blind contained more incidents of friendly speech and thoughts but fewer of friendly acts involving long-term relationships, physical contact, and gift giving.

The study cited more references to body parts and extremities, including the head, and fewer to clothing. Concerning the environment, the study concluded that blind subjects cited fewer incidents of building materials and descriptions of size, including thinness, narrowness, lowness, crookedness, crowding, and vacancy.

Kirtley and Sabo (1979) compared the dreams of visually impaired students, including partially blind, congenitally blind, and adventitiously blind individuals, with those of normally sighted students. The findings revealed that the dreams of the visually impaired group as a whole contained less symbolism than those of the sighted subjects. They concluded that the concreteness of the dreams was a result of the fact that blindness is an internalized stress condition that creates more waking-hour reality problems.

Sabo and Kirtley (1982) discovered that blind subjects tended to dream more often about food and drink; parts of the torso; land areas limited by boundaries such as cities, parking lots, yards, and swimming pools; and construction materials such as bricks, lumber, and boards. They concluded that this is a result of how the blind learn their environment and the limitations surrounding their handicap. The study revealed a significant number of active physical activities such

as running, walking, and climbing but the activities tended to take place in a limited area or space.

Kirtley and Sabo (1983) compared the aggression content of dreams of visually impaired females and normally sighted females and found that the visually impaired women exhibited more verbal and covert aggression. These findings agreed with the Kirtley and Cannistraci (1973) report that found less physical aggression in the dreams of visually impaired persons (both male and female) but a higher incidence of verbal and covert aggression. Rainville (1994) concluded that dreams are extremely important in the rehabilitation of people who are newly blind. They are vital to a person's adjustment to blindness, he says.

Helen Keller described her dreams in her book *The World I Live In* and in the article "My Dreams." Although edited for print, they reflect the images of the visually impaired.

Keller related that her dreams were filled with sensations, odors, tastes, and ideas. She described seeing but not with her eyes and hearing but not with her ears. She explained that she did not often talk with her fingers or read with her fingers in dreams and that she possessed greater freedom of mobility.

She recounted seeing a brilliant light of "flash and glory." Keller mentioned colors such as the "velvety green of moss," "the soft whiteness of lilies," and the "distilled hues and sweetness of a thousand roses."

Keller, Helen. "My Dreams," *Century Magazine,* vol. 77, no. 1 (1908): pp. 134–165.

Keller, Helen. *The World I Live In.* New York: Century Company, 1908.

Kirtley, Donald, and Katherine Cannistraci. "Dreams of the Visually Handicapped: Toward a Normative Approach." *AFB Research Bulletin #27* (April 1974): 111–133.

Kirtley, Donald. *The Psychology of Blindness.* Chicago: Nelson-Hall, 1975.

Kirtley, Donald, and Kenneth Sabo. "Aggression in the Dreams of Blind Women." *Journal of Visual Impairment and Blindness,* vol. 77, no. 6 (June 1984): 269–270.

Kirtley, Donald, and Kenneth Sabo. "Symbolism in the Dreams of the Blind." *International Journal of Rehabilitation Research* vol. 2, no. 2 (1979): 225–232.

Rainville, Raymond E. "The Role of Dreams in the Rehabilitation of the Adventitiously Blind." *Dreaming* (1994): pp. 155–164.

Sabo, Kenneth, and Donald Kirtley. "Objects and Activities in the Dreams of the Blind." *International Journal of Rehabilitation Research,* vol. 5, no. 2, (1982): 241–242.

drugs Topical and systemic drugs are used in ophthalmology to treat eye diseases and disorders, to prepare eyes of examination or surgery, to treat or prevent inflammation, and to diagnose disease or disorders.

Mydriatics are drugs that dilate the pupils. They are generally either sympathomimetics or parasympatholytics. Sympathomimetics imitate or initiate the release of adrenaline and direct the action to the dilator muscle of the iris. Parasympatholytics dilate the PUPIL and retain it in position so that the pupil cannot accommodate its size to changes in light.

Generic sympathomimetics include phenylephrine HCl, hydroxyamphetamine HBr, and cocaine; trade names include Ak-Dilate, Efricel, Mydfrin, Neo-Synephrine HCl, Penoptic, and Paredrine. Generic parasympatholytics include atropine sulfate, cyclopentolate HCl, homatropine HBr, scopolamine, and tropicamide; trade names include Ak-Pentolate, Cyclogyl, Homatrocel, Isopto Homatropine, Isopto Hyoscine, Mydramide, Mydriacyl, and Topicacyl.

Miotics are parasympathomimetics that are used to treat GLAUCOMA and ESOTROPIA. Cholinergic (direct-acting) miotics include the generic carbachol, pilocarpine hydrochloride, and pilocarpine nitrate, and the trade names Carbacel, Isopto Carbachol, Adsobocarpine, Akarpine, Almocarpine, Isopto Carpine, Pilocar, Pilocel, Pilomiotin, Pilopine gel hs 4 percent, Ocusert Pilo, Piloptic, and P.V. Carpine. Anticholinesterasic (indirect acting) miotics include the generic physostigmine sulfate, physostigmine salicylate, demecarium bromide, echothiophate iodide and isoflurophate (DFP), and the trade names Eserine Sulfate, Isopto Eserine, Humorsol, Echodide, Phospholine Iodide and Floropryl.

Ocular infections are treated according whether the infecting agent is bacterial, fungal, viral, or protozoal. Antibiotics are used to treat corneal ulcers and intraocular infections. Antibiotics may be topical or systemic and include the generic ampicillin, bacitracin, carbenicillin, cefazolin, cephalothin, chloramphenicol, clindamycin, colistin sulfate, erythromycin, gentamycin sulfate, lincomycin, methicillin, neomycin, penicillin, polymyxin B sulfate, silver nitrate, streptomycin, sulfacetamide sodium, sulfisoxazole diolamine, tetracycline, tobramycin, and vancomycin. They are known by numerous trade names, including Baciquent, Ak-Lor, Antibiopto, Coly-Mycin S. Ilotycin, Garamycin, Genoptic, Aerosporin, Ak-Sulf, Gantrisin, Achromycin, and Tobrex.

Antifungal drugs are used to treat infections such as fungal KERATITIS and fungal ENDOPHTHALMITIS. Generic antifungal agents include amphotericin B, nystatin, flucytosine, natamycin, miconazole, and ketoconazole.

Antiviral drugs are used to treat infections such as HERPES SIMPLEX. Generic antiviral drugs include idoxuridine, trifluridine, vidarabine (ARA), and acyclovir; trade names for these drugs include Dendrid, Herplex Liquifilm, Stoxil, Viroptic, Vira-A, and Zovirax. Two antiviral drugs, ganciclovir and foscarnet, are used to treat cytomegalovirus retinitis, an infection of the retina associated with AIDS.

Antiprotozoal drugs are used to treat some types of UVEITIS. These drugs include Pyrimethamine, Sulfadiazine, Clindamycin, and corticosteroid preparations.

Anti-inflammatory drugs are used to treat inflammatory disorders such as BLEPHARITIS, CONJUNCTIVITIS, KERATITIS, SCLERITIS, uveitis, and optic neuritis. Corticosteroids are often prescribed under the generic names hydrocortisone, prednisolone, dexamethasone, and progesteronelike compounds. Trade names for these drugs include Hydrocortone acetate, Optef drops, Pred Mild/Pred Forte, Inflamase, Ak-Dex, Decadron, Maxidex, HMS, and FML.

Anesthetic drugs may be topical or regional. They allow the physician to perform procedures on the eye. Topical anesthesia includes the generic cocaine hydrochloride, proparacaine hydrochloride and tetracaine hydrochloride, and the trade names Ak-taine, Alcaine, Ophthaine, Ophthetic, Anacel, and Pontocaine. Regional anesthetics include Tetracaine, Procaine, Hexylcaine, Bupivacaine, Lidocaine, Mepivacaine, Prilocaine, and Etidocaine.

Drugs used to treat glaucoma include sympathomimetics and parasympathomimetics, which increase the flow of AQUEOUS FLUID from the eye; adrenergic antagonists and carbonic anhydrase inhibitors, which decrease the aqueous fluid supply; and hyperosmotic agents, which decrease intraocular pressure.

Adrenergic agents include the generic epinephrine bitartrate, epinephrine hydrochloride, epinephrine borate, dipivefrin hydrochloride, timolol maleate, levobunolol, and betaxolol. Trade names include E, Epitrate, Mytrate, Murocoll, Epifrin, Glaucon, Epinal, Eppy/N, Propine, Timoptic, Betagan, and Betoptic.

Carbonic anhydrase inhibitors include the generic acetazolamide, acetazolamide sodium, dichlorphenamide, and methazolamide, and trade names Ak-Zol, Cetazol, Diamox, Daranide, Oratrol, and Neptazane. Hyperosmotic agents include the generic glycerin, isosorbide, mannitol, and urea and the trade names Glyrol, Osmoglyn, Ismotic, Osmitrol, and Ureaphil.

Artificial tears are used to treat dry eye conditions. These drugs are known by the generic hydroxyethylcellulose, hydroxyproplycellulose, hydroxypropl methylcellulose, methylcellulose, polyvinyl alcohol, and other polymeric solutions. Numerous trade names include Clerz, Lacrisert, Isopto Alkaline, Muro Tears, Methopto, Methulose, Aqua Tears, Liquifilm Tears, aqua-FLOW, Refresh, Adapettes, Comfort Drops, and Hypotears.

Drugs are used in procedures to examine or test the eyes and diagnose disorders. Small strips of paper impregnated with fluorescein dye are used to test the CONJUNCTIVA and corneal epithelium. Sodium fluorescein is injected intravenously to study the circulation of blood in the RETINA and CHOROID.

Rose bengal is a solution used to test the conjunctiva and corneal epithelium for unhealthy cells.

Doctors and scientists are working hard to find new drugs to treat vision disorders, and new uses for existing drugs. One of these promising drugs is Visudyne, approved by the U.S. Food and Drug Administration in April 2000 and used in the treatment of the wet form of age-related macular degeneration. Representatives of the American Academy of Ophthalmology said they are hopeful that Visudyne will be the start of a new era in treating a leading cause of blindness among older people.

American Academy of Ophthalmology Medical Library. *American Academy of Ophthalmology Says Newly Approved Drug, Visudyne, Is Promising.* 2000.

Henkind, Paul, Martin Mayers and Arthur Berger, eds. *Physicians' Desk Reference for Ophthalmology 1987.* Oradell, N.J.: Medical Economics Company Inc., 1987.

dry eye　Dry eye is a condition in which the eye lacks the necessary amount or quality of tears. Tears protect, nourish, and moisturize the eye. Without proper tear function, the CORNEA and CONJUNCTIVA may become dry and develop disorders.

In the normal eye, the tear film is made up of three layers that are produced by the lacrimal gland and accessory lacrimal glands and cells. The lacrimal glands are located in the orbit and inner eyelid. The accessory glands and cells are located in the conjunctiva.

The top layer of tears is formed by the secretion of the meibomian glands and is oily in nature. The second layer is composed of watery tears from the lacrimal glands, and the third layer, which lies next to the cornea, is of mucuslike consistency and is produced by accessory glands. The layers are maintained by constant blinking and are all necessary for proper health of the eye.

Dry eye may occur as a result of poor tear production (called keratoconjunctivitis sicca), poor tear quality, or inadequate blinking, which leaves the eye open to the drying elements or does not properly wet the entire surface of the eye. Conditions that can cause dry eye include sarcoidosis, rheumatoid arthritis, vitamin A deficiency, pemphigoid, trachoma, Stevens-Johnson syndrome, chemical burns, neuroparalytic and exposure keratitis, and aging.

Dry eye may lead to corneal damage, permanent corneal scarring, and opacification. Once the cornea has opacified, vision is lost. Symptoms of dry eye include redness, discomfort or irritation, decreased corneal luster, and loss of visual acuity. Dry eyes can become extremely sensitive to wind, low humidity, heating, air conditioning, and so forth. Excess tearing may occur if the tears produced are inadequate in quality.

Dry eye is diagnosed through a thorough eye examination, including a slit-lamp examination, a Schirmer's test, and a tear film break-up test. The slit lamp is used to examine the tear film for the presence of extraneous microscopic filaments, epithelial cells, and corneal erosion that are apparent and will stain when exposed to rose bengal.

The Schirmer's test involves inserting one end of of a narrow strip of paper into the lower lid. The strip is left in place for five minutes during which time it absorbs tears. At the end of the time, the strip is removed and measured for the amount of tears present. Dry eye may be indicated if the measurement is less than 10 millimeters.

During the tear-film break-up test, the tear film is watched to determine the time needed to break the film once the blinking has stopped. The tears are stained with fluorescein dye and the eye is held open. In cases of dry eye, the tear film may break in less than 10 seconds.

Treatment of dry eye includes treating the underlying cause or disease and the administration of artificial tears. In some cases, antibiotics may be prescribed and the use of home vaporizers or humidifiers advised.

Surgery may be performed to close the tear drainage ducts to ensure better utilization of reduced tear production. If the cornea is severely scarred and vision is lost, a CORNEAL TRANSPLANT or keratoplasty may be indicated. However, those with dry-eye conditions are generally poor candidates for a successful corneal transplantation. Some medications that stimulate tear production are being investigated.

Duxbury Systems, Inc.   A company formed in 1975 to develop braille software for minicomputers. Two of Duxbury Systems's founders, Robert Gildea and Joseph Sullivan, were members of a team that in 1970 developed DOTSYS III, the first braille translator written in a portable programming language. DOTSYS III was developed for the Atlanta Public School system.

In 1975, Gildea, Sullivan, and their partner Anne Simpson developed the Duxbury Braille Translator, which was capable of translating braille in six languages.

Since 1975, Duxbury Systems has become a world leader in software for braille with Windows, Macintosh, DOS, and Unix programs. The Duxbury Braille Translator and MegaDots, a program developed by a company called Braille Planet, originally Raised Dot Computing, continue to be the company's flagship products.

Duxbury acquired the Madison, Wisconsin–based Braille Planet in August 1999. Raised Dot Computing, founded in 1981, produced software that enabled transcribers to produce braille books and create graphics using an Apple computer. It also provided on-line electronic Braille libraries and educational services, and produced and distributed materials relating to blindness issues.

Contact:

Duxbury Systems, Inc.
270 Littleton Road, Unit 6
Westford, MA 01886-3523
978-692-3000 (ph)
978-692-7912 (fax)
www.duxburysystems.com

early intervention A term used to describe programs and services offered to families of visually impaired children and preschools for visually impaired children. They provide information on home management and educational child-development skills and opportunities for children to develop skills and participate in socialization. The programs work closely with parents to maximize the potential for growth and development among these children. Services vary and may include home visitations, small group instruction, and community facilities programs.

The Individuals with Disabilities Education Act was signed into law in 1997. Formerly known as the Education of the Handicapped Act, the law mandates that services, such as early intervention programs, vision services, assistive technology and services, and transportation be provided for three- to five-year-old children with disabilities, including visual impairment.

The intent of the act is to provide appropriate public education to all eligible children. Schools must comply with the regulations of the act in order to receive certain funding.

echolocation See SENSES.

ectropion A disorder of the eyelids in which the lower lid turns outward. Ectropion is generally caused by aging but may result from scarring of the eyelids or nerve palsy. The exposure of the inner lid may cause tearing, irritation, and conjunctivitis.

Ectropion can be corrected with minor outpatient surgery using a local anesthetic. During the procedure, a portion of the sagging lid or scar tissue may be removed. Skin grafting may be required. Corrective surgery for ectropion may result in an over- or undercorrection of the problem. Complications may include bleeding, infection, or recurrence.

education Formal education of the visually impaired prior to the middle 1700s was a private matter, lacking in systematic programs or educational formats. Many who lacked educated advocates or resources were not educated at all.

The first school for blind children, the Institution des Jeunes Aveugles (Institute for Blind Youth), was established in 1784 in Paris by Valentin Hauy. The residential school presented a curriculum orally and through embossed print or enlarged raised letters, read tactually.

In 1824, Louis Braille, one of the school's students, developed the BRAILLE method of communication. Braille is a tactually read language involving a series of configurations of raised dots based on a six-dot cell. The braille method made writing possible and reading more accessible to those with vision impairments and revolutionized the ability of blind students to obtain an education.

In the early 1800s, the first three schools for the blind were founded in the United States. In 1829, the New England Asylum for the Blind, later renamed the Perkins School for the Blind, was incorporated and opened in 1832 under the direction of Samuel Gridley Howe. In 1831, the New York Institution for the Blind, later renamed the New York Institute for the Blind, opened under the direction of Dr. John Dennison Russ. The Pennsylvania Institution for the Instruction of the Blind, now named the Overbrook School for the Blind, was started by Quakers in 1833 under the directorship of Julius R. Friedlander.

The schools were residential, privately financed, and based on the programs offered by the Institute for Blind Youth in Paris. The first students were children of families who could afford to pay the tuition and boarding fees.

The first tuition-free, state-supported school was established in 1837 in Ohio. In the next 45 years, over 30 additional public and private residential schools were established and constituted the sole source of education for visually impaired students.

Most of the current residential schools were established before 1900, and there is now at least one in nearly all of the 50 states. Those states without schools for the blind or visually impaired pay the tuition for students to attend residential schools in other states.

In 1871 at a convention of the American Association of Instructors of the Blind (AAIB), Howe, of the Perkins School, described and advocated a cottage-family-based system of education adopted in 1911 by John Bledsoe at the Maryland School for the Blind.

In Chicago in 1900, in reaction to demands from parents of visually impaired students for education with nondisabled children, Frank H. Hall, superintendent of the Illinois School for the Blind, directed one of his teachers to conduct an integrated program. The teacher, John Curtis, instituted a plan in which the city was divided geographically into grids. One school in each grid taught visually impaired students who attended regular classes and received services from special teachers in typing and braille skills. The grid program was widely adopted throughout the United States in following years.

The education system was altered in the years between 1949 and 1966 by two epidemics, RETINO-PATHY OF PREMATURITY and RUBELLA. Retinopathy of prematurity (ROP), or retrolental fibroplasia (RLF), increased the population of visually impaired children by nearly 40 percent. The vision-destroying disorder was caused by overexposure to oxygen in incubation cradles. Low-weight, premature infants were primarily affected. Rubella epidemics in the mid-1960s caused disabilities to an additional 30,000 children, up to 20 percent of which included visual impairments. Both epidemics created a generation of students with special needs who outnumbered the facilities established to provide them.

The American Foundation for the Blind, the National Society for the Prevention of Blindness and other organizations sponsored conferences, service programs, scholarships for teacher training, and original educational objectives to meet future needs. As a result, day schools grew and expanded to serve over 80 percent of visually impaired students. Residential schools reevaluated their purposes and extended their programs to include multi-handicapped children.

Education of visually impaired children includes all the goals of general education for nondisabled children and encompasses teaching competencies skills to live, work, and play satisfactorily and successfully in society.

Special education is a supplement to general education that meets the needs and provides the skills necessary to achieve general educational goals for disabled students. It supplies adaptations or modifications to the general education curriculum, materials, learning methods, task skills, environmental factors, and teaching techniques.

Education of a visually impaired student is implemented by four major organizational bodies: the federal government, the state department of education, the local education agency, and organizations that serve the visually impaired.

The federal government, through the executive and judicial branches, enacts laws that shape and control education for all students in the United States. One such law, the Education of the Handicapped Act (EHA), also known as the Education of All Handicapped Children Act, ensures all disabled students, including those with visual impairments, the right to a free and appropriate elementary and secondary education in the least restrictive setting from ages six through 21. The law further ensures the right of parent participation in the educational and decision-making process, protects the rights of disabled students and their parents, and ensures the student of an individualized educational program.

The State Department of Education fulfills the requirements mandated by the laws and implements the EHA. A state consultant from the department acts as an advocate and facilitator for quality education for visually handicapped students. The consultant serves as a liaison to the public, the medical community, the U.S. Office of Education, teacher preparation schools, national organizations, and consumer groups.

The Local Education Agency (LEA), such as the school district or residential school, acts to provide the basic curriculum and special education according to the needs of the student. The teacher serves as the primary advocate for the visually impaired student within the school. The district or school program administrator is responsible to obtain services of a qualified teacher, to secure necessary resources to provide the needed services and to evaluate program effectiveness. The residential school in a state or district acts as an additional resource to all districts in the state.

Organizations that serve the visually impaired supply support services, resources, equipment, or materials to visually impaired students. They may supplement or enhance the program offered by the federal government. General or special education begins before the child formally enters school at age five or six. It begins at birth or as soon as possible after the visual handicap has been diagnosed.

Early intervention programs, services to families and preschools for blind and partially sighted children provide information on home management and educational child-development skills and opportunities for skills development and socialization. The programs maximize the potential for growth and development among these children.

Once a child has reached six years of age and is ready to enroll in kindergarten, he must be assured of a free and appropriate educational program. In order to ensure appropriateness, the school may request a formal student assessment to determine whether the student is eligible for special education services.

The assessment is conducted by a professional staff of educational, psychological, and medical experts. It must be complete, nondiscriminatory, and given with consent of the parent. Assessment may follow a regular periodic schedule of once a month to once a year and not less than once every three years.

Once the need for special education has been assessed and determined, an individualized educational plan (IEP) is developed. This written plan is a blueprint for the child's education. It lists the student's present level of educational performance, a statement of annual goals, a list of special educational services to be supplied, the dates the services will begin and end, and the evaluation which will be used to determine whether the goals were met.

The needs and goals stipulated in the IEP will determine the setting where the education will be delivered. The student may have a choice of either a residential setting or a public school.

Those who attend public school are sometimes referred to as "mainstreamed" students. *Mainstreaming* is a term used to describe the practice of educating disabled students, including those with visual impairments, in a standard, public classroom for nondisabled children. Today, although residential schools still provide vital education and training services, the American Foundation for the Blind estimates that nearly 90 percent of disabled students receive all or part of their education in local public schools.

Students may be mainstreamed into a public school program through several models of delivery including the itinerant-teacher model, the teacher-consultant model and the resource-room model. These are three of five basic models or educational plans for the education of visually impaired students that also include the self-contained classroom model and the residential school model.

An itinerant teacher is one who travels to public schools to provide special education modifications to the instructional program of visually impaired children. The visually impaired student lives at home and spends most of the instructional day in a regular classroom.

The itinerant teacher visits every two or three days to work with the student in a section of the classroom, the library, the hall, the office, or any available space. The itinerant teacher provides special equipment, training, and materials adapted to the student's learning needs and consultation services to the regular classroom teacher.

A 1976 study by Moore and Peabody found that itinerant teachers spend just over half their time, 59 percent, working directly with students, while spending the remaining 41 percent of their time driving, in consultation relating to the student, and in administrative duties.

The success of the itinerant-teacher program is dependent on the regular classroom teacher's attitude and willingness to adapt regular teaching practices to the mainstreamed visually impaired child. The model is most effective for students who are self-directed and independent in learning skills and least effective for students who lack academic learning skills and lag in social development in comparison with their peers.

The teacher-consultant is a special educator who advises regular classroom teachers, teacher aides, administrators, and other school personnel in methods that will meet the visually impaired student's needs. The greatest proportion of the work is consultative, rather than instructive.

The teacher-consultant travels from school to school, and often from county to county, to work with personnel. Since traveling time is significant, little time remains for direct instruction with the student.

The teacher-consultant model works best for students who work independently and require minimal skills training. The program is least effective for students who require intensive skills training or lack coping behaviors for study in a regular classroom.

The resource room is a specially equipped room staffed with special education personnel trained to work with blind or visually impaired students. The students live at home and attend public school in regular classrooms and are taught by teachers who provide general curriculum instruction. Students visit the resource room at regularly scheduled intervals or when needed. The resource-room teacher provides specialized skills instruction and counseling relating to vision loss and academic remediation. Special instruction may take place individually or in small groups.

The resource-room model has an advantage over the teacher-consultant and itinerant-teacher models in that it provides instruction or assistance immediately and according to the needs of the student. However, because of its availability, it may foster dependence and restrict growth toward independent working within a self-contained classroom.

The self-contained classroom is a classroom in a public school that is specially equipped and staffed with special-education teachers for the visually impaired. All the students in the class have visual impairments or other disabilities. The teacher of the class provides general curriculum instruction and special education. The program is designed to fit the unique needs of each individual.

Although one-fifth of all programs for visually impaired students centered on self-contained classrooms in the early 1960s, the model has since lost popularity except in large metropolitan areas serving multihandicapped blind students.

In order to achieve maximum enrollment, self-contained classrooms are centered in one or a few schools within a district. This often necessitates busing the visually impaired student to a school outside his neighborhood.

Residential schools are those in which visually impaired students live and receive educational instruction. It is the oldest form of education for the visually impaired and is offered in nearly every state. Many residential schools for the visually impaired share a campus or facilities with schools for the deaf and are referred to as "dual" schools. Residential schools may be either state operated or private. State operated residential schools are funded by state legislatures, are tuition free, and do not charge for room, board, or transportation. Private residential schools charge fees that may be paid by the public school district of the student.

The campus, schoolrooms, and educational program of residential schools are designed and equipped to meet the needs of visually impaired students. The educational materials and curriculum can be designed, or the students may be grouped, to meet each individual's instructional requirements. Trained staff, including houseparents, are on duty 24 hours a day to provide general curriculum instruction, academic remediation, compensatory learning-skills instruction, personal management and independence-skills training, and information counseling concerning blindness.

The residential-school model is superior to many other models in its attempts to meet all levels of student educational needs on an immediate basis. However, because students may return home only on a weekly or monthly basis, some students may suffer from a lack of familial contact or interaction with sighted peers.

The basic curriculum for the visually impaired student is identical to that of the nondisabled student. However, special education may include instruction or counseling in the areas of social-emotional development, living skills, orientation and mobility, communication, and vocational counseling:

- *Social-emotional development* skills work to improve self-adjustment to vision impairment and improve social skills. These may include family counseling, sex education, and preparation for marriage and family life.

- *Daily living skills* center on grooming, hygiene, eating, dressing, and home management skills. These skills may include basic safety measures and skills for using the telephone and identifying money.

- *Orientation and mobility skills* are those that concern orienting the body and moving within the environment. Students are taught the sighted guide technique, cane traveling methods, and other mobility skills. Physical and recreational skills may be taught to ensure participation in physical education courses and recreational activities.

- *Communication skills* include those needed for learning and for interpersonal interaction. Students learn reading, listening, writing, and speaking skills that may include reading and writing braille or use of low-vision aids.

- *Interpersonal communication skills* center on conversation, interviewing, small-group communication, and appropriate language and listening skills. Nonverbal communication skills are introduced that cover facial expressions, touching and body language, personal space, and distracting or unattractive behaviors such as rocking.

- *Vocational counseling* and prevocational counseling presents types of vocations and careers possible for the individual. Prerequisite skills are analyzed and introduced at appropriate stages.

Barraga, Natalie C. *Visual Handicaps and Learning.* Belmont, CA: Wadsworth Publishing Company Inc., 1976.

ERIC Clearinghouse on Handicapped and Gifted Children. *Research and Resources on Special Education: Abstract 13.* Reston, VA: ERIC, 1987.

ERIC Clearinghouse on Handicapped and Gifted Children. *Research and Resources on Special Education: Abstract 14.* Reston, VA: ERIC, 1987.

ERIC Clearinghouse on Handicapped and Gifted Children. *Research and Resources on Special Education: Abstract 19.* Reston, VA: ERIC, 1988.

Mitchell, Joyce Slayton. *See Me More Clearly.* New York: Harcourt, Brace, Jovanovich, 1980.

Scholl, Geraldine, ed. *Foundations of Education for Blind and Visually Handicapped Children and Youth.* New York: American Foundation for the Blind Inc., 1986.

Scott, Eileen P. *Your Visually Impaired Student.* Baltimore: University Park Press, 1982.

Education of the Handicapped Act (EHA) See INDIVIDUALS WITH DISABILITIES EDUCATION ACT.

electronic travel aids (ETA) Visually impaired persons receiving orientation and mobility training may be instructed in the use of electronic travel aids (ETA). These aids are prescribed by an optometrist or ophthalmologist and include canes, hand-held devices, chest-mounted devices, head-mounted, spectacles or control boxes, and devices designed to be mounted on wheelchairs. They require specialized training to use.

Electronic travel aids send out light beams or ultrasonic waves that come into contact with objects in the path. When the beam or waves hit an object, the device responds by vibrating or emitting a sound. The newest ETAs use radio frequency triangulation via timing signals from the worldwide global positioning system, coupled with a digital map database and digital compass.

Electronic travel devices are used by approximately 1 percent of all visually impaired persons and are usually not designed to be used with a dog guide. (See ORIENTATION AIDS.) A listing and description of available ETAs can be found on the Internet at www.noogenesis.com/eta/current/html.

electroretinography (ERG) The study of the function of the RETINA when stimulated by light. An electroretinogram is a test often performed to diagnose RETINITIS PIGMENTOSA and other eye diseases.

Retinitis pigmentosa (RP) is a group of progressive, hereditary diseases that cause retinal dystrophy or degeneration. First the rods, and then the cones, of the retina stop functioning. Early symptoms include night blindness and progressive loss of peripheral vision.

The electroretinogram may be necessary to confirm the diagnosis of RP. The test measures the electrical activity of the retina when exposed to light stimulus. Each eye is tested separately. One eye is first patched to exclude all light. Next, drops are administered to dilate the pupil of the other eye. Anesthetic drops are administered and a contact lens attached to electrodes is placed on the cornea of the eye. The chin is placed on a chin rest, and the patient looks into the test machine. Lights that stimulate the retina are flashed into the eye in both dark and light environmental conditions. The electrodes on the contact lens record the responses of the retina and produce a graph that is interpreted by the ophthalmologist.

employment   The American Foundation for the Blind estimates that there are approximately 4 million working-age, adult Americans who report some type of vision loss that cannot be corrected. Fewer than 50 percent of visually impaired adults are successfully employed. And of those who are employed, one-third feels that they are underemployed and have a monthly pay that is 37 percent less than that of nondisabled workers. Blind and visually impaired people have the highest unemployment rate of any social or economic group in the country. This disparity of unemployment rates between disabled and nondisabled persons may be due to prejudice and misunderstandings concerning the abilities of disabled workers. Disabled workers may be perceived by management as high in absenteeism, difficult to supervise, and a safety risk; however, studies show that this is not true.

This is primarily due to misconceptions and lack of understanding concerning the blind and visually impaired among employers. Efforts are underway to make employers aware of facts such as the following:

- A national poll by Louis Harris & Associates showed that half the employees who hire disabled workers believe those workers have fewer accidents on the job than their non-disabled peers. An additional 25 percent of the employers said there was no difference in safety between the two groups.

- Employer's group health insurance rates do not increase when a visually impaired person is hired. Nor do worker compensation rates increase.

- The Harris poll revealed that 39 percent of employees felt their employees with disabilities were more dependable than their employees without disabilities. Another 42 percent said there was no difference between the two groups.

- Equipment necessary for visually impaired people to do their jobs normally is comparable in cost to that used by workers with normal vision. If special equipment is needed, a state rehabilitation agency will offset the costs.

Because of inequities in the public labor market, some visually impaired employees may work in a protected or sheltered workshop or business enterprise. A sheltered workshop is any protected employment. Many are highly industrialized, produce a variety of goods and pay competitive wages. Sheltered workshops sell the goods to governmental agencies, including the military, through programs outlined and enforced by the Javits-Wagner-O'Day Act.

A business in the Business Enterprise Program (BEP) consists of a vending stand or short order, cafeteria-style stand. These businesses are given a priority for placement in federal buildings and are administered by the State Vocational Rehabilitation Agency under the Randolph-Sheppard Act.

With the advent of new technology that adapts job tasks to the needs of those with limited sight, and in response to recent legislation, visually impaired employees are increasingly seeking work in the competitive marketplace. As stated in federal law, discrimination in hiring due to disability is prohibited in companies that receive federal funds.

While federal agencies and agencies that receive government funds are prohibited by law from discriminating against disabled people in employment, private businesses are encouraged to consider hiring disabled workers, including those with vision disorders.

The American Foundation for the Blind recommends that employers interested in hiring visually impaired workers take the following steps to locate such employees and make the work environment conducive for their success:

- Perform reasonable accommodations to the work place. These may include making changes in the lighting, using e-mail or voice-mail messages among employees instead of written notes and memos, and acquiring software programs that convert the print on a computer screen to large print, Braille, or speech.

- Do not assume that a visually impaired worker cannot do what other workers can. For instance, if a particular job entails travel, do not assume that a visually impaired employee would not be able to handle that position. Canes, guide dogs, and electronic travel aids make travel possible for blind and visually impaired employees.

- Make the job application process accessible to blind and visually impaired potential employees. You can do this by posting the job on your company's Internet site, as well as in a newspaper classified ad. If the application must be completed on site, have someone record or transcribe the visually impaired worker's responses to the questions.

- Focus on the blind person's ability to fulfill the available position, and reflect that focus during the interview process. Do not worry about a visually impaired person being able to locate the rest room or operate the microwave oven in the lunchroom.

There are three federal tax credits available to help employers cover the cost of special equipment necessary for a handicapped worker, or to making the workplace accessible to a handicapped worker. The tax credits for which you may qualify are: the Work Opportunity Tax Credit, the Small Business Tax Credit, and the Architectural/Transportation Tax Deduction. More information about these tax credits is available by contacting the Internal Revenue Service.

If an employee becomes visually impaired or blind while already employed by a company, he or she should be permitted to consult with vocational rehabilitation resources to determine methods and devices that will allow the employee to continue in the same job.

If that is determined to be impossible, the employee and company should work with the rehabilitation resources to locate another job within the company that relates to previous work, requires equal skill, and is of equal status, without resorting to stereotyping. Stereotyping involves placing a visually impaired employee into one type of job that has proven successful for other disabled workers, regardless of the employee's skills, training, and background.

Experts agree that employment of disabled workers benefits all parties involved. Disabled workers who are given the opportunity for employment are able to be self-sufficient and do not have to rely on federal assistance. Businesses benefit by gaining efficient workers and getting a tax credit, and society benefits by the state and federal income taxes contributed by the employee.

Blind prospective employees can get help from the National Federation of the Blind, which operates a program called Job Opportunities for the Blind (JOB) Targeted Jobs Initiative. The program is run in conjunction with major national employers to provide pathways for blind people to find jobs with good salaries and benefits.

Other agencies, such as the Lighthouse for the Blind and the National Industries for the Blind, also provide training programs designed to help blind people find and succeed at employment. (See REHABILITATION ACT, VOCATIONAL REHABILITATION.)

American Foundation for the Blind. *Employment: An Introduction.* www.afb.org/info_document_view, 2001.
National Federation of the Blind. *Job Opportunities for the Blind: Targeted Jobs Initiative.* www.nfb.org/states/newjob.htm, 2000.

employment disincentives Disincentives to employment exist within the disabled community as a result of the structure of federal benefits systems. Many disabled American workers receive federal benefits from the Social Security Disability Insurance (SSDI) program and, of them, a majority do not rejoin the workforce for fear of penalties associated with self-sufficiency.

Reforms, however, are under way to encourage disabled workers to rejoin the workforce. In 1986, revisions to the SSDI program allowed the recipients of SSI benefits to work and continue to receive limited benefits. In 1989, the Social Security Work Incentive Act was instituted, which provided greater opportunities for disabled people to work and still receive some benefits.

In December 1999, the Ticket-to-Work and Self-Sufficiency Program was established with the aim of providing SSI recipients more choices of employment services. The program calls for SSI beneficiaries to receive tickets, which they can then use to obtain vocational rehabilitation services, employment services, or other support necessary to find and keep a job.

The Ticket-to-Work program is being phased in over a three-year period. The first states in which disabled workers received tickets are: Arizona, Colorado, Delaware, Florida, Illinois, Iowa, Massachusetts, New York, Oklahoma, Oregon, South Carolina, Vermont, and Wisconsin.

More information about the Ticket-to-Work program is available from Maximus, Inc., a private firm that has been contracted by the Social Security Administration to serve as the program manager.

Contact:

Maximus, Inc.
866-968-7842 (toll free)
866-833-2967 (TTY) (toll free)

Johnson, Kurt L. *Incentives and Disincentives in the Vocational Rehabilitation Process.* Washington, D.C.: National Rehabilitation Information Center, 1983.
National Institute of Handicapped Research. *Rehab Brief: Work Disincentives.* Washington, D.C.: NIHR, 1980.
Roth, Wendy Carol. "Let Us Work!" *Parade Magazine,* 17 September 1989, pp. 16.
Social Security Administration, Office of Employment Support Programs. *The Work Site,* www.ssa.gov/work/index2.html, 2001.

Enabling Technologies Company Enabling Technologies Company manufactures adaptive equipment for the blind and visually impaired. It was founded in 1969 by three recent college graduates.

The company offers a variety of equipment, including braille printers, embossing, devices, sign makers, and Braille translation software. An online catalogue is available, or one can be ordered by calling the company.

Contact:

Enabling Technologies Company
1601 NE Braille Place
Jensen Beach, FL 34957
800-777-3687 (ph)
561-225-3299 (fax)
www.brailler.com

Employment Assistance Referral Network (EARN) A national toll-free telephone and electronic information referral service created in 2001 by the U.S. Department of Labor. The service matches up employers seeking to hire workers with disabilities with qualified employees. It takes into account employee qualifications, job requirements, and geographic area.

EARN also offers assistance to employers in areas such as tax credits, disability laws, personal-assistance devices, interviewing potential employees, and recruitment and hiring strategies. Interested employers can call EARN Monday through Friday between 9 A.M. and 9 P.M. Eastern Standard Time.

Contact:

Employee Assistance Referral Network
888-695-8289 (ph)
703-820-4820 (fax)
projectear@birchdavis.com
www.earnworks.com

endophthalmitis A condition in which inflammation in the posterior chamber of the eye extends into the center of the globe. This is often the result of severe posterior UVEITIS (inflammation of the CHOROID), which involves the RETINA and VITREOUS.

Severe posterior uveitis may be caused by infections such as TOXOPLASMOSIS and TOXOCARIASIS or by infections following injuries or surgery. Infections such as toxoplasmosis and toxocariasis may be treated with steroids, and those that result from injuries or surgery may be treated with antibiotics. Surgery may be necessary to completely remove the infection.

Once the infection and inflammation spread to the anterior section of the eye, the condition is termed PANOPHTHALMITIS. This condition usually results in the permanent loss of vision, and possibly to removal of the eye.

endothelial cell count An endothelial cell count is a measurement of the number of endothelial cells remaining in the CORNEA. An endothelial cell count is often performed prior to CATARACT surgery to determine the health of the cornea.

Endothelial cells line the inside of the cornea and protect it from the AQUEOUS FLUID of the eye. Loss of endothelial cells through aging or cataract surgery could cause a clouded cornea. The cornea requires enough endothelial cells prior to surgery to allow for cell loss during the procedure.

A presurgical cornea requires approximately 1,000 endothelial cells to function properly after surgery. The cells are counted by an endothelial cell camera, which is similar to a slit lamp or biomicroscope. The test is painless and accurate.

A low endothelial cell count may require surgical techniques to minimize cell loss. In addition, it may prohibit the possibility of an intraocular LENS implantation, a procedure that causes some cell loss.

endothelium The protective inner lining of the CORNEA. It is made up of a single layer of endothelial cells. The cells prevent the AQUEOUS FLUID of the anterior chamber from penetrating the cornea. A reduction of endothelial cells could allow seepage into the cornea resulting in swelling, loss of transparency and loss of vision. Endothelial cells are lost through the natural process of aging and through CATARACT surgery procedures. The cells are generally not regenerated by the eye.

The cornea requires a minimum of approximately 1,000 endothelial cells to maintain adequate vision. The cells can be accurately counted by an endothelial cell camera during an ENDOTHELIAL CELL COUNT. (See FUCH'S ENDOTHELIAL DYSTROPHY.)

Energy Conservation and Production Act The Energy Conservation and Production Act of 1976 established a program to assist in insulating and weatherizing the homes of low income, elderly, and disabled individuals, including those with blindness.

The act provided up to $400 per home and stipulated the use of public-service employees and volunteers and trainees under Comprehensive Employment and Training Act to install the insulation materials. The amount was later increased to cover material and labor costs, program support and administration costs. In the fiscal year 2001, $15.3 million in federal funds were allocated for this program.

U.S. Department of Education. *Summary of Existing Legislation Affecting Persons with Disabilities.* Washington, D.C.: USDE, 1988.

US Department of Energy, Weatherization Assistance Program News Release www.eren.doe.gov/buildings/weatherization, 2001.

enophthalmos An inward displacement of the eye within the orbit. The condition appears as sunken or deep-seated eyeballs. The opposite condition is exophthalmos or proptosis (bulging eyes).

Enophthalmos may be unilateral or bilateral. It may be caused by injuries, tumors, or aging. Injuries may cause orbital fractures that result in enophthalmos. Aging may cause enophthalmos as fatty tissue within the orbit is absorbed and fails to support the eyeball at the former level. In cases that involve continuous DIPLOPIA (double vision) and cosmetic deformity, surgery may be required.

Tumors that cause enophthalmos are usually metastatic, or malignant tumors that originate in other places in the body but spread to the orbit through the blood stream. Metastatic scirrhous carcinomas are a common cause of enophthalmos. These fibrous tumors often originate from breast carcinoma in women and bronchogenic carcinoma in men. Such tumors may be treated with radiation or chemotherapy.

Degrees of enophthalmos may be measured with an exophthalmometer. As the instrument is held up to the eyes, mirrors on the device superimpose a millimeter scale over a side view of the eye. This enables the examiner to measure the distance from the lateral orbital rims to the corneal apices.

Measurement differences between the eyes are often given most importance since general measurements of exophthalmos vary greatly due to individual anatomy. A variance of 2 millimeters between the eyes is considered serious and worthy of further investigation.

entropion A disorder of the eyelid in which the lid turns inward. The lashes of the lid scrape against the CORNEA and irritate it. The condition is generally associated with aging but may occur as the result of an injury, burn, conjunctival scarring, or TRACHOMA.

Entropion usually affects only the lower lid and is most common in those over 50. The disorder may be seen in newborns, but this condition often rectifies itself without treatment during the first few months of infancy. Entropion can be temporary or chronic. In temporary cases, it usually begins in response to something else, such as itchy eyes due to an allergy. The sufferer blinks hard to get rid of whatever is causing the irritation, causing it to become worse.

The condition sometimes respond to a treatment as simple as a piece of adhesive tape placed on the skin of the lower eyelid to prevent it from turning in. Eyelid surgery is performed to correct entropion. The surgery may be performed on an outpatient basis with a local anesthetic. The procedure may involve the removal of sections of the lid or excision of scar tissue with accompanying skin grafts. A TARSORRHAPHY, the placement of stitches to keep the lid in a permanent position, may be performed to hold the lid in an outward position.

enucleation Enucleation is the surgical removal of the eyeball. Enucleation is performed when the eye contains a malignant tumor such as a melanoma, when the eye is blind and causes pain, and when the eye is nearly blind and sympathetic ophthalmia (an inflammation that occurs in both eyes as a result of injury to one eye) is a risk.

Enucleation is performed under general anesthetic. An incision is made in the limbus, the place where the SCLERA meets the CORNEA, and the CONJUNCTIVA is opened. The eye is severed and removed from the optic nerve and the six extrinsic muscles that hold it in place. The vessels are cauterized to stop internal bleeding. The membrane and muscles are tied together and the conjunctiva is stitched closed.

After a period of two or more days, the conjunctiva-lined socket of the eye is fitted with a plastic shell in preparation for an artificial eye or prosthesis. The prosthetic eye is fitted three to four weeks later. A prosthetic eye is generally undetectable from a natural eye.

esophoria A condition of STRABISMUS, or misaligned eyes. Often termed squint or crossed-eyes, strabismus may cause visual problems or loss of vision. Esophoria is a type of convergent strabismus in which the eyes tend to turn toward each other. *Esotropia* is a condition in which one eye turns inward.

As in all strabismus, the eyes view two differing subjects. The brain received the two images and double vision results. Often, in an effort to reconcile the two pictures, the brain may suppress the message received from one eye, reducing the vision of that eye. This results in a condition called amblyopia.

Strabismus is associated with high amounts of myopia (nearsightedness), hyperopia (farsightedness), and ASTIGMATISM. It can develop after a major illness or injury, and some forms of strabismus may also be hereditary.

Treatment may include the prescription of eyedrops, eyeglasses or bifocals, or exercises. Exercises or eye patching may be prescribed if amblyopia is present. Surgery may be necessary to completely align the eyes.

esotropia See ESOPHORIA.

etiquette Courtesy when dealing with visually impaired persons differs little from that involving fully sighted persons. Common sense and sensitivity should be the most important factors in deciding what to do.

Many visually impaired persons, even those who are legally blind, retain some usable vision. Because of this, a visually impaired person may appear to be sighted, especially in familiar sur-roundings. Do not assume that the visually impaired person is totally without sight, and do not assume that because he moves with accuracy and grace that he has abundant vision.

When approaching a visually impaired person or on entering a room, identify yourself to him. If others are present, use his name when talking to him. Unless the visually impaired person has a hearing impairment as well, talk in a normal tone and volume level. Do not avoid using visual words or phrases such as "Do you see what I mean?" or "Look at it this way." Avoid conversations that dwell only on blindness. Keep the conversation as varied as the individual.

When walking with a visually impaired person, do not pull, push, or take his arm. Let him take your arm or elbow, then walk naturally. He will fol-low the motion of your body. Alert him to obstacles in the path or overhead.

When living or working with a visually impaired person, replace furniture and objects to the original resting place. Return doors to their original posi-tion, either fully shut or open. Keep pathways clear and alert him to any changes or additions to the furniture arrangement. When entering new sur-roundings, place his hand on the back of the chair where he is to sit. Familiarize him with the envi-ronment.

In a restaurant, allow the visually impaired per-son to order his own meal. If the visually impaired person reads braille, request a braille menu. If not, offer to read the menu items and prices to him. Tell him the positions of the food on his plate and offer to cut his meat, if applicable. If he is to pay for the meal, guide him to the cashier, but allow him to pay and receive his change.

When taking an order or purchase from a visu-ally impaired person, speak directly to him. Do not communicate through a third party. When return-ing change from a purchase, count the money back to the visually impaired person and identify the denomination of the bills. If necessary, allow time for the customer to fold each denomination of the bills before moving on to the coins.

If you hand more than one item at a time to a visually impaired person, tell him what they are, in the order in which they are placed or stacked.

Do not assume that all blind and visually impaired people use braille. Many do, but others do not.

If a visually impaired person appears in need of help, speak directly to him and ask if he wants assistance. When giving directions, be concise. Tell the number of blocks and turns, right or left, according to the direction he is facing. Do not inter-rupt when someone else is giving him directions.

Do not stop to pet or talk to a working dog guide. The dog needs to concentrate on the job and should not be distracted.

When you take leave of a visually impaired per-son or leave a room, tell him you are leaving. If indoors, ask if you should turn out the lights. If outdoors, let him know whether he is at the curb or near the stairs.

In all situations, keep in mind that the visually impaired person is a unique individual who just happens to have a loss of sight.

American Foundation for the Blind. *What Do You Do When You See a Blind Person?* New York: AFB, 1970.

Braille Institute. *How to Help a Blind Person.* Los Angeles: BI, 1980.

Helen Keller National Center for Deaf-Blind Youths and Adults. *Guidelines for Helping Deaf-Blind Persons.* Sands Point, N.Y.: HKNC, 1988.

National Federation of the Blind. *Do You Know a Blind Per-son?* New York: NFB, 1988.

National Federation of the Blind. *What is the National Fed-eration of the Blind?* New York: NFB, 1988.

San Francisco Lighthouse for the Blind. *At Ease.* San Francisco: SFLB, 1982.

Eustis, Dorothy Dorothy Eustis, born Dorothy Leib Harrison in 1886, founded the first dog-guide training school in the United States. The daughter of a prosperous owner of a sugar refinery, she was educated in Philadelphia and Eastbourne, England. In 1906, she married Walter Abbott Wood Jr., who died in 1915.

In 1923, she married George Eustis and moved to Switzerland to establish a breeding and training kennel to improve the working qualities of the German shepherd breed. She was joined in her work in 1924 by Elliot S. ("Jack") Humphrey, an authority on breeding and genetics.

Dog-guide schools had been established in Ger-many in answer to the need for German shepherd guides for blinded World War I veterans. Eustis became interested in dog-guide training and wrote an article about it for a 1927 edition of the *Saturday Evening Post*.

The article elicited interest in the project, and in 1929 Eustis returned to the United States to found the Seeing Eye, a dog-guide training facility in Nashville, Tennessee. At the time, attitudes in the United States were generally negative toward dog guides but changed toward acceptance as news spread of successful use of the dogs. Today, Seeing Eye Inc. is located in Morristown, New Jersey.

Everest Expedition   An event held in 2001 to promote the attempt of blind mountaineer Erik Weihenmayer to reach the top of Mount Everest, the highest spot on Earth. Sponsored by the National Federation of the Blind, the NFB 2001 Everest Expedition is intended to let the public know that blind people can overcome limits, and should never be considered helpless or dependent. The expedition began in March and the team of climbers reached the summit of Mount Everest on May 25.

exophoria   Exophoria is a condition of STRABISMUS, or misaligned eyes. Often termed squint or crossed-eyes, strabismus may cause visual problems or loss of vision. Exophoria is a type of latent strabismus in which the eyes tend to turn outward, away from each other. Exophoria occurs when binocular vision is lost due to patching of one eye or when the individual is tired. *Exotropia* is condition in which either eye turns outward constantly.

As in all strabismus, the eyes may fail to converge on an object and view two differing subjects. The brain receives the two images, and double vision results. Often, in an effort to reconcile the two pictures, the brain may suppress one completely. This negation may result in a condition called AMBLYOPIA.

Strabismus can be associated with high amounts of myopia (nearsightedness) hyperopia (farsightedness), and ASTIGMATISM. It can develop after a major illness or injury, and some forms of strabismus may also be hereditary.

Treatment may include the prescription of eyedrops, eyeglasses or bifocals, or exercises. Exercises or eye patching may be prescribed if amblyopia is present. Surgery may be necessary to completely align the eyes.

exophthalmos   Exophthalmos, or proptosis, refers to a protruding forward of the eyeballs. The condition is usually accompanied by a retraction of the eyelids and infrequent blinking. The condition may be unilateral, involving only one eye, or bilateral, affecting both eyes. Unilateral exophthalmos may be the result of muscle palsy, a vascular condition, tumors, cysts, edema, or trauma and its accompanying hemorrhage and infection.

Bilateral exophthalmos is usually caused by hyperthyroidism, or Graves's disease. This disease is a disorder of the autoimmune system. It causes the thyroid to overproduce hormones that overstimulate the body's metabolism. Over half of those who develop Graves's disease develop Graves's ophthalmopathy, a condition in which the tissues and muscles of the eye are affected.

Pseudoproptosis (the false appearance of exophthalmos) occurs when the other eye has become sunken due to a fracture or trauma. The normal eye appears to bulge forward in comparison. An overly large eye, as in the case of unilateral high MYOPIA (near-sightedness) may also appear to be exophthalmic.

The amount of exophthalmos can be measured with an exophthalmometer. This instrument determines the degree of protrusion and symmetry between both eyes. Readings beyond the normal range of 12–20 millimeters may indicate exophthalmos.

Other tests may determine the underlying cause. X rays may illuminate a tumor, fracture, or erosion within the orbit. A CAT scan or biopsy may detect a pathology within the eye or orbit, and a culture of any discharge may identify an infection.

Treatment of exophthalmos must include therapy for the underlying cause. This may include antibiotics, steroids, radiation, chemotherapy, radiation iodine treatments, or surgery such as TARSORRHAPHY, a stitching of the eyelid, or removal of the mass causing the proptosis.

exotropia   See EXOPHORIA.

extracapsular extraction   See CATARACT.

eye   The eye is one of the most complex, specialized organs in the body. It is responsible for up to 80 percent of the awareness information we process. The eye can distinguish images, determine distance and depth of those images, and detect their shape, tone, and color. Amazingly, the light-dependent eye can do its job in a brightness range fluctuating from candlelight to brightest sunlight.

Structure

The eye is a globe measuring about one inch long. Its structure has many parts. The front of the eye is a transparent tissue called the CORNEA. The cornea bends and focuses entering light rays. Surrounding the cornea is the SCLERA, the tough, protective, white portion of the eye. The CONJUNCTIVA, a thin layer of membrane, covers the sclera. The cornea and sclera work together to shield the eye much as a watch crystal and case protects a watch.

Just behind the cornea is the ANTERIOR CHAMBER, a space filled with the AQUEOUS FLUID, a clear liquid. The aqueous fluid brings nutrients to the cornea and LENS, and carries away waste.

The IRIS is a thin circle of membrane suspended just behind the anterior chamber and in direct line to the cornea. The iris is the part that gives the eye its color. The hue depends on the amount of pigment contained in the iris. Brown eyes contain the most pigment, blue the least.

In the center of the iris is the PUPIL, a tiny hole through which light passes into the eye. The pupil changes size to accommodate different light extremes. In bright sunlight, it closes down to screen out excess light, in low light it opens up to allow the maximum amount to enter into the eye. The pupil is black because the inside of the eye showing through it is dark. Any change in pupil color is an indication of disorder within the inside of the eye.

The iris and pupil are positioned in front of the POSTERIOR CHAMBER, which, like the anterior chamber, is filled with aqueous. Behind the posterior chamber is the CRYSTALLINE LENS, a transparent, soft

body that focuses the light that enters the eye through the pupil. The lens is held in place by thousands of fibers called ZONULES. These fibers are attached to the ciliary muscle and work with the muscle to help the lens to change shape.

The lens changes shape to correctly focus the light of images at varying distances. To focus on a near object, the lens must bulge forward. To do this, the ciliary muscle contracts, giving the fibers more slack and allowing the lens to bulge into the needed focusing shape. To focus on a distant object, the muscle expands, pulling the fibers taut and flattening the lens.

The large area behind the lens is filled with a clear, gel-like matter called VITREOUS. The vitreous gives the eye its form and substance.

The RETINA, the inner layer of the back of the eye behind the vitreous, contains over 125 million light-sensitive cells that give the retina information about the image. Among these cells are the RODS AND CONES.

The more numerous (by a margin of five to one) rod-shaped cells react to faint light, darkness, shape, and movement. They are located throughout the retina and are responsible for peripheral vision. The cones distinguish color and detail but require high levels of light to be effective. The cones are concentrated into an area called the MACULA.

The macula is in the central section of the retina. It is responsible for straight-ahead or central vision. It is a highly sensitive area of the retina packed with cones. The macula has a small hollow, called the FOVEA, in which the greatest numbers of cones reside. Light is focused directly on the fovea, making it the site of greatest visual acuity.

The CHOROID is a dark tissue layer between the retina and the sclera. Blood circulates through the choroid to nourish the eye. The choroid is a part of the UVEA, the pigmented structures of the eye that also include the iris and the ciliary body. The uvea is a vascularized, pigmented tissue layer that supplies blood to the eye.

The OPTIC NERVE is a cord made up of a collection of nerve cells and fibers. The optic nerve connects each eye to the brain and supplies blood to the retina. The blood enters at the back of the eye and is diverted through vessels over the complete surface of the retina. The blood vessels in the retina are easily viewed through an ophthalmoscope and are the only vessels in the body that can be examined in their natural, unhampered state.

The place where the nerve fibers exit to the retina is called the OPTIC DISC. Since the optic nerve contains no light-sensitive cells, it is blind and renders the optic disc blind as well. This is responsible for the eye's blind spot in the field of vision.

The eyes are protectively placed within the bony depressions of the skull called ORBITS. Each eye is held in place and moved by six extrinsic muscles. Eyelids keep foreign matter out of the eye, close to protect the eye from unwanted light, and blink to encourage tear production. The tears are necessary to maintain a layer of moisture over the cornea.

How the Eye Works

The eye requires light to see. Light falling on an object is reflected to the eye. It passes through the cornea where it is bent and focused to approximately 60 percent of what is needed. The light then enters the lens through the pupil. The lens bends the light the additional 40 percent and focuses a sharp image onto the retina.

The retina transforms the light messages received by the eye into electronic impulses that it sends through the optic nerve to the brain. Since the retinas of each eye receive slightly different images, the impulses sent to the brain vary somewhat. The brain translates and matches the impulses received into a single image, creating a sense of depth.

eye bank   Eye banks are organizations that acquire, evaluate, and distribute eyes from eye donors. The eyes are used for CORNEAL TRANSPLANTS, medical research, and educational purposes.

Donated eyes are necessary for corneal transplantation, or keratoplasty. According to the Eye Bank Association of America, more than 46,000 corneas were replaced by transplants in 2000, 90 percent of which successfully restored vision.

The CORNEA is the clear, curved portion of the eye over the colored IRIS. The cornea bends or refracts light to focus vision. When the cornea becomes clouded or damaged due to injury or disease, vision is decreased. Cornea transplantation replaces the damaged cornea with a healthy one to restore sight.

Eyes are donated anonymously from people who die. Donors may make their intention to donate their eyes known before death by a donor card or the section about organ donation on some state driver's licenses. The Uniform Anatomical Gift Act allows relatives of the deceased to donate the eyes if the donor has not provide written intention. Eye donors are not limited by age or degree of eyesight and pay no fee to donate their eyes.

The eye is enucleated (removed) from the donor as soon as possible after death. It is usually stored in special solutions or fixatives, or in some cases, it may be quickly frozen and stored at low temperatures. Tissue deterioration may occur if the eye is not treated within six to eight hours after death.

The eye bank evaluates the donor's general health, medical history, and the health of the eyes according to strict medical standards. After this evaluation, the cornea is distributed to the corneal surgeon who makes the final determination as to whether the cornea is suitable for transplantation. Tissue and blood typing and matching normally are not necessary in corneal transplantation, except in rare instances, such as cases of major chemical burns or graft rejection.

Corneas that qualify for transplantation are distributed to recipients according to fair, just, and equitable standards. Distribution is made without regard to age, sex, religion, race, creed, color, or national origin.

If the corneas are not suitable for transplantation, or the sight-restoring procedure of epiketophakia, the eyes are used for research and education. Because many sight disorders can not be simulated, donated eyes are valuable in the research of glaucoma, diabetes, retinal diseases, and other eye disorders and conditions.

Eye Bank Association of America   (EBAA)   The Eye Bank Association of America (EBAA), located in Washington, D.C., was established in 1961 by the Committee on Eye Banks of the American Academy of Ophthalmology. It is a nonprofit organization that includes more than 100 member eye banks in 45 states, as well as Canada, Taiwan, India, England, and Saudi Arabia.

The association develops and maintains quality control in eye banking. It develops research programs, professional education and training programs, and public awareness materials. The organization cooperates with other organ and tissue transplant organizations and represents member eye banks in legislative and legal matters.

The EBAA compiles statistics concerning eye banks, transplants, and organ donation, and maintains a speakers bureau. It publishes a newsletter and holds an annual conference.

Contact:

The Eye Bank Association of America
1015 18th Street, NW
Suite 1010
Washington, DC, 20036
202-775-4999 (ph)
202-429-6036 (fax)

eye drops Eye drops are commonly prescribed in the treatment of eye disorders but may be used to treat diseases relating to other organs as well. Eye drops may be used to constrict the pupils in the treatment of diseases such as GLAUCOMA. Such constricting or miotic drops include pilocarpine eye drops. Pilocarpine is a cholinergic medication that constricts the pupils and helps regulate or reduce intraocular pressure. Its most common side effect is miosis, which is a decrease in the size of the pupil. This can cause some loss of sight.

Other eye drops dilate the PUPIL or have a mydriatic effect. These are used during eye examinations. One class is cycloplegic drops that relax the pupil and CILIARY BODY (parasympatholytics) and are used to treat disorders such as acute IRITIS. Atropine, cyclopentolate, and homatropine are common cycloplegic drops. The other class of mydriatic drops are sympathomimetics that stimulate the dilator muscle of the pupil.

Eye infections are often treated with antibiotic drops. Steroids are occasionally used but usually for short periods of time only. ANTIVIRAL DROPS are used to treat viral infections such as HERPES SIMPLEX or HERPES ZOSTER. Idoxuridine, trifluridine, ARA-A, acyclovir, and vidarabine are commonly prescribed antiviral drops.

Other eye drops used to treat glaucoma are beta-blockers, such as brand names Timoptic, Betoptic, OptiPranolol, Ocupress, Betagan, and Carteolol. These drugs lower pressure within the eye by blocking beta adrenergic receptors in the eye. When those receptors are blocked, not as much aqueous fluid is produced. The effectiveness and potentially serious side effects of these various beta-blockers vary, and each patient's case must be thoroughly evaluated before a decision on which one to use is made.

Another type of drop, alpha-adrenergic agonists, also is used to treat glaucoma. Sold under brand names such as Iopidine, Propine, Epifrin, and Alphagan, these drugs lower eye pressure by treating both aqueous production and outflow. There can be side effects to both the eyes and the cardiovascular system from these types of drops.

A newer class of drugs that is used in drops to treat glaucoma is called alpha-adrenergic agonists, and includes the brand names Iopidine, Epifrin, Propine, and Alphagan. They work by decreasing the amount of fluid that is produced and may also help with the drainage of fluid from the eye. They may cause some eye discomfort, as well as some systemic side effects.

Prostaglandin analogs, a new type of drug sold under the brand name Xalatan, work differently to treat glaucoma. Instead of decreasing the amount of fluid produced in the eye, Xalatan, which was approved for use in the United States in 1996, increases the rate at which eye tissue is able to absorb the fluid. This works to get the fluid out of the eye, and reduces pressure. While Xalatan is noteworthy in its effectiveness, and because it has to be administered only once a day, there is a side effect that has prevented it from being more widely used than it is. The drops cause the color of the eye to darken, turning those that are blue, green, hazel, or yellowish to brown. Long-term effects of this pigment change are not known.

These are not the only medicines used to treat glaucoma, but are those commonly found in eye drops.

Before administering eye drops, the hands should be washed. The patient should sit or lie down and tilt the head back. The lower lid should be gently pulled down to form a hollow. A finger can be placed next to the nose to apply pressure and close off the draining tear duct. The dropper should be held close to, but not touching, the eyelid. The prescribed number of drops can then be squeezed into the hollow of the lid. After administering the drops, the eye should be closed for several moments. The dropper or applicator should not be wiped or washed, and the cap should be immediately replaced and tightly shut.

The same medications found in eye drops may be prescribed in ointment form. Ointments are administered in a similar manner to the drops. A line of ointment is squeezed into the hollow of the eyelid. Once the eyelid is closed, the eye should be rolled to spread the medication.

Regardless of what type of eye drop you use, it is important to know that the eye can only hold about one-fifth of one drop. If more than one drop is prescribed, you'll need to wait at least three minutes between applications for the drops to absorb properly. Waiting between applications also helps to avoid the possibility of washing one drop from the eye with another drop.

eye examination A general annual eye exam consists of several examinations of the parts of the eye and tests to determine the health and competence of the eyes. Through examination of the eyes, diseases of the body including hypertension, arteriosclerosis, and diabetes can also be detected.

First, a health history is taken, including questions about general health, medications taken or treatments given, visual history, current visual complaints, and visual needs required by occupation or hobbies. Visual acuity and refraction are tested next. Acuity is tested by reading an eye chart both with and without current prescription lenses. A refraction test to determine which lenses will best correct vision is then given using a PHOROPTOR.

A phoroptor is an apparatus that contains hundreds of lenses within a large base. The patient looks at a wall chart through lens openings in the base. The examiner changes the lenses with a dial to correct the patient's vision. The patient is asked to decide which lenses work best.

The examiner inspects the refractive power of the eyes while shining the light of a RETINOSCOPE

into them. By evaluating the lights and shadows moving on the retina, the examiner can determine whether the eyes are nearsighted, farsighted or astigmatic. The examiner also tests for color perception, depth perception and the ability of the eyes to move freely and work together.

An external examination of the eyes is included. A small flashlight is used to check for abnormalities of the lids, eye muscles and position of the eyes. The light is shined directly into the eyes to test pupil response.

An OPHTHALMOSCOPE, a hand-held lens light shaped like a flashlight, is used to view the inside and back of the eyes. The ophthalmoscope lights and magnifies the RETINA, blood vessels, and OPTIC NERVE of the eye. This is the only place in the body where an examiner can view the nerves and blood vessels in their active state.

A BIOMICROSCOPE (slit lamp) is used to examine the front of the eye. The machine is positioned in front of the patient who places his chin on a chin rest. A bright, vertical beam of light is directed through the CORNEA. The reflected light supplies an illuminated, magnified cross-section of the cornea, IRIS, and LENS.

A TONOMETER is attached to the biomicroscope. After the cornea is anesthetized, it checks the level of intraocular pressure or fluid within the eye when gently, painlessly placed on the cornea.

After the battery of tests is completed, the examiner can prescribe new lenses or treatment. If any abnormalities are found, a referral may be made to a specialist or the patient's physician. (See SCREENING.)

eyeglasses Eyeglasses, or spectacles, are devices that improve sight. They correct the refracting errors of the eye's lens and enable the wearer to see more clearly.

Eyeglasses contain a frame and a pair of lenses. The plastic or metal frame holds the lenses in place in front of the eyes. Side pieces of the frame that fit along the sides of the head and over the tops of the ears are called temples. The section of the frame between the two lenses that rests on the nose is called the bridge.

The lenses are specifically prescribed to correct the individual needs of the wearer. They can improve nearsightedness, farsightedness, astigmatism, and PRESBYOPIA. Lenses to correct nearsightedness, or MYOPIA, are concave in shape. Those prescribed for farsightedness, or HYPEROPIA, are convex. Cylindrical lenses are incorporated into the concave or convex lenses to correct an astigmatism, a nonspherical shape in the eye's lens that causes distortions.

Presbyopia (aging of the eye) results in the inability of the eye's lens to change shape to focus on near objects. Bifocals are eyeglasses that correct this problem. They contain two lenses within each lens frame so that the wearer can adjust to near and distant objects without changing glasses. Trifocals add a third lens designed to help see distances of two to three feet.

Another type of lens, called progressive addition lenses, also contain different prescriptions within the same lens. They do not, however, have seams, as bifocals and trifocals do, which allow your eye to make a smooth movement from one part of the lens to another.

Lenses may be made of glass or plastic and are required by federal law to be shatter resistant. Additional coatings or filters may be added to the lens to screen out light or reduce unwanted glare and reflection.

Eyeglasses are prescribed by an OPHTHALMOLOGIST or an OPTOMETRIST. The type of lenses needed are determined by an eye examination and vision test. The shape and width of the lenses is set by the shape and size of the frame, the length of the bridge, the weight of the lenses, and the shape of the head.

The eyeglass frame must be carefully fitted to the wearer to ensure optimal correction by the lenses. The center of the lenses must be directly in front of the eye, which may not necessarily be in the center of each lens frame. To center each lens, the distance between the pupils of the eyes is measured and recorded. The distance is also measured from the top of the ear to the place where each temple is attached to the frame. This measurement plus two inches is the amount needed for each temple.

New eyeglasses often require adjustment time. Nearsighted wearers may find that things look sharper but smaller with the new lenses. Farsighted wearers may notice that objects seem sharper but larger. Those with an astigmatism may feel off balance because the world looks temporarily slanted or curved. Bifocal wearers may need to develop additional head or eye movements to accommodate the needs of two lenses.

eyelids Eyelids are the eyes' protection from environmental injuries. They shut automatically when an object threatens to enter the eye and provide protection from unwanted light. They blink to produce cleansing tears and have lashes that filter out dust and small debris.

The eyelids are subject to several conditions. BLEPHARITIS is an inflammation of the margin of the lid. The disorder is associated with allergies or dandruff. The lids become red, swollen, and crusty at the base of the lashes. In less severe forms of the disorder, temporary loss of lashes may occur. Severe blepharitis destroys the lash follicles and results in permanent lash loss and deformity of the lid margin.

A HORDEOLUM or sty is an infection of a lash follicle. A spot on the lid margin becomes red, painful, and swollen with pus. The sty eventually ruptures, drains, and heals itself if not treated.

CHALAZION is a swelling of the lid glands. The enlargement grows slowly and painlessly. It may be associated with an inflammation and can become a chronic condition.

PTOSIS is a sagging of the upper eyelid. It may occur as a result of aging or a neurological problem, such as lid muscle paralysis.

ENTROPION is a turning inward of the margin of the eyelid. As a result, the lashes often scrape against the CORNEA and inflame it. Entropion may occur after an injury or burn or as a result of aging.

ECTROPION is a turning outward of the margin of the eyelid. The inner lid is exposed to the elements, which results in tearing and irritation. Ectropion is commonly caused by aging.

Tumorous growths may develop anywhere in the eyelids. Benign cysts and tumors include papilloma, a viral tumor, "strawberry nevus," a reddish tumor, cyst of gland of Moll, a watery, clear cyst, and xanthelasma, a fatty tumor. Malignant tumors most often develop on the lower lid but may be found elsewhere on the lids. These include basal cell carcinoma, squamous cell carcinoma, keratoacanthoma and malignant melanoma.

TRACHOMA is a viral disease that infects the inside of the eyelids, causing scarring of this area, and eventually of the cornea. It is a common cause of blindness in developing countries with limited eye care and sanitation.

TRICHIASIS occurs when the eyelashes grow inward. This may cause a corneal irritation.

DACRYOCYSTITIS is an inflammation of the tear drainage sac caused by an infection. Symptoms include redness, swelling, and pain.

facial expressions See NONVERBAL COMMUNICATION.

facial vision See SENSES.

Fair Housing Act An act that prohibits housing discrimination on the basis of race, color, religion, sex, disability, familial status, and national origin. Most housing, including private housing, state housing, local government housing, and that which receives federal financial assistance, is covered by the act.

The act requires owners of housing facilities to make reasonable exceptions to their policies and operations to afford people with disabilities equal housing opportunities. For instance, a landlord who has a no pets policy may be required to change the policy for a person who uses a dog guide. The act also requires landlords to allow tenants with disabilities to make reasonable access-related modifications to their private living and common-use spaces.

Anyone who feels they have been denied housing on the basis of race, color, religion, sex, disability, familial status, or national origin may file a complaint with the U.S. Department of Housing and Urban Development's Office of Program Compliance and Disability Rights.

Contact:

Office of Program Compliance and Disability Rights
U.S. Department of Housing and Urban Development
451 7th Street, SW
Room 5242
Washington, DC 20140
800-669-9777 (ph)
800-927-9275 (TTY)

Fair Labor Standards Act The Fair Labor Standards Act of 1938 sets the federal standard for minimum wage, work hours, overtime, recordkeeping, and child labor conditions. As amended, the act contains guidelines regarding disabled workers who work in special circumstances such as sheltered workshops.

Section 14 of the act issues minimum wage certificates to those learning a job, including disabled workers, apprentices and students. The certificates are based on individual productivity but require that wages paid to disabled workers must correspond to those paid to nondisabled, certificated workers producing comparable work.

Employers must review the disabled worker's wages every six months and must adjust wages yearly in compliance with those paid to nondisabled employees in the same position. The disabled worker may request a review of wages by the Secretary of Labor. The secretary names an administrative judge to hold a hearing in which the employer must show that the current wage rate is necessary to continue offering the job.

Amendments to the act in 1966 authorized the wages of employees of public or private institutions that serve the handicapped to be included and governed by this act. In 1976, the Supreme Court ruled that such institutions run by federal or state agencies were exempt from this ruling. That decision was overturned in a 1985 Supreme Court decision that determined that federal and local governments must comply with federal standards. Because of the extreme cost of implementation, the Fair Standards Act was amended to allow federal and state governments to offer, instead of wages, one and one-half hours of compensatory time for each hour of overtime worked.

The act was last amended in 1996, when the minimum wage was set at $5.15 per hour. The increase went into effect September 1, 1997.

U.S. Department of Education. *Summary of Existing Legislation Affecting Persons with Disabilities.* Washington, D.C.: USDE, 1988.
Welfare Information Network, Making Wages Work. "Minimum Wage Legislation and Living Wage Campaigns." www.makingwageswork.org/2000.

Federal-Aid Highway Act

The Federal-Aid Highway Act of 1973 approved the use of highway improvement program funds to improve accessibility to physically disabled people. The funds may be used to correct curbs and pedestrian crosswalks and provide accessibility to rest-stop facilities.

U.S. Department of Education. *Summary of Existing Legislation Affecting Persons with Disabilities.* Washington, D.C.: USDE, 1988.

Federal Aviation Act

The Federal Aviation Act of 1958 as amended by the Air Carrier Access Act of 1986 banned discrimination against disabled persons who use air transportation. The Act called for the promulgation of regulations to be issued by the Department of Transportation to ensure nondiscrimination "consistent with the safe carriage of all passengers on air carriers."

The act came under scrutiny in 1999, when a report from the National Council on Disability showed that disabled persons were still experiencing discrimination when using air transportation. The National Council on Disability recommended ways to better enforce the act.

U.S. Department of Education. *Summary of Existing Legislation Affecting Persons with Disabilities.* Washington, D.C.: USDE, 1988.
National Council on Disability. "Enforcing the Civil Rights of Air Travelers with Disabilities." www.ncd.gov/newsroom/publications/acaa, 1999.

Federal Employees Personal Assistants

A 1980 amendment to the Federal Advisory Committee Act allowed federal agencies to hire personal assistants for disabled federal employees. The assistants may work for the employee at the normal work station and on business trips. The assistants may include interpreters for the deaf and readers for the blind.

U.S. Department of Education. *Summary of Existing Legislation Affecting Persons with Disabilities.* Washington, D.C.: USDE, 1988.

federal resources

A myriad of federal agencies exist for the purpose of providing services to individuals with disabilities. These agencies are administered under the U.S. Departments of Education, Health and Human Services, and Labor, plus the Veterans Administration and other agencies. (See Appendix for addresses.)

The U.S. Department of Education encompasses the Center for Libraries and Educational Improvement, which grants funds to states for library services for the blind and physically disabled and administers the Library Services and Construction Act. The Clearinghouse on the Handicapped provides information to the public concerning disabilities.

The Division of Blind and Visually Impaired administers the Randolph-Sheppard Act and aids state rehabilitation agencies in development of methods, standards and procedures. The National Council on the Handicapped develops policy and plans for the National Institute on Disability and Rehabilitation Research. The National Institute on Disability and Rehabilitation Research awards contracts and grants for research and demonstration projects concerning disabilities and directs training and research centers.

The Office of Special Education and Rehabilitative Services supervises the offices of Rehabilitation Services Administration, Special Education Programs and National Institute on Disability and Rehabilitation Research. The Office of Special Education Programs administers the Education of the Handicapped Act, provides funding to the states for the education of disabled students and funds personnel training, research, special program grants, demonstration grants, and scholarships.

The Rehabilitation Services Administration assists state agencies in vocational rehabilitation programs by providing leadership, grants, and demonstration and training programs. It awards independent-living grants for the disabled.

The Department of Health and Human Services contains the Administration for Children, Youth and Families, which operates the Head Start program and advises the secretary of Health and Human Services on issues and programs concerning early childhood education. The Administration on Aging aids states in developing programs for aging citizens and administers the Older Americans Act of 1965.

The Health Care Financing Administration is responsible for the Medicare program and awards state grants for Medicaid. The Health Services Administration/Division for Maternal and Child Health Bureau of Health Care Delivery and Assistance controls state block grants for disabled children's services and maternal and child health services. The National Institutes of Health/National Eye Institute funds eye disease and disorder research and training of researchers.

The Office of Human Development Services administers the social services programs of the Social Security Act and supervises various agencies, including the President's Committee on Mental Retardation and the Administration on Developmental Disabilities. The Social Security Administration dispenses Social Security benefits, including disability insurance and Supplemental Security Income (SSI).

The Department of Labor controls the Employment Standards Administration Branch of Special Employment, which enforces laws concerning disabled workers in sheltered workshops and industry. The Office of Federal Contract Compliance monitors affirmative action as legislated by the Rehabilitation Act of 1973. The U.S. Employment Service controls the federal-state service program.

The Veterans Administration operates the Blind Rehabilitation Service, which administers programs for blinded veterans at Rehabilitation Centers and Clinics. The Department of Medicine and Surgery furnishes outpatient and hospital treatment and nursing-home care in Veterans Administration facilities. The Department of Veterans Benefits administers compensation and pension programs and provides vocational rehabilitation services and counseling.

Other agencies outside these departments include the Office of Civil Rights, which enforces laws prohibiting discrimination on the basis of race, color, national origin, sex, age and disability. It protects the rights of disabled individuals and investigates cases of discrimination due to disability.

The Library of Congress administers the National Library Service for the Blind and Physically Handicapped, which provides free library service to those unable to use standard print materials. The service provides braille and recorded magazines and books, talking book players, and cassette players.

The President's Committee on Employment of People with Disabilities is a partnership of national and state organizations and individuals that work to increase opportunities for the employment of disabled persons.

The Architectural and Transportation Barriers Compliance Board enforces the Architectural Barriers Act of 1968. The Committee for Purchase from the Blind and Other Severely Handicapped administers the purchase of products and services from nonprofit workshops as legislated under the Javits-Wagner-O'Day Act.

The Equal Employment Opportunity Commission monitors and enforces laws that prohibit discrimination on the basis of disability in the federal government. The U.S. Office of Personnel Management Governmentwide Selective Placement Programs Division sets policy for the employment of disabled individuals within the federal government. The Small Business Administration makes loans to small businesses owned and operated by disabled individuals as legislated by the Small Business Act. Contact information for these agencies can be found in an appendix in the back of this book.

financial aid   Financial aid is available to visually impaired individuals to meet the costs of daily living, medical evaluation, public transportation, and rehabilitation and vocational training.

To qualify for many types of financial aid, an individual must be recognized as legally blind. *Legal blindness* is a term for conditions of visual impairment that include either visual acuity of 20/200 or less in the better eye, after correction, or a visual field of 20 degrees or less, in the better eye, regardless of visual acuity. Those who are legally blind qualify for two programs of financial aid under the Social Security Administration. These are termed disability insurance benefits and Supplemental Security Income (SSI).

Disabled individuals are those who have a physical or mental disability that is permanent or long-term (12 months or longer) or one that may result in death.

Disability insurance benefits are authorized under the Social Security Act. They are paid to people who have contributed to the Social Security System but who have become disabled before reaching retirement age. Disability insurance benefits are not affected by financial circumstances or need. Applicants must be unemployed or employed but earning less than a determined amount, and must have a qualifying medical disability according to the ruling of the Disability Determination Service. An applicant must have contributed to the Social Security fund for approximately half of the years since turning 21. Dependents and spouses of an eligible disabled person may also qualify for up to 50 percent of the applicant's rate. In some cases, a divorced spouse also may be eligible for benefits.

The benefits are paid in cash monthly to eligible people and their dependents. The age of the worker when he became disabled, his earned income, and the length of time he was employed determine the amount of the benefit. The amount may be decreased if the worker is a recipient of other state or federal benefits.

After receiving disability benefits for 24 months, the recipient is eligible for Medicare health insurance benefits.

A national policy encourages disabled people receiving Medicare health insurance benefits to try to get back into the workplace, if at all possible. To accomplish this, the government has established laws to provide work incentives and protect disabled people from discrimination in the workplace.

In 1999, Congress passed the Ticket to Work and Work Incentives Improvement Act of 1999. This act provides more opportunities and benefits for disabled people who want to return to work, including a program that provides tickets that dis-

abled people can use to obtain rehabilitation and employment services at an approved employment network. The ticket program was active in 13 states in 2001, with more states expected to be added in 2002. The first 13 states to be included in the program are: Arizona, Colorado, Delaware, Florida, Illinois, Iowa, Massachusetts, New York, Oklahoma, Oregon, South Carolina, Vermont, and Wisconsin.

The 1999 act also encourages disabled workers to find employment by providing work incentives, including cash benefits in addition to Medicare during employment, help with extra expenses incurred as a result of the disability, financial assistance with education or training, or rehabilitation necessary to work. Some of these incentives also apply to people receiving Supplemental Security Income or Medicaid. For more information about the ticket program and work incentives, contact the Social Security Administration at its toll-free number: 800-772-1213 and ask for the fact sheet called "The Ticket to Work and Work Incentives Program of 1993."

Supplemental Security Income provides a minimum income to low-income elderly and disabled individuals. SSI requires that recipients meet requirements of financial need and, unlike Social Security Disability Insurance, does not base eligibility on the amount of taxes paid into the Social Security fund. SSI benefits are funded by general tax revenues, not Social Security taxes, and are available for blind children, as well as adults.

Needy individuals or couples disabled or aged 65 or older may qualify for SSI benefits if financial needs requirements are met.

Monthly cash benefits are paid directly to recipients. The amount of payment is based on a Consumer Price Index figure.

The Work Incentives Improvement Act of 1999 increases the amount of money a disabled person can earn while still receiving benefits.

MEDICAID is the main source of medical-services funding to severely disabled individuals. It allows states to offer coverage not only to those who receive public assistance, but also to eligible needy people who do not qualify for welfare or Medicare.

Medicaid eligibility is determined by financial need. Recipients generally fall into one or more of the three qualifying categories: categorically needy, medically needy, or qualified severely impaired.

The categorically needy receive AID TO FAMILIES WITH DEPENDENT CHILDREN (AFDC) benefits or Supplemental Security Income (SSI) benefits or qualify under specific regulations for their state.

Medically needy persons may have incomes too high to qualify for AFDC or SSI benefits yet cannot afford to pay for necessary medical treatment. States determine a different qualifying income level for those who are medically needy.

Qualified severely impaired individuals are those under 65 who receive SSI benefits because of blindness or disability and are able to be employed but do not have incomes that allow them to pay for healthcare coverage.

MEDICARE offers health insurance benefits to qualified disabled and elderly individuals. Generally, those eligible are 65 years or older and qualify for Social Security benefits. Disabled people may be eligible to qualify for Medicare after a two-year waiting period.

Children's Rehabilitative Services (CRS) is a federal/state program that supplies medical services to disabled children up to age 21. Medical diagnosis and evaluation is free in each state. Additional treatment or hospital costs vary by state but all accept Medicaid, Blue Cross, Blue Shield, and other medical insurance. The program formerly was called the Crippled Children's Services.

The Early Periodic Screening, Diagnosis, and Treatment Program (EPSDT) medically screens children from poor families to determine whether medical treatment or related services are necessary. The program provides remedial and preventative medical care.

Families receiving state Aid to Families with Dependent Children benefits and those in which parents or guardians are receiving Medicaid or local public-assistance benefits qualify for EPSDT services for children up to 21 years old.

Tax deductions are available to legally blind individuals, as well. Married individuals over age 65 and married blind individuals may deduct an additional $850. An elderly or blind spouse also qualifies for the $1,100 deduction. Single elderly or blind individuals are eligible for a $1,100 deduction.

In order to qualify for the deduction, an individual must be LEGALLY BLIND. The individual must attach to the tax return a statement from an OPHTHALMOLOGIST or doctor confirming legal blindness.

Some medical expenses may be deducted from income if itemized. Under the Internal Revenue Code, a deduction is allowed for medical expenses that are above 7.5 percent of the individual's adjusted gross income. Items that are deductible include special equipment and its installation costs, necessary home improvements or renovations, special education tuition, dog guides, and personal items, including prosthetic eyes.

Individuals with disabilities may be eligible for special home loans and rent assistance programs. The Title I Home Improvement Loan is a federally insured loan that can be used to renovate a home to meet the needs of the disabled owner. The loan can be used to finance the removal of architectural barriers or to make necessary improvements. The U.S. Department of Housing and Urban Development (HUD) insures the loans, which are available from banks and other lending institutions.

Low-income disabled individuals may qualify for housing assistance from HUD. Eligible tenants pay approximately 30 percent of their adjusted gross income for rent. HUD pays direct subsidies to the rental unit owners to compensate for the difference between payment and normal rental fee.

Legally blind individuals may mail materials free of postage through a program called Free Matter for the Blind or Handicapped. To become eligible, the individual must present written certification of legal blindness by a competent authority such as a doctor, ophthalmologist, or OPTOMETRIST, to the post office where mailings will be sent and received.

Material eligible for mailing includes books, magazines, musical scores, braille material, 14-point SIGHTSAVING TYPE, records, or cassette tapes. Equipment and parts of equipment used for writing or educational purposes, sound playback equipment for use by visually impaired individuals, and equipment designed or adapted for use by visually impaired persons, such as braille watches and white canes, are also eligible.

Reduced telephone rates may be available to the legally blind. Offerings differ from state to state, but written verification of legal blindness by a doctor or ophthalmologist may in some cases be used to obtain reduced monthly service rates for touch tone dialing and speed calling. Telebraille devices may be offered to those who are deaf/blind and can read braille. Those with low vision may be eligible to receive free 411 information or large-number overlays for the telephone dial.

Interstate bus lines and Amtrak offer reduced fares to legally blind people as do many city public transportation systems. Identification cards may be necessary to obtain the reduced fare and are often issued by the individual transportation agency. An identification card verifying legal blindness can also be obtained from the American Foundation for the Blind.

Legally blind individuals are eligible for state rehabilitation services. Each state supports an agency for the blind under various names such as Department of Rehabilitation, Commission for the Visually Handicapped, State Services for the Blind and Visually Impaired, and Bureau of the Blind.

Services differ from state to state, but most provide home-management skills, orientation and mobility instruction, braille instruction, communication skills, personal-management skills, vocational rehabilitation, counseling services, and adaptive-aids evaluation and selection.

Rehabilitation services are available at little or no cost to the individual. Some aspects of the rehabilitation program may require financial contribution by the individual. In some states, services such as psychological counseling, equipment purchase, transportation to school, or school tuition may be financed by the state or a combination of the state, the individual, and grants or loans.

Disabled individuals may be eligible for low-cost loans or financial assistance to start a small business. Eligibility is determined by the administering agency, the Small Business Administration.

fluorescein angiography   Fluorescein angiography is a type of ophthalmologic photography used to examine the RETINA and CHOROID inside the back section of the eye. The procedure, which is also called fundus photography, allows a more detailed examination than the ophthalmoscope.

In the procedure, fluorescein dye is injected into a vein in the patient's arm. As the dye passes through the retinal vessels and capillaries a specially filtered camera takes photographs every few seconds to record the flow. Analysis of the resulting angiogram can determine the presence of tumors or clogged or leaking blood vessels, diabetic retinopathy, or macular edema. Fluorescein angiography may be used after photocoagulation (sealing of blood vessels with laser treatments) to determine the results of the procedure.

fluorescein eye staining   Fluorescein eye staining is a procedure performed to examine the CORNEA, the transparent covering of the eye. The test allows the examiner to look for suspected scratches, irritations, or infections.

The examiner applies fluorescein dye into the eye by touching the lower eyelid with a fluorescein-laden paper strip. The dye covers the cornea and settles into any cuts or scratches of the surface. The excess dye is washed from the cornea with the natural tearing process.

The examiner observes the eye under an ultraviolet light. The fluorescein dye glows bright green, illuminating any irregularities such as cornea abrasions, ulcers, burns, or overexposure to light.

Food Stamp Act   The Food Stamp Act of 1967, as amended, authorizes food coupon allotments to low-income families and individuals. The food stamps can be used to buy food in retail stores, to pay for the delivery of prepared meals to elderly or disabled people or to purchase meals or food served in small, group-living residences by disabled persons receiving Social Security or SSI benefits. Allotments are made based on net income and family size.

The current food-stamp program was initiated by President Kennedy in 1961 in a few low-income areas of the country and was expanded in 1964 as a formal Food Stamp Act. Its roots, however, go back to 1939, when the food stamp plan was started to help needy depression-era families. In 1973, amendments were made to encompass numerous regional and federal food programs and to expand the program to include the entire country.

The Food Stamp Act of 1977 revised the program to regulate eligibility and to issue the stamps at no charge to qualified recipients. It further expanded on the program by lifting restrictions on certain elderly people living in federally subsidized housing, institutionalized persons and those completing drug or alcohol residential treatment programs.

The act simplified the application process by allowing some governmental assistance agencies to qualify applicants for food stamps. This allowed applicants the opportunity to apply for food stamps while applying for other benefits such as Aid to Families with Dependent Children, Social Security or SSI. The act directed state Food Stamp Program agencies to alert SSI recipients to the Food Stamp Program and launched a system in which food stamp values could be paid in cash to families whose members are all 65 years or older or who all receive SSI benefits.

Amendments made in 1979 increased the spending limit for the program and eliminated some housing and medical deduction constraints. They allowed disabled persons, including the blind, receiving Social Security or SSI benefits and living in nonprofit group-living residences of no more than 16 people to be eligible for food stamps. The stamps could be used to buy food or to pay for prepared meals.

In 1982, the Omnibus Budget Reconciliation Act authorized certain disabled individuals over 60 living in a household to be regarded as a separate household and eligible for food stamps. The Food Security Act of 1985 continued the cash payment program and redefined disabled persons to include those receiving SSI and other federal or state disability benefits.

The food stamp program served 17.2 million people each month during fiscal year 2000, at a cost of $21.2 billion. The all-time high in program participation occurred in 1994, with 27.97 million people served.

U.S. Department of Education. *Summary of Existing Legislation Affecting Persons with Disabilities.* Washington, D.C.: USDE, 1988.

Foundation Fighting Blindness   The Foundation Fighting Blindness is a national eye research foundation that was founded in 1971. It was formerly known as the RP Foundation Fighting Blindness Retinitis Pigmentosa Foundation, Inc.

The goal of the Foundation Fighting Blindness is to find the cause, treatment, cure and prevention for retinitis pigmentosa (RP), Usher's syndrome, and other associated retinal degenerative diseases. The organization is the largest voluntary nongovernmental sponsor of research to cure RP, macular degeneration and other retinal disorders. Since 1971, the foundation has raised $150 million for retinal degenerative disease research.

In 2000, it formed a cooperative agreement with the National Eye Institute that devotes a larger percentage of NEI budget increases to research in retinal degenerative disease.

The Foundation Fighting Blindness serves as a clearinghouse of information for RP specialists, professionals, patients and families. It compiles statistics, directs extensive public education and human services programs and maintains a national and international membership. Among its programs are a national registry and retina donor program. The foundation also publishes a newsletter and provides free information about retinal diseases.

Contact:

The Foundation Fighting Blindness
Executive Plaza I, Suite 800
11350 McCormick Road
Hunt Valley, MD 21031-1014
888-394-3937 (toll free)
800-683-5551 (TDD)
www.blindness.org

fovea   A small hollow or indentation in the macular section of the RETINA. The retina is an inner layer of the eye behind the VITREOUS. The retina contains millions of light-sensitive cells, including RODS AND CONES. These cells give the retina image information that it sends to the brain.

The MACULA is the central section of the retina, which is packed with cones, the cells that distinguish detail and color. The fovea is in the center of the macula. It contains the highest concentration of cones. Light is focused directly on the fovea, making it the site of greatest perception.

Freedom Scientific Inc. A company that offers a variety of assistive technology products for people with sensory impairments and learning disabilities. It was formed in April 2000 when Henter-Joyce, Blazie Engineering, and Arkenstone merged.

Henter-Joyce was a leading software company specializing in products for blind people. Blazie Engineering was a manufacturer of Braille computers, software, and embossers. Arkenstone was a nonprofit organization that provided technical solutions to visually and reading-impaired individuals.

Freedom Scientific continues to design, produce, and market the products and services for which Henter-Joyce, Blazie, and Arkenstone were known. Among those products is an extremely popular screen reading software called Job Access With Speech (JAWS). The user moves the JAWS cursor anywhere on the screen to activate a speech synthesizer. Another product is Braille 'n Speak, a compact computer with a Braille keyboard that can be used as a talking computer terminal, a Braille-to-print transcriber, a word processor, a talking clock and calendar, and a talking calculator.

The product is extremely popular because it allows blind users to take notes, keep an address book, and update a personal calendar without the use of pen and paper. There are now five different models of the Braille 'n Speak.

Freedom Scientific has its corporate headquarters in Carlsbad, California, and facilities in St. Petersburg, Florida. About 30 percent of the company's work force is visually impaired. In January 2001, the company acquired the accessibility division of OMNI PC Systemintegration, GmbH, a German PC software distributor and consulting company. The new division of Freedom Scientific will oversee the distribution in Europe of all the company's products.

Contact:

Freedom Scientific, corporate office
760-602-5232
www.hj.com

Freedom Scientific Blind/Low Vision Group
11800 31st Court North
St. Petersburg, FL 33717
www.freedomscientific.com

free matter for the blind and handicapped See MAILING PRIVILEGES.

freezing method See CRYOSURGERY.

Fresnel prism See PRISMS.

Fuch's endothelial dystrophy Fuch's endothelial dystrophy is a hereditary disease in which the corneal endothelium is destroyed. It is a leading cause of corneal transplantation in the United States.

The endothelium is the protective inner lining of the CORNEA made up of a single layer of endothelial cells. The cells prevent the AQUEOUS FLUID of the ANTERIOR CHAMBER from penetrating the cornea. A reduction of endothelial cells allows seepage into the cornea, resulting in swelling, loss of transparency, and loss of vision.

The disease usually becomes apparent when a person is in his or her 40s or 50s. It is more common in women than in men. It is diagnosed from a slit-lamp examination by dystrophic spots in the endothelium. As the condition progresses, CORNEAL EDEMA or fluid retention and swelling develops, the cornea thickens and vision is lost. In later stages, blisters form on the epithelium, resulting in painful ruptures.

Early treatment of Fuch's endothelium dystrophy may include CORNEAL TRANSPLANTATION (keratoplasty), or replacement of a disk of healthy cornea for a disk of diseased cornea. Keratoplasty is not effective for later-stage dystrophy. Severe, painful forms of this disease are treated with cryotherapy; a cryoprobe is applied to the sclera of the CILIARY BODY to alleviate the pain.

Washington Academy of Eye Physicians and Surgeons. Fuch's Corneal Endothelial Dystrophy. On the Internet at: www.wa-eyemd.org, 2001.

fundus The term for the back section of the inner eye. It contains the RETINA, the CHOROID, and the OPTIC NERVE.

The retina is the section of the eye where light information is processed and sent to the brain where it is transformed into an image. The choroid is the pigmented layer behind the retina that supplies the eye with blood. The optic nerve is the cord of nerve fibers that acts as a conduit to transmit information from the eye to the brain.

The fundus can be viewed with an instrument called an OPHTHALMOSCOPE. This handheld instrument lights and magnifies the fundus for examination. Examination of the fundus, called funduscopy or ophthalmoscopy, allows the examiner to detect disorders within the eye and to determine other diseases of the body, such as hypertension, diabetes, and arteriosclerosis.

fundus photography See FLUORESCEIN ANGIOGRAPHY.

galactosemia A rare, congenital disease that prevents infants from metabolizing galactose, a sugar found in milk. Galactosemia occurs in about two of every 100,000 births. As a result of the inability to process the galactose, it accumulates in the blood and lens of the eye. The galactose in the lens absorbs water and disrupts the lens fibers forming vacuoles, or pockets of liquid in the tissue. Bilateral CATARACTS form from these vacuoles.

Cataracts may be avoided or reduced in severity by early removal of milk and milk products from the diet. Dense opacities may be surgically removed within the first month. Early extraction limits the possibility of developing amblyopia.

genetics the study of genes, segments of DNA located on the chromosomes that carry information for all inherited characteristics. Genetics explores the heredity and variation of organisms and the conditions that affect them. Genetic disorders are diseases caused by gene abnormalities or irregularities. Genetic disorders may be evidenced at birth as congenital diseases or may surface as a disease or disorder later in life.

Over 3,000 major and minor hereditary disorders have been identified, 30 percent of which affect the eye. Hereditary and congenital diseases cause one in every five cases of blindness in the United States. Thousands more are affected by these visual disorders to a less severe degree. Genetic factors are the major cause of blindness for children from birth to six years. The cost of health care, aid to disabled persons, and lost income due to visual disorders, many of which are genetic diseases, is in the billions of dollars.

RETINITIS PIGMENTOSA (RP), a retinal degenerative disease, is the most common of all inherited retinal disorders. It affects approximately 100,000 persons and roughly one of every 80 persons carries the recessive gene for RP. The disease most often is diagnosed during childhood or young adulthood and may lead to blindness or severe visual impairment.

USHER'S SYNDROME occurs when those with RP are also born deaf. Usher's syndrome is the leading cause of deaf-blindness and accounts for more than half of all adults seeking rehabilitative services for deaf-blindness.

There is no treatment or cure for RP or Usher's syndrome. Low-vision aids may be helpful, and genetic counseling may help define the risks to relatives and future offspring.

Inherited MACULAR DISEASE, also called macular dystrophy, is almost always a genetic disorder that appears at birth or up to age six. This disorder destroys the MACULA, or center of sharpest vision of the RETINA. Although the disorder blurs and eventually may eliminate central vision, most patients retain some peripheral vision. There is no medication or cure for macular degeneration but a small number of patients may benefit from laser treatments.

Genetic CATARACTS appear at birth or later in childhood as infantile or juvenile cataracts. The lens may be partially or completely opaque at birth. Surgery to remove dense cataracts may occur following the neonatal period, but it is often postponed until the density threatens to affect the child's performance at school or home. After surgery, patients may develop AMBLYOPIA or RETINAL DETACHMENTS.

Some corneal dystrophies are genetic and may appear early in life or in middle age. Corneal dystrophies lead to the formation of opacities and may result in blindness or vision impairment. Treatment may include corneal transplantation.

SICKLE-CELL DISEASE is a single cell disorder that affects one in every 400 Americans of African descent. The trait is present in one of every 10 Americans of African descent. Sickle-cell disease may cause blockage of the blood vessels in the CONJUNCTIVA, CHOROID, or RETINA. Sickle-cell retinopathy and vision loss may result. There is no cure for sickle-cell disease. Visual complications are treated with varying results using scleral buckling and photocoagulation therapy.

Tumors may be genetic and congenital. RETINOBLASTOMA is the most common intraocular tumor in children. The malignancy is usually present at birth and may be inherited. It may occur in one or both eyes. Treatment often involves enucleation, or removal of the eye, but in less severe cases may include radiation, chemotherapy, or cryotherapy treatments.

Color blindness is a single gene disorder predominant in males. The inherited characteristic is transmitted by the male chromosome. The disorder does not affect the visual field or visual acuity.

Other diseases and conditions that result in visual impairments or blindness are genetic in nature. These include albinism, galactosemia, Marfan's syndrome, and Down's syndrome. Diabetes may also be linked to genetic defects that react to environmental or other factors.

Genetic research with an emphasis on the eye and vision continues. Recombinant DNA technology is producing new knowledge about gene function, diseases and treatments of the eye. The research strives to identify and confine the underlying genetic defects in cataracts, retinal degenerations, color vision disorders, and inherited ocular tumors.

Genetic counseling may determine the risk of disease for future children by determining the chances for recurrence. Genetic counselors also describe methods of diagnosis (such as amniocentesis) and recommend reproductive options. (See CONGENITAL DISORDERS.)

Galloway, N. R. *Common Eye Diseases and Their Management.* Berlin: Springer-Verlag, 1985.

Kaiser-Kupfer, Muriel I., and Julian Morris. "Advances in Human Genetics—The Long Range Impact on Blindness and the Visually Impaired." *Yearbook of Association for Education and Rehabilitation of the Blind and Visually Impaired.* Vol. 2 Alexandria, VA: Association for Education and Rehabilitation of the Blind and Visually Impaired, (1984, 1985): pp. 46–49.

Maumenee, Irene. "Discoveries in Genetic Eye Disease." *Sight-saving* vol. 53, no. 4 (1984–85): 14–15.

glaucoma   Glaucoma is group of eye diseases responsible for over 8.5 million cases of blindness in the world. It is estimated that 3 million Americans have glaucoma, and about 67 million people worldwide. It is the second most common cause of blindness in the United States and the most common cause among African Americans. According to Prevent Blindness America, approximately one of every seven blind Americans is blind as a result of glaucoma.

The disease affects roughly 1 percent of people over age 40. Those at most risk of developing glaucoma are those with a family history of glaucoma, those over 40, blacks, diabetics, extremely nearsighted individuals, and those with undersized, farsighted eyes.

Glaucoma is characterized by an abnormal rise in intraocular pressure, a condition affected by the AQUEOUS FLUID. The ANTERIOR CHAMBER of the eye is filled with aqueous fluid, a watery fluid that brings nutrients to the avascular CORNEA and LENS and removes waste material.

The ciliary epithelium constantly produces new aqueous that circulates through the anterior chamber and drains from the eye at the anterior angle. The aqueous passes through a meshwork grill called the trabecular meshwork, into the Schlemm's canal, and out of the eye. When the eye overproduces aqueous or the drainage systems of the eye inhibit the drainage of the aqueous, the pressure inside the eye increases.

As the pressure builds, it affects the function of the RETINA and OPTIC NERVE. The blood supply to these organs is reduced, nerve cells and fibers are destroyed and blindness results if not treated.

There are many types of glaucoma, but the two most common forms are open angle (also called wide-angle or chronic glaucoma) and angle closure (also called narrow-angle or acute glaucoma).

Open-angle glaucoma accounts for approximately 70 percent of all cases of glaucoma. It occurs when the angle of drainage is open, but the aqueous fluid is unable to percolate through the mesh-work. It is bilateral, may be inherited and rarely affects those under age 40.

The disease progresses slowly, painlessly, with few, transient symptoms. As the disease develops, it destroys the optic nerve, constricts peripheral vision, which causes tunnel vision, forms scotomas, or blank spots, in the field of vision and eventually destroys central vision.

Angle-closure glaucoma accounts for roughly 5 percent of all glaucoma cases and occurs when the drainage angle is blocked by the IRIS. Angle-closure glaucoma usually develops in small, farsighted eyes, which tend to have shallow anterior chambers. Angle-closure glaucoma may be occasionally brought about by dilating drops.

Angle-closure glaucoma happens suddenly, reducing vision and often producing pain. Symptoms of angle-closure glaucoma include pain, redness, pupil distortion, blurred or clouded vision, and halos around lights.

The disease may progress to rapid and permanent vision loss. Although the condition is not always bilateral, approximately half of patients with angle-closure glaucoma affecting one eye will develop the condition in the unaffected eye without preventative surgery.

Glaucoma may be diagnosed during a routine ophthalmologic examination by symptoms of raised intraocular pressure, cupping of the OPTIC DISC, and visual field loss. Three tests—tonometry, GONIOSCOPY, and perimetry—may be performed in the screening, diagnosis, and treatment of glaucoma.

Tonometry is a simple, painless method of measuring intraocular pressure. An instrument called a TONOMETER is gently touched to the open eye and records the amount of pressure that is within the eye. It is recommended that all individuals over 40 be screened for glaucoma with tonometry on a yearly basis.

Gonioscopy is a test to examine the angle of the anterior chamber. The examiner looks through a mirrored lens called a gonioscope to estimate the angle of the chamber. The procedure indicates abnormalities or changes in the angle of the chamber and assists the examiner in prescribing treatment.

Perimetry is a test that measures and maps the field of vision. The patient looks into a bowl-shaped device. Points of light are flashed into the bowl and the patient indicates when the lights appear.

Glaucoma can be controlled but not cured. Treatment of glaucoma may include medication, surgery or laser therapy. Open angle glaucoma may be treated with drops that reduce the size of the pupil, inhibit production of aqueous or increase the outflow of the drainage system.

Medications used to treat glaucoma may be topical, such as eye drops or ointments, or oral. Medications that increase the outflow of aqueous from the eye are called miotics, and include Isopto Carpine, Ocusert, Pilocar, and Pilopine. Other drugs that increase the outflow of aqueous fluid from the eye are called epinephrine compounds. These include Epifrin and Propine.

Beta-blockers and carbonic anhydrase inhibitors help reduce the amount of aqueous produced in the eye. Beta-blockers include Betagan, Betimol, Betoptic, Ocupress, Optipranalol, and Timoptic. Carbonic anhydrase inhibitors include Alphagan, Iopidine, and Trusopt.

In 1996 the U.S. Food and Drug Administration approved a new glaucoma medicine called latanoprost. Marketed as Xalatan, it works near the drainage area of the eye to increase the secondary route of aqueous outflow.

Oral medications used to control glaucoma include Daranide, Diamox, and Neptazane. These are carbonic anhydrase inhibitors, which work to slow the production of aqueous fluid in the eye.

Surgery is indicated if the medication fails to correct the increase in intraocular pressure of open-angle glaucoma, and in cases of angle-closure glaucoma that cannot be corrected with medication. Two major forms of surgery are IRIDECTOMY and filtering surgery called TRABECULECTOMY.

An iridectomy is a surgical procedure in which a portion of the iris is removed with a laser to eliminate the blockage of closed-angle glaucoma and prevent further attacks. It may be performed preventively on an unaffected eye that is predisposed to the condition.

A trabeculectomy is performed when the damage to the drainage angle has occurred due to angle-closure or open-angle glaucoma. It bypasses the damaged meshwork and creates a new drainage tract to allow the aqueous to flow from the eye.

Laser therapy may be employed in a laser trabeculoplasty, which opens the drainage area located where the cornea meets the iris. A series of 100 laser burns are placed in the drainage area, which causes scarring and opens the meshwork of drainage channels. The fluid drains more easily from the eye, and intraocular pressure is reduced. A fairly new program called seton placement is being used to treat glaucoma, and involves placing a tube-like device into the eye, allowing fluid to drain.

Secondary glaucoma may occur as a result of another disease or disorder such as vascular eye disease, UVEITIS, tumors, trauma, eye surgery, or in reaction to drugs such as local or systemic steroids or dilating drops.

Congenital glaucoma is a rare and often inherited condition. The raised intraocular pressure level may be present at birth or develop some months after. This type of glaucoma is caused by a defective development or formation of the angle of the anterior chamber.

Symptoms of congenital glaucoma include bulging eyes, photophobia, and CORNEAL EDEMA. The treatment involves goniotomy, a surgical procedure that opens the trabecular meshwork. (See LASERS.)

American Foundation for the Blind. *Understanding and Living with Glaucoma,* New York: AFB, 1984.

Blacker, M. M., and D. R. Wekstein, eds. *Your Health after Sixty.* New York: E.P. Dutton, 1979.

Cooley, Donald G. *After 40 Health and Medical Guide.* Des Moines, Iowa: Better Homes and Gardens Books, 1980.

International Association of Lion's Clubs. *Glaucoma.* Oak Brook, Illinois: IALC, 1987.

Medem Medical Library. "Important Facts About Glaucoma." www.medem.com, 2000.

Prevent Blindness America. *Glaucoma: Sneak Thief of Sight.* New York: NSPB, 1985.

Reynolds, James D. *Glaucoma.* HealthNet Library. Columbus: CompuServe, 1989.

Reynolds, James D. *Glaucoma Surgery.* HealthNet Library, Columbus: CompuServe, 1989.

gonioscopy   Gonioscopy is a test to determine the width of the angle of the eye's ANTERIOR CHAMBER. This angle, formed by the CORNEA and the IRIS, is the place where fluid drains from the eye. If the angle becomes narrow or blocked, the fluid cannot drain effectively, pressure builds up within the eye and GLAUCOMA may develop.

The angle of the chamber is examined with a *gonioscope,* sometimes called a gonioprism. This instrument is a mirrored lens, which the examiner holds up to the patient's eye. Gonioscopy is performed during glaucoma screening and the routine eye examination of a person with glaucoma. The procedure detects abnormalities or changes in the angle of the chamber and assists the examiner in prescribing treatment.

Gonioscopy is a routine part of a presurgical eye examination for those undergoing CATARACT surgery. The surgeon may administer cycloplegic or dilating drops prior to surgery, which could further restrict a narrow angle and cause complications. In addition, if an anterior chamber INTRAOCULAR LENS (IOL) implant is planned, the gonioscopy could indicate the amount of space, or lack of space, available to accommodate the implant.

Gonioscopy may be performed on any patient prior to the application of cycloplegic drops. During an examination or other procedure, cycloplegic drops may be used in a patient with a narrow angle if care is taken to ensure that the PUPIL has returned to normal size after the procedure.

gonorrhea   A type of venereal or sexually transmitted disease. It is the most frequently reported communicable disease in the United States. Approximately 1 million cases of gonorrhea are reported each year, a figure that the Centers for Disease Control estimates to be roughly only half of all cases contracted in the United States annually.

Gonorrhea is caused by the gonococcus bacteria and may result in blindness when contracted congenitally. The disease is passed from mother to child during birth. As the child moves through the birth canal the eyes come into contact with the gonococcus bacteria growing in or near the cervix and become infected.

The infection, called gonococcal ophthalmia, or ophthalmia neonatorum in the case of newborns, causes severe conjunctivitis. Early symptoms include swelling and redness of the CORNEA, CONJUNCTIVA, and eyelids. Without treatment, the condition may progress to damage the cornea and result in blindness.

Adults may contract gonococcal ophthalmia by exposing the eyes to anything carrying the bacteria. Adults exhibit more severe signs and symptoms than newborns, including a copious pus-like discharge. Blindness can result from untreated cases. Gonorrhea in adults may be diagnosed from a Gram's stain or a cervical culture.

Treatment for gonococcal ophthalmia involves use of local antibiotic drops or ointments such as penicillin or tetracycline. Systemic or injected antibiotics may also be prescribed.

At one time, congenital gonorrhea was the leading cause of blindness in children. The passage of laws in all states requiring the administration of silver nitrate drops, or comparable antibiotics, to the eyes of all newborn infants has drastically reduced its incidence. Many doctors also recommend that pregnant women be tested for gonorrhea before giving birth.

grants   Grants are available from the federal government to disabled individuals and agencies serving the visually impaired. The grants may be in the form of formula grants, block grants, or discretionary grants.

Formula grants are funds allocated to local and state governmental agencies rather than individuals or institutions. They provide support for established major state programs concerning the disabled. The amounts of the grants are determined by criteria such as population, per capita income, unemployment rate, and percent of population made up of disabled individuals or disabled veterans.

Block grants also provide ongoing support for programs for the disabled but are specially designed to fund programs that have been consolidated into another program and were formerly separately funded. Although states are allowed great discretion in dividing the block grant funds among the various consolidated programs, general guidelines of percentages are usually set.

Discretionary grants are distributed to state and local governments and dispersed to other institutions, including universities and private organizations. Unlike formula or block grants, discretionary grants fund small, undiversified programs. They are administered by a federal agency and often include grants for training, research, experimentation, demonstration, evaluation, planning, construction, fellowships, and scholarships.

The Office of Management and Budget publishes the *Catalog of Federal Domestic Assistance,* which describes federal programs, projects, and services that provide public assistance or benefits. The catalog lists goals, guidelines, eligibility requirements, application process, and specific interest location indices. The catalog is available from the Superintendent of Documents, U.S. Government Printing Office, Washington, DC 20402 (202-783-3238). It can also be accessed on the Internet at the Catalog of Federal Domestic Assistance website at www.cdfa.gov.

The *Federal Register* is a daily periodical that informs the public of all federal agency regulations, funding information, and policy changes. It provides information concerning federal grant background data, eligibility requirements, and funding information.

The *Federal Register* is available in public libraries and in many organizations that serve the disabled. It can be obtained through the Superintendent of Documents for subscription and is available on DIALOG Information Services and System Development Corporation. It can also be found online at the National Archives and Records Administration website at www.access.gpo.gov/su_docs/aces/aces.

Graves's disease   Graves's disease or hyperthyroidism is a disorder of the immune system. The Irish doctor Robert Graves first described the disease in 1835.

The disease is hereditary and affects approximately one of every 1,000 people. It is often diagnosed among young women and teenage girls or among late-middle-aged persons of either sex.

The disease was once thought to be caused by stress but is now recognized as a disorder of the autoimmune system. In this disorder, the immune system produces antibodies against cells in the thyroid gland causing it to overproduce hormones. The hormones, which regulate the body's metabolism, increase the metabolism in many of the body's tissues causing the symptoms of nervousness, weight loss, sensitivity to heat, and tremors.

Graves's disease is treated with medication or radioactive iodine treatments. Drugs such as methimazole, pills that block thyroid hormone production, may be prescribed. As a side effect, they may rapidly destroy the body's white cells and are therefore generally used for short periods only.

Radioactive iodine treatments involve drinking a liquid solution containing radioactive iodine. The iodine treatments destroy the thyroid gland after two to three months. After the thyroid gland ceases to function, a daily hormone supplement pill is taken to sustain appropriate hormone levels. The radioactive iodine treatments have been used successfully for 40 years and have relatively few side effects. In some cases, surgery to remove most of the thyroid gland is performed.

In some cases, Graves's disease may also develop into Graves's dermopathy or Graves's ophthalmopathy. Graves's dermopathy is a rare condition in which the skin becomes inflamed due to a dysfunction in the immune system.

Over half of all patients with Graves's disease develop Graves's ophthalmopathy. It is a condition in which the immune system attacks the muscles and tissues of the eyes.

Symptoms of Graves's ophthalmopathy may include mild conjunctivitis, tearing, eyelid retraction, protruding eyeballs, and impaired or constricted vision. Eyelid retraction and protrusion of the eyeballs may lead to exposure keratitis, an inflammation of the cornea and corneal ulceration.

Symptoms of Graves's ophthalmopathy may be exhibited in the absence of other symptoms of Graves's disease. It may be seen in patients previously treated with radioactive iodine or in those who are without thyroid dysfunction. The condition is serious, and although it may spontaneously resolve itself after three or four years, it can cause blindness before resolution if the condition is not treated.

If the symptoms are mild, the disease may be treated with antibiotic ointments for keratitis and tarsorrhaphy, a stitching of the lids, to improve lid retraction. In more severe cases, steroids may be prescribed to reduce swelling. Muscle surgery and surgery for decompression of the orbits may become necessary.

It is recommended that people with Graves's ophthalmopathy care for their eyes by applying cool compresses to sooth them. Also, wearing sunglasses protects vulnerable eyes from ultraviolet light and bright light, which can be uncomfortable. Lubricating eyedrops may relieve dry, scratchy sensations on the eyes. And elevating the head to keep the head higher than the body reduces the blood flow to the head and may relieve pressure on the eyes.

Guide Dog Foundation for the Blind, Inc.   Guide Dog Foundation for the Blind, Inc., founded in 1946, is a nonprofit organization that breeds and trains dog guides for qualified blind clients.

Qualified clients must be legally blind, physically ambulatory, and in good physical health and a minimum of 16 years old. The applicant must be able to provide adequate food, housing, and care for the dog.

The organization breeds golden retrievers and Labrador retrievers. The dogs and their new owners receive training together over a 25-day in-residence instruction period.

The dog, training in its use and care, and in-residence services are provided free of charge. The foundation receives no governmental aid but relies on corporate and private contributions.

Contact:

Guide Dog Foundation for the Blind, Inc.
371 E. Jerico Turnpike
Smithtown, NY 11787
631-265-2121 or 1-800-548-4337 (ph)
631-361-5192 (fax)

The organization can be located on the Internet at www.guidedog.org.

Guide Dogs for the Blind, Inc.   A nonprofit organization founded in 1942 that provides trained dog guides for use by qualified blind individuals. The school breeds and trains German shepherds,

Labrador retrievers and golden retrievers and provides in-residence training for blind individuals in the use of dog guides. It has placed more than 7,500 dogs with people since its start.

Licensed instructors from the school provide dog-guide recipients with a 28-day training course in dog-guide use, grooming and care and provide follow-up services to clients. Qualified recipients must be legally blind, over age 16, and physically and temperamentally suited to use a dog guide.

Guide Dogs for the Blind, Inc. is supported by voluntary contributions in the form of memberships, memorial and honorary gifts, grants, and bequests. Clients are not charged a fee for the dog, the in-residence training in the dog's use, transportation to and from the school, dog handling equipment, or follow-up services. The organization has training facilities in San Rafael, California, and Boring, Oregon. Its headquarters are in San Rafael.

Contact:

Guide Dogs for the Blind, Inc.
P.O. Box 151200
San Rafael, CA 94915
415-499-4000 or 800-295-4050
www.guidedogs.com

Guiding Eyes for the Blind (GEB) A nonprofit training school and breeding farm of dog guides. Founded in 1954, GEB breeds and trains Labrador retrievers, German shepherds and golden retrievers, and provides in-residence training to qualified blind clients from around the world. It has matched more than 5,000 dog/people teams.

Dog-guide applicants must be 16 years of age, legally blind, ambulatory, self-motivated, and physically and psychologically able to care for a dog. GEB accepts applications from those with multiple handicaps, and there is no maximum age limit. Dog-guide recipients receive in-residence training over a 26-day period. Services are provided at no charge.

Students provide their own transportation to and from the school, but GEB may pay transportation costs or find a sponsor to pay if the applicant cannot afford to do so. GEB receives no governmental funding and is supported by corporate and personal contributions.

Contact:

Guiding Eyes for the Blind, Inc.
611 Granite Springs Road
Yorktown Heights, NY 10598
800-942-0149 or 914-245-4024 (ph)
914-245-1609 (fax)
www.guiding-eyes.org

Guide Horse Foundation Founded in 1999 by Janet Burleson, a former horse trainer, the Guide Horse Foundation trains small horses known as dwarfed, or pigmy, horses to assist visually impaired people with travel.

Burleson decided to begin training small horses to assist blind people after she and her husband, Don, rented and rode standard-size horses during a visit to Central Park in New York City. They were extremely impressed with the horses' ability to remain calm even in heavy traffic and with how they understood that they could turn right on a red light. When Burleson returned to her home in Kittrell, North Carolina, she taught her pet dwarfed horse, Twinkie, to lead a blind woman through the local mall.

The program is still very new, and horses are just beginning to be placed with visually impaired people. The foundation depends on volunteers to donate, train, and deliver trained horses to those who need them and has a waiting list of more than 30 people who would like to have a trained horse for assistance.

Contact:

Guide Horse Foundation
2729 Rocky Ford Road
Kittrell, NC 27544
252-433-4755
www.guidehorse.com

guide horses Used in much the same way as guide dogs, guide horses are a mobility alternative for visually impaired people. They typically are small horses, known as dwarfed or pigmy horses. Although horses have been recognized for their ability to guide and lead for many years, they only recently have been trained to assist visually impaired people.

The Guide Horse Foundation, located in North Carolina, trains horses that meet the criteria to be a guide horse and provides the animals free of charge to visually impaired people who qualify. The horses must pass a physical examination by an equine veterinarian and are tested for intelligence. They must be no more than 26 inches high at the withers, must have structurally sound legs, and demonstrate good stamina.

Guide horses are recommended for rural or suburban use. They are popular among blind people who are allergic to dogs or afraid of dogs, those who love horses, and those who want an animal with a longer life span than a dog has. Dwarfed horses typically live to be between 25 and 35 years old and have been known to live to be 50. Advocates say that horses are easier for people who have physical disabilities to use than dogs are, due to the docile nature of the dwarfed animals. And, some people prefer using horses because they can be housed outside. Horses are natural guide animals, have good memories, and remain calm in difficult situations when trained to do so. Because their eyes are located on the sides of their heads, they have a very wide range of vision. They also have very good night vision. They are trained to wear special sneakers so they do not skid on smooth surfaces.

The Guide Horse Foundation reports that dwarfed horses are very clean and can be housebroken. They do not get fleas, and horses shed only twice a year. Although the organization recognizes that guide horses are not right for everyone, it claims that many people do extremely well with the small animals and are able to move very confidently with them. More information about guide horses can be obtained by contacting:

Guide Horse Foundation
2729 Rocky Ford Road
Kittrell, NC 27544
252-433-4755

Hadley School for the Blind The Hadley School for the Blind, founded in 1920 by William A. Hadley, offers over 100 accredited home-study instruction courses for blind and visually impaired individuals throughout the world. Courses range from those for high school diploma and college preparation to adult-education courses.

The courses cover six categories of education, including academic, vocational, personal enrichment, parent/child, compensatory, and rehabilitation and technical. Course materials are available in braille or cassette textbook form by mail or telephone. Some also are available online.

Hadley School courses are available tuition free to legally and functionally blind individuals, those with a hearing impairment with prognosis of visual loss, and sighted professional, paraprofessional, or family members interested in assisting blind and deaf-blind students enrolled at Hadley. Students must be able to read and understand course material written at high school level.

Contact:

Hadley School for the Blind
700 Elm Street
Winnetka, IL 60093
800-323-4238 (ph)
847-446-0855 (fax)
www.hadley-school.org

handicap There is no complete consensus on terms concerning the topic of blindness and vision impairment, since experts in the field (educators, rehabilitation specialists, doctors) define the TERMINOLOGY according to their own preferences and viewpoints. In recent years, those involved in the field of blindness and vision impairment have made efforts to standardize terms such as handicap to eliminate confusion or misinterpretation.

The word *handicap* stems from "cap in hand," a reference to beggars. Because of this negative connotation, the word *disability* is often the preferred term. When the term *visually handicapped* is applied to a child it usually refers to the requirement for special educational provisions due to the sight loss.

Hansen's disease See LEPROSY.

haptic sense The haptic sense refers to the sense of touch. It is used extensively by blind and visually impaired individuals to gather information. The other senses of hearing, taste, smell, and sight are associated with a central organ to receive the information and transmit it to the brain. The haptic sense is not centrally located but receives information throughout the body via the skin.

The haptic sense defines temperature, shape, size, texture, moisture and consistency, movement, and presence. It is used as a compensation for sight, as in the performance of tasks, or perceptually, as in reading braille or using an abacus. Early stimulation of the haptic sense is especially important to blind infants and children. It helps to link the infant to the surrounding world and indicate the presence of a protective or loving person.

Blind infants and children rely heavily on the haptic sense for developmental progress. Since the lips and hands of the body have large concentrations of sensitive haptic receptors, blind children tend to mouth and handle objects longer than sighted children in an effort to gain information. Blind and visually impaired children rely on the haptic sense for aid in movement and exploration, essential developmental activities. Tactual experiences such as fondling a stuffed animal may be stimulating for a blind child and alleviate the need to develop self-stimulating behaviors such as rocking.

Factors such as the ability to move the hands, finger dexterity, wrist flexibility, and motor control may affect the effectiveness of the haptic sense. If the haptic sense itself is impaired, information gathering may be impaired. Those who have lost sensitivity of touch in the fingertips due to diabetic neuropathy may be unable to feel the detail necessary to read braille, and those with motor-control problems may be unable to direct the hands in place to gather information.

heat cautery   See PHOTOCOAGULATION.

Helen Keller International (HKI)   An American, nonprofit, voluntary organization that works with foreign countries to prevent blindness, treat eye disorders and assist those who are permanently blind. It was founded in 1915 by Helen Keller and others to assist European servicemen blinded in World War I. It has since offered aid to 80 nations but now works exclusively in developing countries.

HKI provides aid to countries developing eye-care components to basic health services. It works with governments and voluntary organizations to improve blindness-prevention programs by providing managerial and material aid.

The agency trains and sends eye-care professionals to rural areas and eye surgeons to urban hospitals. The personnel diagnose and treat eye disorders and refer patients for additional care.

The organization distributes vitamin-A capsules to fight blindness resulting from malnutrition. It conducts programs that offer nutritional education and food fortification to alleviate vitamin A deficiency in the diet.

HKI works to integrate permanently blind children and adults into the activities of their families, villages, and towns. The organization trains counselors, fieldworkers, and schoolteachers in the development of community-based education and rehabilitation programs. Programs include counseling parents of blind children, education of school-age children, daily living skills training, and adult vocational training.

The agency surveys the causes and rates of blindness in an area and maintains data on the effectiveness of the treatment provided. Recent studies by the organization have concluded that vitamin A distribution has not only alleviated blindness due to malnutrition, but has also helped to improve child survival rates.

Contact:

Helen Keller International
90 West Street, 2nd Floor
New York, NY 10006
212-766-5266 (ph)
212-791-7590 (fax)
www.hki.org

Helen Keller National Center for Deaf-blind Youths and Adults (HKNC)   A comprehensive rehabilitation, research and training facility established in 1967 by an act of Congress. HKNC is funded by annual Congressional appropriations and is operated by Helen Keller Services for the Blind, under supervision of the Rehabilitation Services Administration.

The HKNC program consists of training and research headquarters in Sands Point, Long Island, New York, 10 Regional Offices, and extensive Affiliated Agency Programs. The residential school at the headquarters offers instruction in orientation and mobility, communication skills, speech, auditory and low-vision training, basic education, work-experience programs, psychological and medical services, industrial arts, daily living skills, home management, industrial arts, creative arts, leisure activities, and horticulture.

The Regional Offices support state and local agencies serving deaf-blind persons by offering assistance and consultation services. Regional Representatives locate and refer deaf-blind persons to appropriate services, aid in resettlement, assist in finding employment opportunities, and serve as an advocate for services to the deaf-blind population.

HKNC provides temporary financial support to Affiliated Agency Programs, public or private agencies that work to develop or expand services to deaf-blind individuals throughout the country. The center acts as a clearinghouse and resource center of information for the deaf-blind, their families, and professionals working in related fields. It maintains a National Register of deaf-blind individuals to provide statistics concerning the deaf-blind population that are used in planning appropriate services.

HKNC designs and improves sensory aids, maintains a National Training Team that works in the field, offers training seminars to rehabilitation workers, and sustains a Community Education Program to educate the public as to the needs and abilities of deaf-blind persons.

Contact:

Helen Keller National Center for Deaf-Blind
   Youths and Adults
111 Middle Neck Road
Sands Point, NY 11050
516-944-8900 (ph)
516-944-8637 (TTY)
516-944-7302 (fax)
www.helenkeller.org/national

helping blind people   See ETIQUETTE.

hemianopsia   A loss of vision in one-half of the eye. This results in a loss of the right or left half of the field of vision. Objects or people in the field of vision may appear to be cut in half.

Hemianopsia is a common symptom of migraine headaches. It occurs during the preheadache or prodrome stage. The loss of vision may be accompanied by shimmering zigzag light patterns and blind spots called scotomas. Hemianopsia accompanying migraines usually lasts from five minutes to one hour. The lost vision generally returns with the onset of the headache.

Retinal migraine occurs when a spasm occurs in the blood vessels in the retina of one eye. One half of the vision of the affected eye is lost but the unaffected eye retains full vision. The condition is temporary and abates with the migraine.

Hemianopsia is also associated with strokes. As a result of a stroke, vision may be blurred or lost in one half of the field of vision, or the entire vision in one eye may be lost. Recovery of this visual loss depends on the damage done during the stroke and the progress made during recovery.

As a result of a focal transient ischemic attack, a temporary disruption of the flow of blood to the brain and eye, the vision may be lost and then may suddenly return in a matter of minutes. Usually, the vision lost due to these attacks is completely recovered within 24 hours.

herpes simplex   A virus that causes most corneal blindness due to infection in the United States. According to the National Institutes of Health, 500,000 cases of ocular herpes simplex are diagnosed each year. Herpes simplex is the most common virus found in humans.

Herpes simplex is one of four types of herpes virus that also include HERPES ZOSTER, cytomegalovirus, and Epstein-Barr virus. Herpes simplex may infect the genitals, skin, brain, and eyes. All herpes viruses contain a central core of DNA, the genetic code of the organism, enveloped by a layer of protein. The organism cannot reproduce itself but must obtain reproduction molecules from a healthy host human cell. The virus invades a healthy cell and uses its molecular properties to reproduce. After prolific reproduction, the host cell may burst.

Herpes simplex virus cells usually enter the body through the mouth, genitals, or eyes. In the past, those infections that occurred above the waist were commonly referred to as Type I, and those below the waist were referred to as Type II. However, the above and below the waist categorizations are used less commonly since Type I herpes is now frequently seen below the waist and Type II is increasingly diagnosed above the waist.

Approximately 90 percent of the population has been exposed to and infected by herpes simplex. Most first infections are generally Type I and usually infect the mouth. The symptoms of fatigue and a low-grade fever may go unnoticed. Others may have a more severe infection that is called primary herpes. In each case, the infection appears to run its course, and the symptoms disappear.

After the symptoms subside, the virus has not been killed. Herpes simplex Type I passes through nerves in the mouth or skin to deep nerve tissue centers, called ganglia, located the base of the brain and upper spinal cord. Herpes Type II travels through nerves to the ganglia at the base of the spinal cord. Here the virus lies dormant. The virus may remain dormant or reactivate and reinfect the body. During latency, healthy host cells are not infected, and the virus cannot be passed to others.

Herpes simplex may infect the eyes in one of three ways: congenitally, primarily, or recurrently. Congenital herpes is contracted by infants during birth. If the mother has active genital herpes, the infant may become exposed to the virus when the water breaks or when traveling through the birth canal. It is estimated that 1 of every 7,000 births involves infection of the newborn from the maternal reproductive system.

Congenital herpes is a serious disease that carries a fatality rate of 50 percent. Survivors may retain permanent damage to the eyes, brain, liver, or kidneys. Damage to the eyes usually concerns the retina but may also entail the CONJUNCTIVA, OPTIC NERVE, LENS, and CORNEA.

If the mother is aware of an active case of genital herpes, a Caesarean section delivery may avoid newborn infection. However, mothers are often unaware of the infection when the symptoms are mild or hidden, or when the virus is a first infection. In these cases, congenital herpes may be unpreventable.

Primary herpes infection of the eyes is rare in adults and generally occurs only in children or adolescents. The symptoms include fever, fatigue, swollen eyelids, CONJUNCTIVITIS, and a blistering rash around the eyes. The infection is usually mild and short-lived. It can be treated with antiviral eye drops or ointments.

Recurrent ocular herpes is an eye infection, usually involving only one eye, which happen as a result of a reawakening of the herpes virus. The virus, which may have first infected the mouth, travels to the fifth nerve ganglion, the trigeminal, where it remains dormant. The fifth ganglion has connecting fibers to the upper part of the face, including the eyes. On reactivation, the virus travels back up these fibers and infects the eye.

A recurrent infection is typified by redness, pain and a watery discharge of the eye. Herpes keratitis, or corneal infection, iritis, an infection of the iris, glaucoma, and cataracts may result from this infection. As the eye attempts to heal itself, corneal scarring may develop, followed by loss of vision. Each recurrence increases the possibility of scarring and vision loss.

Most patients do not experience a recurrence after an initial recurrent attack. A patient has a 25 percent chance of a new recurrence within five years of the first and the possibility of additional recurrences increases with each attack. However, the virus is unpredictable, and the recurrences may suddenly discontinue for no known reason.

Herpes keratitis is treated with the drugs vidarabine, trifluridine, idoxuridine, acyclovir, and antiviral eye drops or ointments. These drugs are not a cure for herpes. They stop the reproduction of viral cells but cannot rid the body of the virus. During periods of dormancy, the drugs are ineffective in fighting the virus.

Severe scarring is treated with cortisone eye drops. Cortisone is a steroid that may actually worsen the herpes infection and is therefore used only for short periods of time. Severe vision loss due to scarring may in some cases be corrected with a CORNEAL TRANSPLANT, or keratoplasty.

U.S. Department of Health and Human Services. *Vision Research: Report of the Corneal Diseases Panel.* vol. 2, part 2, NIH Publication No. 83-2472 (1987) Washington, D.C.: USDHHS.

Review of Optometry Online. "Handbook of Ocular Disease Management, Herpes Simplex Keratitis." www.revoptom.com/handbook/sect3m: 2001.

herpes zoster   Herpes zoster, or shingles, is a painful skin disease that may involve the eye. It is caused by the same virus that causes chicken pox or varicella. According to the National Institutes of Health, it is responsible for roughly 7 percent of all skin disorders, a substantial amount of which affect the eye. If you have shingles on your face to any extent, it is extremely important to see your eye doctor promptly.

Generally, only one eye is affected. Complications may include corneal ulcers, scarring and cataracts, which can cause loss of vision. Additional conditions may include recurrent KERATITIS (corneal inflammation), increased eye pressure resulting in GLAUCOMA, UVEITIS, secondary infections, and eye-muscle paralysis.

Treatment of eye disease caused by zoster is problematic. Corneal ulcers are often treated with soft contact lenses that remain on the affected eye for a period of months until the ulcers heal.

Keratitis is treated with antiviral drops or ointments. These drugs are effective only when the virus is active. During periods of latency, they are impotent. Since the virus is not destroyed, it may become active again and the keratitis may recur.

Glaucoma is treated with medication or eye drops and CATARACTS may eventually be removed. Eye muscle paralysis is not treatable with medication or therapy but usually heals itself in time.

Zoster scarring causes unique problems. Vision loss caused by zoster scarring cannot be corrected by corneal transplantation. The scarred cornea becomes vascularized, a condition in which blood vessels invade the cornea and interfere with post-transplantation healing. In addition, there may be lid abnormalities and epithelial or tear function disorders as a result of the scarring, which further complicate a transplant. An unsuccessful cornea transplant may develop complications during healing that could result in the loss of the eye.

U.S. Department of Health and Human Services. *Vision Research: Report of the Corneal Diseases Panel,* vol. 2, part 2, NIH Publication No. 83-2472 (1987). Washington, D.C.: USDHHS.

Herplex   See IDOXURIDINE.

Higher Education Act   Enacted in 1965 to encompass and expand existing federal laws such as the Morrill Act, the GI Bill, and the National Defense Education Act.

Originally, the act provided grants and guaranteed loans for tuition and financial aid for instructional materials or equipment. Additionally, the act supported college libraries and community support services, founded the Teacher Corps, and included policy-making language that increased accessibility of handicapped and educationally disadvantaged students to higher education.

Amendments made in 1972, 1976, 1980, and 1998 to revise the act included the creation of new grants and loans. Some of the accompanying conditions and stipulations of the loans aided disabled students.

Under Part E, Title IV, low-interest Perkins loans were authorized for students lacking financial means. These loans, awarded through universities and colleges, could be canceled after the student's graduation if the student entered a public-service field. These fields included teaching full time in a public or nonprofit school for disabled students. A portion of the loan is canceled for each year of public service. Loans awarded through the National Defense Student Loan Program are also eligible for cancellation by these amendments.

Under Title VII, the act addresses accessibility and usability of university and college buildings by disabled students. The Rehabilitation Act of 1973 and the Architectural Barriers Act of 1968 prohibit discrimination toward disabled people in federally funded programs, including barring access to institutions or buildings. Title VII funds reconstruction or renovation grants that can be used to correct barriers in existing buildings or to construct new buildings in accordance with the Architectural Barriers Act of 1968.

U.S. Department of Education. *Summary of Existing Legislation Affecting Persons with Disabilities.* Washington, D.C.: USDE, 1988.

Hoover, Richard E.   Richard E. Hoover is credited with developing the long cane foot travel system, a method of independent traveling using a long cane as an aid.

Born in 1915, Hoover began as a teacher and physical training coach at Maryland School for the Blind. At the time, there was no comprehensive system for teaching blind people how to use the existing cane of the time, the white cane. Hoover found the white cane too short, heavy, and awkward for efficient mobility use.

As an army sergeant (and later lieutenant) in World War II, he was transferred to the Valley Forge General Hospital in Phoenixville, Pennsylvania, to work as the eye center's director of physical reconditioning, orientation, and recreation. Convinced that the men needed a lighter, longer cane, he experimented with several adaptations of the white cane until he developed the prototype for the long cane. The new cane was made of metal with a plastic tip and a crook at the top. It was up to 10 inches longer than the white cane, half the diameter, and weighed only seven ounces.

Hoover developed a series of techniques for using the long cane in sweeping arc movements, low, in front of the body, rather than by the side. The techniques were incorporated into the orientation and mobility program that was then transferred to the Veterans Administration Hospital at Hines, Illinois, where word of its achievements spread.

Today, the Hoover methods and the long cane are universal components of orientation and mobility programs. Hoover entered medical school after World War II and became a distinguished ophthalmologist. He died in 1986.

hordeolum   An infection on the outside or inside of the eyelid, also called a sty. An external hordeolum is an infection of an eyelash follicle. As the sty begins to form, the entire lid swells and becomes painful. A localized area on the lid margin then becomes red and swollen with pus. If untreated, the sty eventually bursts, drains, and heals itself.

An internal hordeolum is a sty on the inside of the eyelid. It is the result of an infection of a gland. If untreated, the hordeolum becomes inflamed and swollen, and is called a chalazion. These chalazia normally do not affect vision unless they are located in the middle of the upper eyelid, where they can flatten the central cornea and distort sight. Sties can be treated by holding a warm, damp cloth over the site for 20 minutes, three or four times a day. Most sties and chalazia go away on their own, without medication.

Housing Act of 1949   As amended, the Housing Act of 1949, Title V, allows direct, insured loans for the establishment and renovation of rural housing. The Housing and Community Development Amendments of 1977 allowed people with disabilities to participate in the program. A "handicapped" person, as described in Title V, is anyone with a permanent or long-term impairment that obstructs independent living and whose ability would be improved by better housing. Those with developmental disabilities are considered eligible by the act.

Two major programs offered by Title V affect disabled people. These housing-assistance programs are established under Section 515 and Section 521 of the act.

Section 515 offers guaranteed or insured loans to owners of rural property rented by elderly or disabled persons. The loans may be used to purchase or construct new property, to improve existing property, to add special designs or equipment such as ramps or grab bars to aid the elderly or disabled, or to fund recreational or related services or facilities. The loans are disallowed for nursing homes or special-care institutions.

The loans may be granted to individuals, partnerships, cooperatives, nonprofit organizations or trusts. Loan recipients must have sufficient security and income to repay the loan and be able to accept all related loan obligations.

Section 521 of the act establishes direct rent subsidies for low-income families, including disabled or elderly persons. The families must live in rural rentals, rural cooperative housing, or farm-labor housing. Families pay up to 30 percent of their net income toward rent. A subsidy payment is made to the landlord to compensate for the difference between this payment and comparable rental housing prices.

The Housing Act of 1949 was celebrated and commemorated on its 50th anniversary. Ceremonies were held November 3, 1999, at the National Building Museum in Washington, D.C., to mark the anniversary.

U.S. Department of Education. *Summary of Existing Legislation Affecting Persons with Disabilities.* Washington, D.C.: USDE, 1988.

Housing Act of 1959   The Housing Act of 1959, Section 202, establishes direct long-term federal loans to build, renovate, or manage rental housing for disabled and elderly people. The loans are granted to private nonprofit organizations or corporations and consumer cooperatives at below-market interest rates. The funds may be used to construct basic housing units or related facilities such as cafeterias, recreation halls, or medical-services buildings.

Families are eligible for such housing if their household consist of one or more persons who are disabled or 62 years of age or older. Rental subsidies described under Section 8 of the Lower Income Housing Program of the United States Housing Act of 1937 are available for this housing.

The Supportive Housing Demonstration Program is also described and funded by this act. The program contains transitional and permanent housing projects for homeless disabled people. A homeless disabled person is described by the act as one who has a handicap and is homeless or at risk of becoming homeless or is living in a transitional home.

The transitional program supplies temporary housing and assistive services for homeless people. The program strives to find permanent housing for residents within 18 months. Services of this program include housing location, medical and psychological care, child care, vocational training, transportation, and other support.

The permanent housing program provides long-term community-based housing and assistive services. Homes must not exceed the resident limit of eight disabled persons.

Assistance for both programs fund the purchase, rehabilitation, or renovation of existing facilities, grants for modest renovation, transitional program operating costs and HUD technical support.

Section 232 of the Housing Act establishes federal mortgage insurance to finance or renovate board-and-care homes, intermediate-care homes, or skilled-nursing facilities. This loan insurance may be used to fund construction or rehabilitation of facilities sheltering 20 or more people who need skilled-nursing services or who require limited, continuous services by skilled or licensed personnel.

U.S. Department of Education. *Summary of Existing Legislation Affecting Persons with Disabilities.* Washington, D.C.: USDE, 1988.

Housing and Community Development Act of 1974

The Housing and Community Development Act of 1974 authorized block grants as federal aid to urban areas. The grants are administered under a program called the Community Development Block Grant program or CDBG. The grants finance a variety of projects, including those that benefit people with disabilities.

Under Title I of this act, cities and urban counties may apply for entitlement grants. A formula based on the population, income level, and availability of housing in the area is used to determine qualification. Title I funds may be used to improve conditions for disabled people by financing improvement of access to buildings, removal of architectural barriers, and renovation or construction of facilities, including public centers for disabled persons.

The funding application outlines area housing and development needs and specifies long- and short-term goals to meet these needs. A list of necessary actions, their locations, the resulting costs, and contributing resources is included. Maps are added to show areas in which ethnic groups or low-income families are concentrated.

The application requires a Housing Assistance Plan that outlines the area's available housing and evaluates future housing-assistance needs for low-income families. From these figures, one-year and three-year housing assistance goals are determined and listed. The plan suggests locations for construction of new facilities or renovation of existing facilities.

Title I outlines nonentitlement grants as well. These grants fund urban community-development and housing projects for non-entitlement areas. The funds may finance a variety of services, including the construction or purchase of public works facilities, urban or economic renewal projects, and housing renovation or code enforcement.

The act was amended in 1999 to establish and sustain affordable housing in rural and remote areas affected by very low income levels and excessive outmigration.

U.S. Department of Education. *Summary of Existing Legislation Affecting Persons with Disabilities,* Washington, D.C.: USDE, 1988.

Howe Press

The Howe Press of Perkins School for the Blind was established as a printing department of the Perkins School for the Blind in 1835. It was renamed the Howe Memorial Press in 1879 after the founding director, Dr. Samuel Gridley Howe, and is commonly called the Howe Press.

The goal of the Howe Press initially was to produce books for the blind in Boston line type, a raised and enlarged Roman alphabet. As braille became the standard medium for books for the blind, the Howe Press began to produce books in braille.

The Howe Press began producing braille writing machines (braillers) in 1900. The Perkins Brailler was developed in 1939 by David Abraham, a Perkins shop teacher. The Howe Press began producing the Perkins Brailler after World War II, and it now concentrates on the manufacture of approximately 5,000 Perkins Braillers per year.

The Howe Press sells the braillers, brailler accessories, brailling slates, slate accessories, handwriting aids and games, mathematical aids, music, maps, and braille paper by mail-order catalog.

Contact:

Howe Press of Perkins School for the Blind
175 North Beacon Street
Watertown, MA 02172-2790
617-924-3490 (ph)
617-926-2027 (fax)

Howe, Samuel Gridley   Samuel Gridley Howe was born in 1801 in Boston. He graduated from Harvard Medical School in 1824 and offered his services for six years as a soldier and surgeon to Greece during the Greek War of Independence against Turkey. He continued to raise money for relief shipments after his return to America in 1831.

In 1829, the New England Asylum for the Blind, the first school for the blind in the United States, was incorporated. In 1831, the state of Massachusetts hired Howe to serve as director. Howe journeyed to Europe to study prototypes and returned in 1832 with two teachers. He opened the school in his home with six pupils. The school was renamed the New England Institution for the Education of the Blind and finally the Perkins School for the Blind after a wealthy philanthropist, Thomas Handasyd Perkins, who donated a mansion to house the school.

Howe developed new methods and devices for instruction of the blind, including a variation of raised-letter printing and textbooks on geography, grammar, and spelling. He became internationally renowned for his successful instruction of Laura Bridgman, a deaf-blind girl who became his student in 1837.

Howe founded a school printing department in 1831 to produce reading materials for the students. In 1879, three years after his death, the printing department was named the Howe Memorial Press in his honor.

Throughout his 44 years as director of Perkins School, he maintained an activism in the abolition of slavery and reform of public schools, prisons, and treatment of the insane. In 1843, he married Julia Ward, author of the words for "The Battle Hymn of the Republic." He died in 1876.

HumanWare, Inc.   HumanWare Inc., formerly Sensory Aids Corporation, is a company that manufactures products and tailors services for use by both disabled and nondisabled individuals. The goal of the company is to make technology more accessible to the nontechnical person while providing features attractive to those with highly developed technical skills.

Located in Loomis, California, the company is a unit of Arianne Beheer B.V. of the Netherlands. Arianne Beheer is owner of several companies that together make up the world's largest manufacturer of low-vision devices. HumanWare is a major distributor of print-access products for people who are blind or have reading and learning disabilities. It works closely with the Overbrook School for the Blind in Philadelphia to implement advanced classroom technology for Overbrook students and staff.

HumanWare print-access products include braille terminals, braille printers, CCTVs, talking palmtop organizers, specially configured talking computers, scanners, and reading systems. The firm also provides reading and writing software and self-contained reading systems incorporating speech synthesis for people with learning difficulties or low reading competency. The company recently introduced Braille Note and Voice Note, new Windows CE-based personal note takers, and Braille Voyager, a new kind of braille terminal.

A complete listing, descriptions, and prices of HumanWare's products are available on the company's website at www.humanware.com.

Contact:

HumanWare, Inc.
6245 King Road
Loomis, CA 95650
800-722-3393 or 916-652-7253 (ph)
916-652-7296 (fax)

hyperopia   Hyperopia is farsightedness. This occurs when the CORNEA and LENS cannot clearly focus an image onto the RETINA. This is the result of weak focusing power or eyes that are too "small" or "short" for their refracting capabilities.

Farsighted people generally see far objects more clearly than near objects. Convergent or convex corrective lenses are usually prescribed for either eyeglasses or contact lenses. In some cases, surgery can be performed to correct farsightedness.

Babies are often born farsighted because of their small eyes. They maintain strong focusing power to offset the problem, and seldom require correction except in severe cases or in the presence of additional eye disorders.

hypertensive retinopathy   The name given for the effects of hypertension on the eye's RETINA. The retina is the light-sensitive layer in the back of the eye that receives light and encodes it into electrical impulses. The impulses travel from the OPTIC NERVE to the brain, where they are translated into an image.

Hypertension is a term for high blood pressure. It is a condition commonly associated with aging and occurs when the small arteries of the body lose elasticity and become clogged, a condition called ARTERIOSCLEROSIS. The blocked arteries become smaller in diameter, and the blood flows slower and less smoothly.

As the blood supply is decreased to vital organs, serious consequences may result. Heart attacks and heart failure, strokes, angina, kidney disease, and poor circulation are often attributable to hypertension and arteriosclerosis.

Hypertension and arteriosclerosis can affect the blood vessels in the retina. The vessels may become constricted, causing bleeding or fluid leakage. The condition may lead to infarcts, localized areas of tissue-cell destruction due to lack of oxygen. In severe cases, the damage to the retina may destroy vision.

Hypertension tends to run in families and may be hereditary. It is also associated with obesity, smoking, and lack of exercise. Many cases of hypertension and the accompanying retinopathy exhibit few outward symptoms of the condition. The patient may be unaware of the hypertension and may be first alerted to it during a routine medical or ophthalmologic exam. Since hypertensive retinopathy has few symptoms in the early stages, the condition rarely requires therapy. The underlying cause of hypertension is treated with medication, diet and exercise.

hypertropia   A condition of STRABISMUS, or misaligned eyes. Often termed squint or crossed-eyes, strabismus may cause visual problems or loss of vision. Hypertropia is a type of strabismus in which one eye turns upward. *Hypotropia* is condition in which one eye turns downward. As in all strabismus, the eyes fail to converge on an object and view two differing subjects. The brain receives the two images, and double vision results. Often, in an effort to reconcile the two pictures, the brain may suppress one completely, causing partial vision loss. This results in a condition called AMBLYOPIA.

Strabismus is associated with high amounts of MYOPIA (nearsightedness), HYPEROPIA (farsightedness) and ASTIGMATISM. It can develop after a major illness or injury, and some forms of strabismus may also be hereditary.

Treatment may include the prescription of eye drops, eyeglasses or bifocals, or exercises. Exercises or eye patching may be prescribed if amblyopia is present. Surgery may be necessary to completely align the eyes.

hyphema   A bleeding into the ANTERIOR CHAMBER of the eye. Hyphemas may occur as a result of an injury or following intraocular surgery such as CATARACT removal. Hyphemas may appear spontaneously due to diabetes-related neovascularization, tumor, juvenile xanthogranulomatosis, or previous vascular occlusions.

Hyphemas due to injury are caused by damage to blood vessels in the IRIS or CILIARY BODY. In most cases, the bleeding slows and then ceases, and the blood is reabsorbed within the eye over a period of a week. Secondary bleeding that starts one to five days following the injury may fill the anterior chamber and elevate intraocular pressure.

The raised intraocular pressure of secondary bleeding may cause secondary glaucoma, a serious result for which children are particularly at risk. The CORNEA may also become permanently blood-stained, causing an opacity or clouded area.

Hyphemas due to surgery are common but much less likely to result in secondary bleeding. The bleeding generally recedes within days, and no further treatment of hyphema is necessary.

Hyphemas are treated initially to prevent secondary bleeding and its consequences. Treatment varies according to the practitioner. Patients may be admitted into the hospital, confined to bed rest for several days, treated with cycloplegics, which widen the pupil, or with steroids or undergo patching of the eyes.

Secondary bleeding may be treated surgically. Medication is given to reduce intraocular pressure. The hyphema may be removed or flushed out of the eye with a saline solution.

hypotropia   See HYPERTROPIA.

hysterical blindness   An emotionally caused condition of blindness. The blindness occurs as a result of the need to physically resolve an emotional upset or shock. It also is called psychogenic or psychic blindness.

The blindness is usually bilateral and often occurs suddenly. Often the blindness is not total and is restricted to a particular field. Additional symptoms of hysterical blindness include lack of regard for the loss of sight, ability to travel within surroundings, and normal blink response.

An eye examination is necessary to diagnose hysterical blindness. The examination reveals that the pupils react normally, and the fundus (back of eye) appears normal, discounting damage to the optic nerve, cortical blindness, chiasmal lesions, or other ocular disease. The condition is usually diagnosed in light of information gathered through the eye examination and study of the patient's psychological history.

Treatment of hysterical blindness may include reassurance to the patient that the condition will right itself, presentation to the patient of ability to see, and placebo medicine therapy. The patient may recover from the hysterical blindness only to replace it with another physical illness. Psychiatric counseling is often recommended to address the underlying emotional problem.

Hysterical blindness is not to be confused with malingering, a condition of feigned blindness often undertaken as an attempt to receive continued compensation for an accident or injury.

IBM International Business Machines Corporation (IBM) has established itself as a leader in providing information, training, and assistive devices for people with vision, hearing, speech, and mobility impairments; learning disabilities; and mental retardation. In January 2000 the company opened the IBM Accessibility Center and the IBM Accessibility Research Institute, both based in Austin, Texas. Previously, IBM operated the IBM National Support Center for Persons with Disabilities, located in Atlanta. That organization was integrated with the Accessibility Center, and the Atlanta facilities closed.

The goal of the Accessibility Center is to enable people with disabilities to compete equally in today's electronic society by making sure they have equal access to information, e-business services, and education. The center has facilities and operations in Austin, Japan, and Europe. The IBM Accessibility Research Institute was created to explore emerging technologies and ongoing research generated by IBM's research laboratories and to refer any applicable technology to the Accessibility Center. The Accessibility Center will continue to invest in new technology for assistive devices and will focus on the development of tools that generate accessible applications and middleware software, which could be integrated with IBM products to enhance accessibility. It also will continue working to improve existing assistive devices, such as the Home Page Reader. The Home Page Reader is a talking web browser, which allows users who are blind or visually impaired to fully explore the Internet and take advantage of e-business opportunities. The Home Page Reader software provides JavaScript support, which enables it to speak all information contained on a webpage. The software recognizes and speaks nine languages: English, French, Italian, German, Spanish, Japanese, Chinese, Portuguese, and Finnish.

IBM has developed other products for visually impaired users, such as the Screen Reader, the Page Scanner, Book Manager, and TextReader. More information about these and other products is available on the company's website at www.ibm.com/able. The website also contains information for human resource professionals who are responsible for making information more accessible to employees with disabilities.

Contact:

IBM Accessibility Center
11400 Burnet Road
Building 901, Room 5D-014
Austin, TX 78758

idoxuridine An antimetabolite drug used in the treatment of ocular HERPES. It is also called IDU, Herplex, Stoxil, and Dendrid. It was one of the first drugs developed for the treatment of herpes keratitis, a disorder involving corneal inflammation.

Idoxuridine is activated by enzymes contained in healthy human cells and cannot differentiate between viral and healthy cells. Therefore, while it is effective in destroying viral cells, it unfortunately may attack and destroy healthy cells. Because of the toxicity, idoxuridine cannot be taken intravenously; possible side effects could cause potentially dangerous disorders.

Idoxuridine is available in ointment or eye-drop form. Normal dosing for the ointment is to apply it five times per day. The eye drops normally are administered every hour during the day and every two hours during the night. The period of use for either form is roughly two to three weeks. Dosing varies from patient to patient, however, so the doctor's instructions should be followed.

Idoxuridine is not a cure for herpes keratitis. It is only effective once the virus is active. During periods of latency, the drug is ineffective against the virus. Its ocular side effects include redness and swelling of the conjunctiva and possible irritation of the cornea.

illumination   The density of light falling on a surface. Illumination is a factor in visibility, and control of illumination may result in improved vision for those with impairments.

To properly control illumination, type of light source, intensity of the light source, distance from the light source, surface the light falls on, diffuseness, the amount of glare, and environmental changes must be considered. The best lighting situations involve properly intense, diffuse light from overhead (or the side of usable vision if reading with one eye only) that causes the least amount of shadows and glare.

Light sources commonly include daylight, incandescent light, and fluorescent light. Daylight varies according to time of day and weather conditions. Incandescent lights simulate daylight but in a constant, steady flow. Fluorescent lights may flicker but can be linked and adjusted to eliminate the flicker.

Specially designed lights may be used to maximize residual vision. The BLBS (Better Light Better Sight) lamp is a study lamp constructed according to requirements of the Illuminating Engineering Society of America and incorporates ideal lighting components.

Tensor-type lamps are intense lights that can be adjusted for maximum illumination with limited glare. Small clip-on lamps are available that attach to the sides of spectacle frames.

The intensity of light is measured in footcandles. One footcandle equals the intensity of light that falls on one square foot of a surface located one foot from one international candle.

The intensity of light on an object is controlled by the distance from the light to the object. A lamp two feet from the reading page has four times the light intensity as a lamp four feet away.

The surface the light falls on affects the visibility. An uneven surface may contribute to uneven diffuseness of light, and a smooth, reflective surface may increase glare.

Diffuseness is the distribution of light. Shadows and spotlights may decrease visibility. Glare results from an excess of light, a concentration of light, or an uneven distribution of light, and may decrease visibility.

Illumination may be controlled or manipulated by making changes in the environment as well as the light source. Light transmission, reflection control, and contrast enhancement may be used to maximize available illumination.

Light transmission is improved through lenses, filters, and absorptive lenses that reduce glare and highlight contrast for those with light sensitivity, or photophobia. Lenses, filters, and absorptive lenses are available in a wide range of degrees of protection from simple filters that reduce glare to photochromic lenses that use gray, green, and amber filters to block all ultraviolet light.

Reflection is controlled by visors, side shields, specially treated lenses, and typoscopes. Visors may be supplied by the brim of a hat or can be a filtering visor lens attached to the spectacle frame. Sideshields are filters that attach to the sides of spectacle lenses to control the light on the sides of the eyes.

A typoscope is a slit reading device that isolates one line of type at a time, thus reducing glare from the light reflected from the page. Typoscopes are especially helpful for those with cataracts.

Contrast is enhanced by using highly contrasting colors near one another such as black ink on white or yellow paper or fluorescent strips on stair risers. Contrast for reading pale or bluish print may be improved by using pale yellow tinted lenses or by placing a clear yellow or amber sheet over the page.

Lighting requirements vary according to the age of the individual and the cause of the visual impairment. As the eyes age, they need greater amounts of illumination to function properly. Sixty-year-old eyes need twice as much light to complete a task as 20-year-old eyes.

Eye disorders and conditions may create a need for either reduced or increased light. Those who function best in low light include persons with ALBINISM, ANIRIDIA (lack of IRIS), CATARACT, and corneal opacities. Those who function best in maximum light include those with GLAUCOMA, OPTIC ATROPHY, surgical aphakia (lack of natural lens), MYOPIA, COLOBOMA, and MACULAR DISEASE.

impairment   There is no complete consensus on terms concerning the topic of blindness and vision impairment. Educators, doctors, rehabilitation specialists, and other leaders in the field define TERMINOLOGY according to their own preferences but have recently made efforts to standardize terms such as impairment to eliminate confusion or misinterpretation.

An impairment refers to a recognizable defect or malfunctioning of an organ or any part of the body, such as an eye. The defect or malfunction can be diagnosed and defined by a medical doctor. A visually impaired person may include an individual with no sight as well as someone with low vision.

independent living aids   See ADAPTIVE AIDS.

Independent Living Aids, Inc.   A mail-order company that provides adaptive aids and devices for disabled persons, including visually impaired individuals. Through its catalog, the company offers watches, magnifiers, braille items, canes, writing guides, medical and health related items, adaptive tools and appliances, cooking aids, adaptive games and toys, large-print books, talking items, and portable electronic magnifying viewers.

Contact:

Independent Living Aids, Inc.
200 Robbins Lane
Jericho, NY 11753-2341
800-537-2118
www.independentliving.com

independent-living center   A program of services or a facility that provides a variety of independent living services for persons with disabilities. The services are directed to provide resources, training, counseling, and assistance to promote the independence, productivity, and quality of life of persons with disabilities. They may be supported by federal, state, local, or private funds.

These services may include counseling to determine the individual's need for independent living services, individual counseling, referrals and counseling regarding attendant care, and peer counseling.

An independent living center may offer attendant care and training, advocacy services, legal services, independent living skills training, job-seeking skills training, equipment training, and housing and transportation referral and assistance.

The center may provide community group-living arrangements, health-maintenance programs, education and training for living in the community and participating in community activities, social and recreational activities, interpreter services for deaf and deaf-blind individuals, and reading services for blind individuals.

independent living skills   See DAILY LIVING SKILLS.

Individuals with Disabilities Education Act (IDEA)   Formerly known as Public Law 94–142, this law guarantees that all children between the ages of three and 21 who need special education and services due to a disability will have access to a free and appropriate public education. The law provides money to assist states in providing an individualized education program (IEP) for each student. The IDEA was formerly known as the Education of the Handicapped Act (EHA). The original act—EHA—was implemented in 1975 and changed to IDEA in 1991. IDEA was amended in 1997.

Before 1975, about 1 million disabled children did not have access to public schools, and thousands more did not receive appropriate education in the schools. Ninety percent of children with serious disabilities used to be housed in state institutions and did not attend public schools.

IDEA states that school administrators, teachers, and parents should be involved with developing an individualized education program for each student who needs one. The 1997 amendments to the act, signed into law by President Bill Clinton on June 4, include the following:

- Changes in the formula for distributing federal money to states
- Instruction in braille and the use of braille for visually impaired students, unless braille is not considered by the IEP team to be in the best interests of the child
- More freedom for school districts to serve disabled children who attend private schools
- Requirement for a state to set performance goals for disabled children and a means for mapping progress
- More flexible, but more frequent re-evaluations of children with individualized programs
- Changes in the way in which disputes between the parents of a disabled child and the local education agency are handled
- Changes in the way in which discipline problems involving disabled students are to be handled
- Children with disabilities must be included in statewide and district-wide assessments
- Regular education teachers must be included in IEP teams if there is any possibility that a disabled child will participate in regular class
- Children with disabilities must be given access to the regular curriculum

Office of Special Education and Rehabilitative Services, the U.S. Department of Education. *IDEA '97 Amendments, Final Regulations*. www.ed.gov/offices/OSERS, 2001.

injuries   According to the National Society to Prevent Blindness, nearly 1.3 million people suffer eye injuries each year in the United States. Injuries are responsible for 4 percent of all cases of blindness and 3 percent of all new cases of blindness in the United States each year. Currently, approximately 1 million people have sustained some vision loss due to injuries. Nearly half of these injuries occurred in or around the home in product-related incidences.

Four product groups—construction materials, home products, personal products, and workshop tools—account for more than half of these injuries. Construction materials include nails, metal parts, lumber, and any other building matter. Home products are those used to maintain a household and include bleaches, chemicals, glues, and acids. Personal products consist of items such as contact lenses, sun lamps, combs, and brushes. Home workshop materials encompass tools and machinery, wet cell batteries, and welding gear.

In order of severity, the most hazardous materials are metal debris, contact lenses, and automobiles, followed by batteries, sun lamps, and adhesives or glue. Among children aged five to 14, most accidents involve metal debris, baseball gear, workshop apparatus, and adhesives. Injuries for those aged 15–24 most often involve contact lenses, metal debris, sun lamps, automobiles and batteries. Injuries for those 25–64 generally include metal debris, automobiles, and contact lenses.

Sports or recreational injuries are responsible for nearly 40,000 eye treatments in hospital emergency rooms each year according to the National Society to prevent blindness. The society estimates as many as 100,000 such injuries each year, although not all are reported. Nearly one third of those treated are children five to 14 years of age. Generally, baseball and basketball account for most injuries, followed by racquet sports and football.

It is estimated that 90 percent of all injuries can be prevented if proper precautions are taken to wear protective safety goggles and to store harmful chemicals and spray cans. When a chemical or acid injury occurs, the National Society to Prevent Blindness suggests gently flushing the eyes with water for 15 minutes and immediately obtaining a medical examination. Do not use an eye cup or bandage the eye.

When specks or debris enter the eye, lift the upper eyelid outward and down over the lower lid. If the tears do not wash out the particle, do not rub the eye, keep it closed, bandage it lightly and see a doctor.

When an impact to the eye occurs, apply cold compresses for 15 minutes and each successive hour until pain and swelling are reduced. If the eye becomes discolored, see a doctor.

In the case of a puncture or cut to the eye, do not wash with water or try to remove a foreign body. Bandage the eye lightly and see a doctor immediately.

National Society to Prevent Blindness. *Vision Problems in the U.S.: Facts and Figures.* New York: NSPB, 1998.

Internal Revenue Code See TAX BENEFITS.

International Guiding Eyes, Inc. (IGE) A nonprofit dog-guide training facility founded in 1948. The organization breeds and trains dog guides and provides in-residence training in dog-guide use and after care for qualified blind individuals. The organization also is known as, and conducts business as Guide Dogs of America.

IGE breeds and trains male and female Labrador retrievers, German shepherds, and golden retrievers. The school has graduate dog-guide users working in 24 states and four foreign countries.

Recipients of the dog guides must be 16 years old, physically healthy and able to walk freely, and desire independence. An applicant must be able to afford food for the dog and have received orientation and mobility training before qualifying. Recipients attend a one-month in-residence course of instruction with the dog guide at the facility. The dog guide, dog harness, and in-residence training are provided without cost to the recipient.

IGE receives no government or state funding. It is supported by corporate and private contributions.

Contact:

International Guiding Eyes, Inc.
13445 Glenoaks Boulevard
Sylmar, CA 91342
818-362-5834 (ph)
818-362-6870 (fax)
www.guidedogsofamerica.org

intracapsular extraction See CATARACT.

intraocular lens See IOL SURGERY.

Intrastromal Corneal Ring (ICR) Segments Thin, crescent-shaped segments that can be implanted into a patient's cornea in order to reduce myopia (nearsightedness). The segments are made of a specialized polymer, and the thickness required depends on the level of nearsightedness present in the patient. The greater the degree of nearsightedness, the thicker the implant needs to be. Two segments are implanted into each eye. The ICR segments, which recently were approved by the U.S. Food and Drug Administration, reduce nearsightedness by reshaping the cornea without having to cut or remove tissue from the central optical zone.

The central optical zone is the most critical area for clear vision. The segments can be removed if necessary or desired, leaving the eye in the same state it was before they were implanted. So far, ICR segments can only be used to treat mild to moderate cases of myopia. They cannot be used at present to treat farsightedness, astigmatism, or high levels of nearsightedness. The procedure of implanting an ICR segment is performed under topical, numbing eye drops. A normal implantation on one eye typically would take between 10 and 15 minutes, with only a tiny incision made at the base of the cornea. Recovery time generally is rapid, with vision improving in a short time. Few side effects or complications have been noted, although a small percentage of ICR segment patients have experienced problems, including decreased night vision, glare, halos, and blurry vision.

Eyesearch.com, Inc. "Intrastromal Corneal Ring Segments (INTACS) are the first FDA-Approved Non-Laser Surgical Technique for Correcting Nearsightedness," 1999.

IOL surgery Intraocular lens implants, or IOL surgery, is the implantation of a small, clear plastic lens in the eye to replace the section of natural lens lost in CATARACT removal surgery. As a permanent substitute for the lens, it enables the CORNEA to focus light onto the RETINA and produce a distinct image.

The intraocular lens is made up of two parts. The optic is the center portion of the lens that does the job of focusing. It is approximately one-quarter of an inch long and is made of PMMA plastic. The portion called the haptic holds the lens in place.

The power of the IOL is determined by two tests. KERATOMETRY is a test that determines the curvature of the cornea. More curved corneas require incrementally weaker implants. An ultrasonic A-scan determines the length of the eye. The longer (more nearsighted) the eye, the weaker the implant needed. An A-scan may determine that an IOL is unnecessary.

Intraocular lens implantation can be performed in either intracapsular or extracapsular cataract removal. Significant advances have been made in the technology of IOLs. They are smaller than they used to be and can be folded and placed into the eye through a tiny incision. There are three implantation methods: ANTERIOR CHAMBER, POSTERIOR CHAMBER, and IRIS supported. The lens is placed in front of the iris in the anterior method behind the iris in the posterior method and is clipped or sewn to the iris in the almost obsolete iris-supported method. Most ophthalmologists prefer the posterior method, claiming the lenses are more secure there and in a better position to help restore eyesight. IOLs provide constant, immediate improvement in vision and require no ongoing care. Patients may require normal glasses or bifocals as a supplement.

IOL surgery is often restricted to older patients since long-term side effects are unknown. It is recommended that the surgery not be repeated if an implant was unsuccessful in one eye or in the presence of other serious eye problems.

iridectomy The surgical removal of part of the eye's IRIS. The procedure is often performed as treatment for narrow-angle GLAUCOMA, a condition in which AQUEOUS FLUID builds within the eye due to a pupillary block and causes a rise in intraocular pressure.

The removal of the section of iris creates a passageway between the posterior and anterior chambers of the eye and eliminates an iris bombe, a condition in which the iris is abnormally bowed forward due to the increased intraocular pressure. The procedure allows aqueous fluid to pass from the posterior to ANTERIOR CHAMBER and thus reduces intraocular pressure.

The surgery is performed under general or local anesthetic. Traditionally, a small incision is made at the limbus through the CORNEA and SCLERA, into the anterior chamber of the eye. Since the iris is malleable, the incision allows a peripheral portion of the iris to prolapse out of the eye. The prolapsed section is held with forceps and excised with scissors. The iris bombe sinks backward into the eye. Often, the condition or blockage requires only a cut to be made rather than a removal of the iris. The cut is called an iridotomy. The cut or incision may be made surgically or with an argon laser, which burns a hole in the iris through the closed eye. Iridectomy or iridotomy is usually performed at the initial attack of narrow-angle glaucoma after treatment with medication has begun. It is used as a treatment and as a prophylactic measure to prevent recurrent attacks of narrow-angle glaucoma.

iridocyclitis A condition of the IRIS and ciliary body in which these two portions of the eye become inflamed. Because of the close proximity of the CILIARY BODY to the iris, inflammation and infection pass easily from one body to the other. Since the iris and ciliary body are located in the front portion of the uveal tract, which also includes the CHOROID, the condition is also called anterior UVEITIS, or inflammation of the uveal tract.

Symptoms of iridocyclitis may include pain, especially when focusing on near objects, redness, light sensitivity, and changes in the appearance of the pupil. The inflammation irritates the sphincter muscle of the pupil, which causes it to constrict, appear misshapen, or develop spasms. As a result of iridocyclitis, posterior SYNECHIAE may occur. This is a condition in which the pupil adheres to the underlying lens.

Iridocyclitis may be caused by IRITIS, which in turn is caused by injuries, viruses, HERPES ZOSTER, funguses, parasites, arthritis, and sinus or tooth infections. The condition may be treated with cycloplegic, or dilating, drops, local steroids, and medications for underlying causes. The condition may last for two weeks or more and carries a tendency to recur. Several recurrences may raise the possibility of CATARACT development.

iridodonesis A trembling of the iris. This condition is frequently seen with a subluxated (displaced) lens or following CATARACT surgery. It also is associated with MARFAN'S SYNDROME.

iris The thin circle of membrane suspended behind the ANTERIOR CHAMBER and in front of the CRYSTALLINE LENS. As a part of the uveal tract (the IRIS, CILIARY BODY, and the CHOROID), it is pigmented and gives the eye its color. The hue depends on the amount of pigment in the iris. Brown eyes have the most pigment, blue the least. The PUPIL is the black dot in the center of the iris. The pupil is a hole through which light passes into the eye. The iris opens the pupil wider in low light and shuts it down in bright light.

The iris is subject to several conditions or disorders. Iritis is an inflammation of the iris and often involves the adjacent ciliary body. Symptoms include pain, redness, and sensitivity to light. The pupil may become misshapen or constricted, as well. Iritis may be caused by injuries, viruses such as HERPES ZOSTER, funguses, parasites, or arthritis. When iritis spreads to the adjoining ciliary body, the condition is termed IRIDOCYCLITIS, or anterior uveitis. Iritis is present in the condition uveitis, an inflammation of the uveal tract.

SYNECHIAE is a condition that often follows iritis in which the iris bonds to the crystalline lens. Symptoms include pain and a misshapen pupil. The iris may also become attached to the CORNEA as a result of an injury or ophthalmologic surgery.

COLOBOMA is a defect in which the iris is missing a part. This can be due to a birth defect, eye surgery, or an injury.

Cysts or tumors may grow in the iris. They may be benign or malignant.

IRIDODONESIS is a condition in which the iris trembles uncontrollably. It is caused by a missing or displaced crystalline lens.

Heterochromia is a harmless condition in which one iris differs in color from the other. The iris may change color through contraction of iritis, but generally the condition is due to a birth defect.

iritis An inflammation of the IRIS. Symptoms of iritis may include pain, especially when focusing on near objects, redness, light sensitivity, and changes in the appearance of the pupil. While the CORNEA remains clear, the pupil may appear constricted or misshapen and develop spasms.

Because the iris is part of the uveal tract, iritis may be present in UVEITIS. Other causes may include injuries, viruses, HERPES ZOSTER, funguses, parasites, arthritis, and sinus or tooth infections. When the inflammation of iritis spreads to the adjoining CILIARY BODY, the condition is termed IRIDOCYCLITIS, or anterior uveitis.

Iritis is most often treated with cycloplegic, or dilating, drops and local steroids. The condition may last for two weeks or more and carries a tendency to recur. Several recurrences may increase the possibility of CATARACT development.

Ishihara Test See COLOR BLINDNESS.

Isopto Carpine An ophthalmic solution used in the treatment of GLAUCOMA. The main ingredient, pilocarpine hydrochloride, is also contained in the equivalent products known as Adsorbocarpine, Adarpine, Almocarpine, Akarpine, Ocusert Pilo-20, Ocusert Pilo 40, Pilocar and Pilopine HS. The medicine causes the pupils to constrict and lowers pressure within the eye.

The dosage is administered in drops. Some patients may suffer side effects. Minor side effects may include headache or aching in the brow, loss of night vision, blurred vision, and twitching eyelids. Major side effects may include diarrhea, nausea, difficulty urinating, stomach cramps, sweating, palpitations, shortness of breath, muscle tremor, nearsightedness, or other changes in vision.

Isopto Carpine should not be taken by those with a pilocarpine allergy. It should be used with caution by those with a history of heart disease, asthma, thyroid disease, peptic ulcer, gastrointestinal spasms, urinary tract blockage, Parkinson's disease, or seizures.

itinerant teacher The itinerant-teacher form of education or model is a model of education commonly used for visually impaired students. Other education models include the residential-school model, teacher-consultant model, resource-room model, and self-contained classroom model.

An itinerant teacher is one who travels to public schools to provide special education modifications to the instructional program of visually impaired children. The visually impaired student lives at home and spends most of the instructional day in a regular classroom.

The itinerant teacher normally visits every two or three days to work with the student in a section of the classroom, the library, the hall, the office, or any available space. The itinerant teacher provides special equipment, training, and materials adapted to the student's learning needs, and consultation services to the regular classroom teacher.

The success of the itinerant-teacher program is dependent on the attitude of the regular classroom teacher and his willingness to adapt regular teaching practices to the mainstreamed visually impaired child. The model is most effective for students who are self-directed and independent in learning skills and least effective for students who lack academic learning skills and lag in social development in comparison with their peers.

Javits-Wagner-O'Day Act The Javits-Wagner-O'Day Act of 1971 was enacted as an amendment to the Wagner-O'Day Act of 1938. The Wagner-O'Day Act mandated a program in which federal agencies may buy specific products from qualified workshops for the blind in an effort to improve employment opportunities.

In 1971, the Wagner-O'Day Act was renamed the Javits-Wagner-O'Day Act and amended to include severely disabled workers and add services as well as products. The products for sale to the federal government are approved by the Committee for Purchase from the Blind and other Severely Handicapped, a presidentially appointed committee that oversees the act.

A study in 1998 concluded that the Javits-Wagner-O'Day Act contracts have the potential to provide significant cost savings to the federal government.

The committee is composed of 15 members; 11 are representatives of federal agencies, three are representatives of the general public, and one is a private citizen representative of the disabled community. The committee determines and lists the products and services reasonable for purchase from qualified workshops, decides the fair market price for such products and services and sets the rules and regulations to execute the act.

U.S. Department of Education. *Summary of Existing Legislation Affecting Persons with Disabilities.* Washington, D.C.: USDE, 1988.

Job Accommodation Network (JAN) An international information clearinghouse and consulting resource established by the President's Committee on Employment of People with Disabilities. It provides guidance on practical methods of job accommodations.

JAN counsels employers, rehabilitation professionals, and individuals with disabilities seeking job-accommodation solutions. It provides additional information on accessing available programs such as the Job Training Partnership Act, Projects with Industry, Supported Employment, Targeted Jobs Tax Credit, and Barrier Removal incentives.

Employers with questions or concerns about job accommodation may call JAN. A Human Factors Consultant takes the information request, including details about functional requirements of the specific job, functional limitations of the worker, and environmental factors involved. The consultant accesses the computer for information based on these facts and provides matching or similar situation solutions. Additional addresses and phone numbers of resources are provided.

The service is free, but the user is requested to provide information about resulting accommodations for the computer files.

Contact:

Job Accommodation Network
West Virginia University, 809 Allen Hall
P.O. Box 6080
Morgantown, WV 26506-6080
1-800-JAN-PCEH (526-7234) (voice and TDD)
http://janweb.icdi.wvu.edu

Job Training Partnership Act (JTPA) The Job Training Partnership Act (JTPA) of 1982 was designed to revise the existing Comprehensive Employment and Training Act (CETA). Its purpose is to set up programs that will prepare youth and unskilled adults to enter the workforce, and to provide job training. The new act eliminated federal funding for public-service employment, involved the private sector through a series of incentives, transferred additional administrative authority to the state, demanded improved accountability, included community organizations, targeted specific populations, and extended the program by broadening the eligibility requirements.

The act established vocational training and placement programs for economically disadvantaged people, including those with disabilities. The term "economically disadvantaged" includes those who qualify for or receive welfare payments or food stamps, live within a family whose income is below the poverty level, or receive local or state payments as a foster child.

Although income is the chief criterion for qualification, the JTPA program may fund handicapped individuals, regardless of economic means, so long as the percentage of such recipients does not exceed 10 percent of the total. According to the act, the term *handicapped* includes physical and mental disabilities that form a barrier to employment.

The act is divided into five titles. Title I describes structure and planning guidelines. Title II establishes conditions for adult and youth training programs. Title III approves funding for training and employment services through formula or discretionary grants. Title IV authorizes human services research and development programs, the Job Corps, and Veterans' Employment Programs. Title V contains stipulations pertaining to other federal laws.

Title II-A establishes a grant program to maintain training services. The program is administered by the state and executed through agreements between local and state governmental agencies and the private sector. These formula grants support 28 services, including vocational counseling and training, transitional counseling and training, custom job development or training with the agreement to hire, and postemployment follow-up services.

Title IV provides grants for national pilot-demonstration programs. These programs support and encourage job training and related aid to those disadvantaged in the employment market, including persons with disabilities. Additional research grants in Title IV fund training and job market studies used to develop improved training methods and placement programs.

Title IV, Part B, establishes the Job Corps program, a national education, job training, and counseling program. Job Corps centers, both residential and nonresidential, provide trainees with the skills necessary to become employable. Trainees are most often between the ages of 14 and 22 but older, disabled individuals may be allowed to participate in the program.

U.S. Department of Education. *Summary of Existing Legislation Affecting Persons with Disabilities.* Washington, D.C.: USDE, 1988.

juvenile retinoschisis   An inherited disease that causes progressive loss of central and side vision due to degeneration of the retina. Loss of sight usually occurs at about age 13. The condition, which also is known as X-linked retinoschisis, almost always occurs in males.

The condition begins at birth, but there usually are no symptoms until about the age of 10, when a decline in vision begins. Other early signs of the disease include involuntary eye movements and the loss of ability to focus both eyes on an object. Blindness sometimes occurs within three years of diagnosis, while other people with the disease retain some vision into adulthood.

Juvenile retinoschisis is genetically passed along by the X-linked pattern of inheritance, because the gene for the disease is located on the X chromosome. There is no treatment or cure at this time for juvenile retinoschisis, but surgery can be performed to repair retinal detachments, which often occur as part of the disease. People with the disease may benefit from the use of low-vision aids, orientation and mobility training, and so forth.

Keller, Helen Helen Keller is perhaps the best-known figure in history associated with blindness. Born sighted in 1880 in Alabama, she contracted a fever at 18 months, which left her deaf and blind. The infant grew into a wild and unruly child with few methods for communication with others. Her father, Captain Arthur Keller, editor of the *North Alabamian*, sought advice from Alexander Graham Bell in his search for help for his daughter. Bell suggested that Captain Keller write to the Perkins Institution for the Blind to request a teacher for Helen.

In 1887, Anne Mansfield Sullivan arrived to teach the child. Sullivan taught her to fingerspell the words for objects, but Keller showed no understanding of the connection between the spelling and the object. The breakthrough came one day at the well when water gushed onto Keller's hand as Sullivan spelled W-A-T-E-R. Keller continued to study with Sullivan, mastering the alphabet in both manual and raised print.

Keller entered the Cambridge School for Young Ladies in 1898 in preparation for Radcliffe College. She enrolled in Radcliffe in 1900 and graduated with a bachelor of arts degree cum laude in 1904. Sullivan remained at Keller's side throughout Keller's studies, translating lectures and textbooks.

Keller began a writing career while studying at Radcliffe. In 1902, her autobiography, *The Story of My Life*, was published. The book was written with the assistance of John Macy, a critic and socialist reformer. When Sullivan married John Macy in 1905, Keller went to live with the couple.

Keller worked for the interests of blind and deaf-blind individuals throughout her life by appearing before legislatures, writing articles and books, and lecturing. She became a member of the first board of directors of the Permanent Blind Relief War Fund (later named the American Braille Press, the American Foundation for Overseas Blind and Helen Keller International) in 1915.

She was a member of the staff for the Foundation of the Blind from 1924 until her death in 1968, serving as an adviser on national and international relations. In 1924, she founded the Helen Keller Endowment Fund to benefit the foundation. She established the foundation's special-service program for deaf-blind individuals in 1946.

In 1946, when the American Braille Press became the American Foundation for Overseas Blind, she became a counselor on international relations for the organization. She embarked on speaking tours that covered 35 countries on five continents between 1946 and 1957. Her last speaking tour, at age 75, covered over 40,000 miles in Asia.

Keller received honors during her lifetime for her work benefiting blind persons. Honorary degrees include those from Temple University, Harvard University, and the Universities of Glasgow, Berlin, Delhi, and Johannesburg. Awards bestowed on her include the Presidential Medal of Freedom, Brazil's Order of the Southern Cross, Japan's Sacred Treasure and the Philippines' Golden Heart. She was elected to the National Institute of Arts and Letters and named a Chevalier of the French Legion of Honor.

Versions of Keller's life have been the subject of stage and film productions. The documentary *Helen Keller in Her Story* and the play and movie *The Miracle Worker* all chronicle the events of her life.

Sullivan, long separated from Macy, died in 1936. Polly Thomson, who joined the two in 1914 when Sullivan's eyesight deteriorated, continued to serve as Keller's interpreter and companion. In 1961, Keller retired from public life to her home,

Arcan Ridge, in Westport, Connecticut. She died in 1968 at the age of 87.

keratitis An inflammation of the CORNEA caused by viruses, bacteria or, infrequently, fungi. Keratitis can occur as a result of a corneal abrasion caused by CONTACT LENSES or by an injury. Elderly persons, diabetics, those with poor tear functions, and those treated with corticosteroid drugs may be more likely to develop keratitis after an abrasion.

Keratitis is a serious infection and should be treated by a physician. Symptoms of keratitis include redness, sharp pain, tearing, impaired vision, light sensitivity, and dulled or milky corneal surface.

Simple viral keratitis is generally the least serious type. Patients are usually treated with medication on an outpatient basis. However, herpes keratitis is a very serious viral infection that can result in scarring and permanent visual impairment.

Bacterial keratitis is more dangerous than viral types and often must be treated in a hospital. The infection is treated with antibiotics and cortisone-based steroid drugs. Bacterial keratitis can permanently scar the cornea and cause vision loss. Bacterial keratitis may be contracted congenitally as in syphilis.

The most common forms of fungal keratitis are caused by yeasts. Fungal keratitis may require hospitalization and treatment with antibiotics. Scarring frequently results, despite treatment, and causes vision impairment. Another type of keratitis is exposure keratitis. This sometimes occurs when the eyelid cannot cover the eye because of bulging, as found in some thyroid conditions. Exposure keratitis can vary from mild dry spots to ulcers on the cornea.

keratoconus A degenerative disorder of the CORNEA in which the central part of the cornea thins and bulges forward into a cone shape. As the cornea thins, vision becomes distorted. As a result of further stretching, the cornea may break at the peak. The cornea will heal itself, but scar tissue will form at the break, causing vision loss.

It is a chronic, progressive disease. The exact cause of kertatoconus is not known, but it is thought that there is a genetic predisposition to the disorder. Most researchers agree that there probably is more than one factor involved in the cause in the disorder, and there is a "trigger" that sets off a series of events in the tissues of the eye that eventually result in keratoconus. It is most often diagnosed in children or adolescents and usually presents symptoms when they are near 10 years of age. The National Keratoconus Foundation estimates that one of every 2,000 people will develop the disorder.

Keratoconus may be diagnosed during the routine ophthalmologic exam. Examination with the BIOMICROSCOPE, or slit lamp, will reveal thinning of the central cornea or presence of the Fleischer ring, a narrow, greenish-brown ring in the cornea. Later stages of keratoconus, in which the cornea has markedly bulged forward, can be seen without benefit of examination instruments.

This disorder progresses slowly and affects both eyes. Milder forms of the condition are often corrected with spectacles or special CONTACT LENSES that cover the cornea and part of the SCLERA. More serious and advanced forms are corrected surgically or by a CORNEAL TRANSPLANT, called keratoplasty.

Keratoconus is a prime reason for keratoplasty in the United States. It is a highly successful procedure since, in cases of keratoconus, the cornea remains vessel free.

keratometer See KERATOMETRY.

keratometry Measurement of the curvature of the CORNEA with an instrument called a keratometer. The exact keratometer measurement is used to determine the power of an INTRAOCULAR LENS to be implanted during CATARACT surgery.

The greater the degree of corneal curvature, the more nearsighted is the eye. Higher degrees of nearsightedness require weaker implants. The curvature measurement and the length of the eye, measured with an ultrasonic A-scan, are analyzed by a computer that determines and prescribes the precise power of the implant.

keratoplasty   See CORNEAL TRANSPLANT.

keratotomy   A procedure in which incisions are made in the cornea to change its curvature over the pupil. There are two kinds or keratotomies: radial and astigmatic. Radial keratotomy, done to reduce myopia (nearsightedness), was introduced in North America in 1978. During the procedure, the surgeon makes several deep incisions in the cornea to change the curvature of the cornea over the pupil. The incisions are made in a spokelike, or radial, pattern. No cuts are made in the optical zone, which is the portion of the eye that you see through. The surgeon measures the thickness of the cornea to determine how deep to make the incisions, then, under a microscope and using a calibrated diamond blade, the surgeon will make the precise cuts.

Normal pressure within the eye causes the areas around the incisions to bow, which results in a flattening of the center of the cornea. The flattened area reduces the refractive power of the cornea and allows light rays to focus on the retina, thus reducing nearsightedness. Radial keratotomy is an outpatient procedure that normally takes no more than 30 minutes to perform. Approximately 85 percent of people who have this type of surgery can pass a standard driver's license exam that requires 20/40 vision without corrective lenses.

Astigmatic keratotomy is a similar procedure that is used to reduce astigmatism. The incisions used in astigmatic keratotomy are made in a curved, rather than a radial, pattern. Astigmatic keratotomy sometimes is used in combination with radial keratotomy to reduce myopia with astigmatism.

The cornea heals slowly after keratotomy is performed, and there may be side effects such as fluctuating vision, a weakened cornea, infection, temporary pain, or difficulty in getting contact lenses to fit. Rarely, patients develop cataract, serious infection, or experience rupture of an incision. In extreme cases, loss of vision may occur.

American Academy of Ophthalmology. *Radial and Astigmatic Keratotomy.* www.eyenet.org, 1997.

Kurzweil Educational Systems Group   A company that develops reading software for people who are blind or visually impaired, have learning disabilities, or difficulty with reading, such as with dyslexia. Kurzweil Education Systems Group is a division of Lernout & Hauspie, an international company based in Belgium that specializes in speech and learning products.

The Kurzweil company was first known for its Kurzweil Reading Machine, which was introduced in 1977. It now offers two new products for blind or visually impaired users. The Kurzweil 1000 is an advanced scanning and reading tool that scans documents into a computer and converts them to speech. The MagniReader is a scanning and reading software package designed for people with low vision. It displays scanned documents on a computer screen in large print. The print can either be scrolled for reading, or converted into speech.

Contact:

Lernout & Hauspie Customer Support Center
3984 Pepsi Cola Drive
Melbourne, FL 32934
888-483-6266 (toll free)
www.lhsl.com

large print Large print is a low-vision aid that benefits visually impaired individuals who have some usable vision but cannot read conventional print. Large print, 18-point type is roughly 3/16 of an inch high and therefore easier to read than standard print.

In the United States, large print originated in 1913 in sight-saving classes. In order to help their students who could not read conventional print, teachers began to hand-print enlarged text. In 1914, the early large-type books were printed, and by 1935 the American Printing House for the Blind began to publish large-print textbooks for children.

Today, large-print books, magazines, and literature are available through publishers, visual-aids catalogs, and public libraries. There also is computer software available to get large print on a computer screen.

laser cane An electronic traveling device. It is prescribed by an ophthalmologist or optometrist, and it requires specialized training from an orientation and mobility instructor.

The laser cane is a long cane that sends out three thin beams of invisible infrared light. The beams detect objects within 20 feet at face level, waist level, and ground level. It can detect changes in the terrain of the path, including drops down to five inches below surface, such as curbs and potholes. When the laser light hits an obstacle, it sets vibrating pins into motion and/or sends out an auditory signal.

The signal is pitched according to the height of the obstacle. When the beam touches an obstacle at face level, the auditory signal is a high-pitched beep. When it hits a center or waist-high obstacle, the beep is pitched lower. When it hits a ground-level obstacle, the pitch is low.

The laser cane requires from 30 to 40 hours of training with a qualified instructor to operate. (See ELECTRONIC TRAVEL AIDS.)

laser in situ keratomileusis (LASIK) A procedure that combines the vision-correcting techniques of automated lameller keratoplasty (ALK) and photorefractive keratectomy (PRK) to correct moderate to extreme nearsightedness, farsightedness, and astigmatism. Sometimes referred to as laser assisted in situ keratomileusis, the name refers to the use of a laser to reshape the cornea without affecting surrounding cells. *In situ* is from the Greek, meaning "in the natural or normal place." In medical terms, "in situ" refers to the site of origin without invasion of neighboring tissues. *Kerato* is the Greek word for cornea, and *mileusis* means "to shape."

LASIK surgery has become increasingly popular since it was first performed in U.S. clinical trials in 1991. It is now the most commonly performed refractive procedure in the United States. The procedure has been done internationally for more than 10 years. While LASIK is relatively new, ophthalmologists have been reshaping the cornea for more than half a century. So, while the LASIK procedure is new, the concept of it is not.

In the LASIK procedure, a MICROKERATOME is used to make a thin, shallow incision in the cornea. The incision is made from the side and produces a hinged flap. During surgery, the flap is opened, and an EXCIMER LASER is used to remove small amounts of corneal tissue. The flap is then removed, generally eliminating the need for a protective contact lens to be worn after surgery. The excimer laser is extremely accurate and does not disturb surrounding tissue. LASIK surgery normally is performed using only topical drops to numb the eye. In some cases, patients may be given a mild sedative to help them relax. The procedure does not take very long—only 15 to 30 minutes for both eyes.

While some surgeons perform the procedure on both eyes during the same visit, others prefer to operate on one eye and then wait for anywhere between a few days and several months before doing the other. If you are considering LASIK surgery, you should discuss this matter with your doctor. Some patients prefer having both eyes done at the same time because they feel it is more convenient than having to return for a separate procedure. Others like a waiting period between procedures. If the procedure is done on only one eye, it may be uncomfortable to use both eyes together until the vision in the other eye is corrected. If both eyes are not operated on at the same time, the patient may need to wear a contact lens in the uncorrected eye in order for it to be able to work in concert with the corrected eye.

Because the eye's natural surface is merely pulled away and then returned to its original position after surgery, there is generally less discomfort than with photorefractive keratectomy, during which the surface layer of the eye is removed. Some patients report a mild burning sensation in their eye following surgery. For this reason, patients often are encouraged to sleep for several hours following the procedure, after which time most of the discomfort will have abated. Patients may experience blurred vision for several hours following the procedure, but most are able to return to work and drive a car the following day.

LASIK surgery is widely recognized and the quality of the procedure continues to improve. Most patients who undergo the LASIK procedure enjoy improved vision as a result. More than 90 percent of those with low to moderate nearsightedness achieve at least 20/40 vision, which is considered good enough in most states to drive without wearing corrective lenses. Many patients achieve 20/20 vision or better as the result of LASIK. Those with more severe cases of nearsightedness, however, or with severe farsightedness, may not achieve the same results. Although LASIK is generally considered to be very safe, it is not recommended for everyone.

Patients with a strong desire to be less dependent on glasses or contacts they must wear due to nearsightedness, farsightedness, or astigmatism, are considered candidates for LASIK, provided they fully understand the potential risks of surgery. Also, people who are bothered by wearing glasses but cannot tolerate contacts are considered to be good candidates. Patients considering LASIK should have no eye diseases and should have had stable vision for at least two years.

While the effects of LASIK do not wear off, changes that may affect vision can still occur within the individual. For this reason, LASIK is not recommended for patients under the age of 18, whose eyes are still undergoing many changes. Performing the procedure after internal eye changes have slowed down or stopped increases the chances for long-term, continuing correction.

Possible side effects of the LASIK procedure include temporary glare, scratchiness, and mild discomfort. In some cases, overcorrection or undercorrection could occur, meaning that the procedure would have to be redone in order to fix the problem. Infection also is a remote, but a possible side effect. Because LASIK is considered to be elective surgery, the procedure is not covered by most insurance companies. Some U.S. companies, however, will offset or cover the cost of the procedure. Also, the cost may be able to be deducted from your federal income taxes as a deductible health expense. The cost varies greatly, depending on patient circumstances, the surgeon, and the area in which the procedure is being conducted.

The LASIK Institute, Boston, MA. *LASIK Surgery.* www.lasikinstitute.org, 2000.

Florida Eye Institute. *Laser In Situ Keratomileusis (LASIK),* www.fleye.com/laser/lasik, 2000.

EyeSearch. *Lasik.* www.eyesearch.com/lasik/lhtm, 2000.

Federal Trade Commission in cooperation with the American Academy of Ophthalmology. *Basik Lasik: Tips on Lasik Eye Surgery.* www.ftc.gov/bcp/conline/pubs/health/lasik.htm, 2000.

lasers The word *laser* stands for Light Amplification by Stimulated Emission of Radiation. Lasers use natural oscillations of atoms to amplify or generate electromagnetic waves of visible light. The light energy produced by a laser contains great power since the photons (units of light) are all the same wavelength and are moving in the same direction. This allows the light to be concentrated into a very bright, focused beam.

The first laser, which used a ruby as its active medium, was built by Theodore Mainman and introduced in 1960. Later lasers included the argon, the CO_2 or carbon dioxide, the krypton and the neodymium: yttrium-aluminum-garnet or ND-YAG laser.

Lasers affect living tissues in one of three ways: to burn, cut, or destroy tissue. Laser light directed into and absorbed by tissue causes energy to be released in the form of heat or a burn. Lasers are used to create an acoustical wave that disrupts or cuts tissue and can be directed to break down or vaporize tissue. All three laser techniques are used surgically. Low-level laser energy is used in imaging tissue and is nondestructive.

Laser therapy is often used to treat DIABETIC RETINOPATHY, a leading cause of blindness in the United States. A complication of diabetes, diabetic retinopathy occurs as a result of damage to retinal blood vessels that leak or hemorrhage. The retinal tissue loses oxygen normally brought by the vessels and develops new vessels (neovascularization) that tend to be weak and bleed. Continuous leaking and the formation of retinal scars may lead to blindness.

Lasers such as the ARGON are used to treat diabetic retinopathy in a process called photocoagulation. The laser is directed into the eye with a special lens. The light passes through the transparent structures of the eye and is stopped when it reaches the pigmented layer of the retina. The energy of the laser is converted to heat that coagulates or congeals the tissue. Several burns are placed in the tissue surrounding the bleeding vessel. The tissue develops scars that form a ring to enclose the vessel and stop the bleeding.

If neovascularization has occurred, unhealthy, oxygen-deprived tissue is treated with the laser. The directed energy of the laser causes scarring and prohibits the tissue from forming new, weak vessels.

Lasers are used to treat subretinal neovascularization, a disorder caused by AGE-RELATED MACU-LOPATHY (ARM), a major cause of blindness associated with aging. ARM produces scarring of the MACULA, the region of the retina that allows for sharpest vision. Subretinal neovascularization is caused by a break in the pigment epithelium, a layer below the retina. A collection of blood vessels below the retina bleeds into the retina through the break and causes scarring.

An argon or krypton laser is used to treat the disorder. The blue-green light of the argon laser is absorbed by the pigment of the inner retina. The red krypton laser is absorbed only in the melanin pigment of the deepest layers of the retina where the neovascularization occurs. Treatment with the krypton laser is preferred because it allows the inner, unaffected retinal layers to remain untouched while treating only the deep, affected layers.

A laser treatment called photodynamic therapy is used for some patients with the wet form of ARM. This therapy, which was approved by the Food and Drug Administration in April 2000, involves a special dye that is injected into the patient and absorbed by the abnormal blood vessels in the eye. Once the dye has been absorbed, a low-level laser is used to activate it, causing the dye to block the abnormal blood vessels. This can be done without damaging other areas of the eye, which makes it a significant breakthrough in the treatment of ARM.

Another use of lasers in ophthalmology is to repair retinal holes, which, if left untreated, can cause retinal detachment. A laser can be used to seal a hole in the retina before detachment occurs. If the retina does detach, a retinal reattachment operation would be performed, and a laser may be used to secure the retina.

Laser therapy may be an alternative to surgery in the treatment of GLAUCOMA, a disease in which the intraocular fluid fails to properly drain from the eye, accumulates, and causes elevated intraocular pressure. The procedure is called laser trabeculoplasty.

When medication fails to lower the intraocular pressure, laser trabeculoplasty is often used to open the drainage area located where the CORNEA meets the IRIS. A series of laser burns are placed in the drainage area, which causes scarring and openings within the meshwork of drainage channels. The fluid drains more easily from the eye, and intraocular pressure is reduced.

Lasers are used postoperatively in CATARACT extraction. After a cataract is removed in an extracapsular procedure, the capsule of the lens remaining in the eye opacifies in approximately 20 percent of all cases and impairs vision. In the past, a second intraocular operation, a posterior capsulectomy, was required to remove the capsule. That surgery has been replaced by a procedure performed by the ND-YAG laser.

The physician focuses the YAG LASER to a fine point on the capsule and releases a series of 500,000 watt explosions of energy that destroy the capsular matter. Because the laser can be so minutely focused, the physician can aim the beam accurately and avoid surrounding tissue or an intraocular lens resting on the opaque capsule.

The YAG laser is unique in its ability to perform this procedure since, unlike other lasers, it is not dependent on pigmented tissue to be effective. The argon and other lasers depend on pigment such as that found in the iris of the eye or in blood flowing through blood vessels in retinal tissue. The pigmented tissue absorbs the energy from the argon laser and is destroyed. However, cataracts or their remaining capsules contain no pigmentation and are immune to the power of the argon laser.

A relatively new type of laser—the excimer laser—also is being used in ophthalmology. Excimer laser light is a beam that is produced when two gases—argon and fluorine—are mixed. It is referred to as a "cold" laser. The beam has the ability to remove tiny layers of tissues with very little or no heat damage to the surrounding tissue. The excimer laser is important because of its precision, and it is being considered for new uses and applications.

The excimer laser currently is used in photorefractive keratectomy (PRK) to permanently reshape the cornea by removing tiny amounts of tissue. It also is used in LASIK surgery and in phototherapeutic keratectomy (PTK). PTK is another surgical procedure that is used to remove cloudy scar tissue from the cornea. Lasers also are used to help manage tumors within the eye and for cosmetic surgery involving the eye or area surrounding the eye.

All laser treatments are administered in a similar manner. The therapy is usually performed without anesthesia but a topical anesthetic or dilating drops may be administered. A contact lens may be placed on the eye to aid in properly focusing the beam. The patient sits in a dimmed room with the chin placed on the chin rest in front of the slit lamp or biomicroscope. The patient may be asked to direct his vision to a specific point in the room.

The surgeon focuses the laser and then administers several bursts to the affected area. The patient may see flashes of colored light. The procedure is usually painless, but some mild discomfort or short, intense painful moments may occur. The procedure may take from five to 30 minutes. After the procedure, some discomfort may be felt for a day. If a local anesthetic was applied, the vision may be blurred for a few hours. If the eyes were dilated, it may take several hours for the PUPILS return to normal size. The patient should be able to walk or drive home. After a week, the patient may have a follow-up examination.

Complications due to laser therapy include damage to surrounding healthy tissue, loss of focus, bleeding, cataract, neovascularization, opacification of the VITREOUS, inflammation, temporary intraocular pressure elevation, and vision loss.

While lasers have many uses and great promise for more uses and applications in the future, doctors warn that they should not be viewed as a means of miracle cures. Lasers are tools that doctors can use to work more precisely and effectively. They are not, however, cures in themselves.

Berland, Theodore, and Richard A. Perritt. *Living With Your Eye Operation*. New York: St. Martin's Press, 1974.

Eden, John. *The Eye Book*. New York: Penguin Books, 1978.

Krames Communications. *The Retina Book*. Daly City, California: KC, 1987.

Reynolds, James D. "Lasers in Ophthalmology," HealthNet Library. Columbus: CompuServe, 1989.

Shulman, Jules. *Cataracts*. New York: Simon and Schuster, 1984.

Wavikar, C. M., M.D. "Lasers in Ophthalmology." www.exicom.org, 1999.

laser trabeculoplasty See LASERS.

legally blind Legally blind or legal blindness are terms used by the Internal Revenue Service and other governmental agencies to determine whether an individual is eligible for federal or state benefits. This classification is determined by measuring visual acuity (how much detail one sees at a specific distance) and visual field (the area of vision).

A person is classified as legally blind if the visual acuity of the better eye, with correction, is 20/200 or less. This involves a loss of central vision.

One may also be termed legally blind if the visual field of the better eye, even with 20/20 vision, is limited to 20 degrees or less. An individual with loss in the visual field may experience peripheral or central vision loss. Loss in the peripheral, or side, vision may result in tunnel vision. Loss in the central, or straight-ahead, vision may result in difficulty in seeing an object in the center or direct line of sight. Because the classification involves measurement of the better eye only, people who are blind in one eye are not considered legally blind.

Legally blind people should not necessarily be considered totally blind. The term includes a wide range of visual abilities. Two individuals with 20/200 visual acuity or 20 degree visual fields may have vastly different vision levels.

Current statistics show that there are approximately 500,000 legally blind people in the United States. Of these, over 75 percent have some remaining vision. They are often able to utilize their remaining vision to work, read, travel, and continue their daily routine by using adaptive devices or by developing accommodating body or head movements.

Individuals who are classified as legally blind may be eligible for financial aid. The Social Security Administration offers two programs authorized by Titles 2 and 16 of the Social Security Act. The first program offers assistance based on contributions made to the Social Security System. The second, also called Supplemental Security Income, or SSI, is based on financial need. Benefits vary according to one's income and financial resources.

Medicare programs available to legally blind people provide assistance with medical and hospital bills. Tax deductions, reduced public transporta-tion fares and telephone rates, heating and insulation reductions, as well as other benefits that vary by state are available to the legally blind.

American Macular Degeneration Foundation. AMDF Bulletin Board, Re: Legally Blind. www.macular.org, 2001.

Legal Services Corporation A nonprofit organization established by Congress in 1974 to provide funding for a variety of legal services to needy individuals including representation, advice and referral. The Legal Services Corporation Act amendments of 1978 allowed disabled persons to become eligible for these services.

Under the new amendments, the corporations were directed to consider the needs of potential clients to determine priorities, giving particular priority to those most needy, including those with disabilities and the elderly. However, Congress restricted the powers of the legal service corporations in 1981 when it reauthorized the Legal Services Corporation. It prohibited participating attorneys from bringing a class-action suit against any government agency.

The Legal Services Corporation does not provide services directly but provides grants to independent local programs. In 1997 grants went to 269 such programs.

U.S. Department of Education. *Summary of Existing Legislation Affecting Persons with Disabilities.* Washington, D.C.: USDE, 1988.

Legal Services Corporation. What is LSC? www.lsc.gov, 1999.

lens See CRYSTALLINE LENS.

leprosy A disease with complications that causes between 50,000 to 100,000 cases of blindness throughout the world. In 1997 there were estimated to be 1.2 million leprosy patients in the world, as reported by 91 countries. About half a million new cases are detected each year.

Leprosy is widespread in 60 countries. The 16 rated "most endemic," which account for 90 percent of all leprosy cases throughout the world, are Bangladesh, Brazil, Cambodia, Ethiopia, Guinea, India, Indonesia, Madagascar, Mozambique,

Myanmar (Burma), Nepal, Nigeria, Philippines, Sudan, Tanzania, and Democratic Republic of the Congo (formerly Zaire). India, and Nepal account for nearly 70 percent of all cases.

Leprosy is a chronic infectious disease caused by *Mycobacterium leprae,* a bacillus that reproduces very slowly and mainly affects the skin, nerves, and mucous membranes. If untreated, it leads to progressive damage of the skin, eyes, and limbs. Visible symptoms might not appear for five to 20 years after a person has contacted the disease.

Advances are being made in controlling leprosy, and public health officials are hopeful that the disease will soon be eliminated. A combination of drugs has been found to be effective in treating leprosy.

World Health Organization. *A World Without Leprosy.* www.who.int/lep/index.html, 2000.

Lernout & Hauspie   One of the world's largest providers of speech- and language-technology products. Headquartered in Belgium, Lernout & Hauspie has offices in Massachusetts, Connecticut, and Florida.

Founded in 1987 by Jo Lernout and Pol Hauspie, the company provides advanced speech and language technologies to industries, individuals, educational facilities, government agencies, and other customers. Its products include the Kurzweil 1000, an advanced scanning and reading tool that scans documents into a computer and converts them to speech. Lernout & Hauspie's products and service stem from four technologies: automatic speech recognition, text-to-speech, digital speech and music compression, and text-to-text (translation).

Contact:

Lernout & Hauspie World Headquarters
Flanders Language Valley 50
8900 Ieper, Belgium
+32-57-228-888 (ph)
+32-57-208-489 (fax)
www.lhsl.com

Library of Congress   See NATIONAL LIBRARY SERVICE FOR THE BLIND AND PHYSICALLY HANDICAPPED.

Library Services and Technology Act (LSTA)   An act passed by Congress on September 30, 1996, to replace the Library Services and Construction Act. The act provides federal funding for libraries in the United States and guidelines for library programs and services.

The goal of the LSTA is to enhance technology in America's libraries, including that which will benefit people who are blind or visually impaired. Some of the aims of the LSTA are to establish or enhance electronic link-ups among or between libraries; link libraries electronically with educational, social, or information services; help libraries access information from electronic networks; buy computers and telecommunications equipment for libraries that do not have them; provide library services in areas that do not have them; and provide services for everyone who wishes to use them, including blind, visually impaired, and learning impaired persons.

The original act to fund libraries in the United States was the Library Services Act, which went into effect in 1956. It was replaced by the Library Services and Construction Act in 1964. In 1966, the act was amended to authorize special library-access programs and services, including those that benefit blind or visually impaired people.

Contact:

The American Library Association. Highlights of the Library Services and Technology Act. www.ala.org.washoff/lstahigh.html, 2000

Lions Clubs International   A service group founded in 1917 by Melvin Jones, a Chicago businessman. The goals of the organization are to provide service to the community and around the world. The group has a membership of 1.3 million business and professional men and women. The organization operates over 39,000 clubs located in 164 countries and geographical areas.

In 1925, Helen Keller challenged the Lions to promote the cause of the visually impaired. As a result, Lions Clubs established GLAUCOMA screening and detection centers, eye research foundations, eye banks, dog-guide training facilities, rehabilitation centers, and other service enterprises for the visually impaired. The organization runs the Lions

Recycle for Sight program, which collects used eyeglasses that are sent around the world to people who need them.

The organization is also involved in drug-awareness programs, environmental health, international understanding, diabetes research and education, international youth camps, educational, recreational, social and citizenship programs, and the Leo Clubs, a young adult organization.

The American Council of Blind Lions, an organization made up of legally blind members of the Lions Clubs International, was established in 1970. The group informs the public about the abilities and needs of blind people.

Lions Clubs International issues four publications, the Lions Magazine, Club President's Update, District Governor's Update, and Lions Club Community Activities Bulletin. The organization holds an annual convention.

long canes   The long cane or prescriptive cane is the travel aid most commonly used by visually impaired people. The American Foundation for the Blind estimates that about 109,000 people in the United States use long canes to get around. The lightweight fiberglass or aluminum shaft of the cane is roughly one-half inch in diameter. The length of the cane is individually prescribed by an orientation and mobility expert according to the user's height and length of stride.

The cane is usually white and covered in one section with a reflective material. The tip of the shaft is red and made of steel or nylon. The handle of the cane is usually a rounded crook shape underneath which is a rubber grip.

The cane is also available in collapsible folding or telescoping models. These are made of fiberglass, aluminum, or wood, and have crook, rounded, or straight handles with a rubber grip, or wrist loop. Collapsible canes are often shorter and less durable than the prescription length but are used in the same manner.

The cane user swings the cane in front of his body in wide sweeping arcs. The tip of the cane touches the ground and alerts the user to obstacles or changes in terrain. Cane use cannot alert the user to obstacles overhead. The user is taught cane use techniques by trained orientation and mobility experts. The user learns to employ all the senses in conjunction with cane techniques to travel safely.

Low Income Home Energy Assistance Act   The Low Income Home Energy Assistance Act of 1981 is a state block-grant program of the Omnibus Budget Reconciliation Act of 1981. The grant established a program in which tax credits and emergency federal payments are made to states and individuals to compensate for the rise in home heating costs.

Individuals receiving SSI or AFDC benefits, Food Stamps, and specific income-related veterans benefits are eligible for the assistance. Also eligible are those whose household income is less than 150 percent of the federal poverty level or 50 percent of the state median income. In fiscal year 2000, 84,122 U.S. Households received an average of $414 each in energy assistance grants.

U.S. Department of Education. *Summary of Existing Legislation Affecting Persons with Disabilities.* Washington, D.C.: USDE, 1988.
U.S. Department of Health and Human Services. Low Income Home Energy Program. www.acf.dhhs.gov, 2001.

low vision   A term generally used to describe a level of vision that is below normal after correction. It is a serious vision loss that cannot be corrected with lenses, surgery, or treatment and that interferes with the performance of daily activities at home or work. A person with low vision is also sometimes referred to as partially sighted, partially seeing, visually impaired, visually limited, or visually handicapped.

According to the American Foundation for the Blind, there are approximately 11 million adults and children in the United States who have vision below normal, even with correction. Of these, almost 1.5 million can be classified as having low vision. Unless their vision loss is severe enough to enable them to be classified as legally blind, they do not qualify for federal or state benefits.

Although there is no legal term for low vision, ophthalmologists and other eye care professionals define low vision by visual acuity and visual field measurements. Visual acuity is the amount of detail a person can see at a set distance, and visual field is the amount of area, measured in degrees, that a person can see.

A person with a visual acuity measurement of 20/50 or less and a visual field of 20 to 40 degrees or less in the better eye, with correction, is considered to have low vision. Someone with a visual acuity of 20/200 and a visual field of 20 degrees or less in the better eye, with correction, is termed legally blind.

Most legally blind people have some usable vision. Because of this, and since the word "blind" is involved in the legal classification, a misconception exists about what blind people can actually see. Therefore, many agencies for the blind suggest that the word "blind" be used to describe only those with no usable vision and that the words "low vision," "visually impaired," and "partially sighted" be used to describe people with some remaining usable vision.

Low vision may be caused by injury, birth defects, disease or aging. The most common vision-limiting diseases or disorders are GLAUCOMA, AGE-RELATED MACULOPATHY, CATARACT, OPTIC NERVE ATROPHY, and DIABETIC RETINOPATHY. A stroke also can result in low vision.

Some conditions limit the vision by blurring or clouding the general or central vision. Others block out or blur specific areas within the entire field of vision. In the latter, a person might experience tunnel vision, the illusion of looking through a straw, or randomly blocked vision, giving the illusion of looking through a web or tree branches.

Those with low vision may seek low-vision services. Low-vision programs provide specialists who examine the patient's eyes, evaluate how the patient uses his vision and how it affects his daily activities, provide specific counseling and training, and prescribe low-vision aids or devices.

Cockerham, Paul. *Low Vision Questions and Answers.* New York: American Foundation for the Blind. 1987.

National Society to Prevent Blindness. *Vision Problems in the U.S.* New York: NSPB, 1980.

American Foundation for the Blind. *What Is Low Vision?* www.afb.org/info, 1999.

low-vision aids Low-vision aids or devices are optical lenses or nonoptical devices that help those with low vision to enhance their sight. A low-vision aid may be as simple as a stronger lightbulb to better illuminate the subject or as complex as a talking computer. Emerging technologies promise even more exciting and complex aids, such as electrodes that can be implanted to transmit signals from a video camera directly to the brain. However, most aids either enlarge the image of the object, enlarge the object itself, illuminate or improve contrast or enhance an object or task.

Many aids magnify the image of an object. An enlarged image spread out over the RETINA helps the viewer to overcome any blind spots in the field of vision. Those that magnify the image include MAGNIFIERS, telescopic devices, and electronic devices.

Magnifiers improve close vision for reading and writing tasks. These aids range from the inexpensive dime-store magnifying glass to sophisticated, expensive video equipment. Hand-held or stand magnifiers are available in a wide range of sizes and strengths and come with or without built-in illumination.

A loupe, or spectacle magnifier, is a convex lens that clips onto an eyeglass frame. The lens is attached to the frame by a thin, metal arm and swings down into position just in front of the eyeglass lens. Two or more loupes can be simultaneously mounted on the frame to accommodate work or reading done at different distances.

Telescopic devices increase distance vision. They can be used with one or both eyes and may be hand-held or spectacle mounted. Telemicroscopic lenses or reading telescopes improve intermediate distance vision. These lenses are clipped or mounted onto one or both of the eyeglass lenses.

Other lens systems include filters and prisms. Filter shields worn over eyeglasses reduce glare and ease bright lights for those with light sensitivities. Prisms incorporated into spectacle lenses adjust the image to a different section of the retina to take advantage of functional vision and avoid blind spots.

Electronic magnifying systems are more complex and expensive. Video magnifiers such as CLOSED-CIRCUIT TELEVISION (CCTV) enlarge an original print image up to 60 times and display the image on a large viewing screen.

A low-vision aid that magnifies the object, rather than its image, is LARGE PRINT. This enlarged print enables some people with low vision to read with or without additional magnifying aids.

Many low-vision aids adapt or enhance an object to compensate for the loss of vision. These ADAPTIVE AIDS include communication and writing aids, household devices, and health-care instruments. Low-vision aids for computers also are available.

Low-vision aids are available through low-vision clinics and adaptive aids catalogs. Many of the magnification aids should be prescribed by a low-vision specialist through the services offered at low-vision clinics.

low-vision clinics   Low-vision clinics provide special services to people with low vision. They may be located in clinics or hospitals or medical, rehabilitation or optometric centers. Many ophthalmologists and optometrists specialize in low-vision services and offer them through private practice.

Low-vision services vary. Most offer vision assessment, low-vision eye examinations, training in techniques to help maximize remaining vision, and prescription of aids or devices to enhance vision.

Some low-vision clinics extend this basic program and offer pediatric low-vision exams, genetic counseling, and contact lens evaluation and disbursement. Others add rehabilitation experts to train patients in orientation and mobility instruction and counsel them in vocational and financial matters.

A standard low-vision eye exam includes an assessment interview, specialized examination of the eyes, assessment of remaining vision use, evaluation of vision needed to complete daily tasks at work and home, counseling, and prescription for and training in the use of adaptive devices or aids.

The assessment interview may be conducted by a social worker, rehabilitation or mobility instructor, psychologist, counselor, nurse, or other professional worker in the low-vision field. The oral-assessment interview consists of questions that determine how the patient feels about loss of vision and how it interferes with daily living. The patient may be asked about general health, living conditions, traveling needs, and job tasks.

Next, the eye examination is performed by an optometrist or an ophthalmologist. The examiner uses specifically designed eye charts and carefully monitored light levels to assess the patient's distance vision. Powerful lenses and magnifiers are used to evaluate the patient's near vision and reading skills. The examination may take many sessions to complete, and each session may last up to an hour in length.

After the eye examination, the patient receives training in visual techniques and/or the use of low-vision aids. The instruction is given by a rehabilitation counselor or professional low-vision clinician. During the lesson, the patient is taught skills for using his vision efficiently and is introduced to appropriate devices or aids. These may include optical lenses such as magnifiers, clip-on loupes, and telescopic devices or nonoptical aids such as lamps, reading stands, filters, or large print. The patient may take the aids home for a trial period. The half-hour lesson may be repeated until the proper prescription can be made. An additional recheck examination is usually scheduled after six months.

A patient may be referred to other professionals in the field such as an orientation and mobility instructor or a vocational rehabilitation counselor for additional training. These specialists may direct the patient back to the low-vision clinic at any time during training to reevaluate the patient's vision or aids.

LS&S Group, Inc.   A mail-order company that specializes in products for the visually impaired. Through its catalog, the company offers adaptive aids and electronic equipment.

Items offered include talking and braille watches and clocks, large-print, braille, and speech computer systems; reading machines; personal computers; talking calculators; large-print and braille translation software; speech synthesizers; closed-circuit television systems (CCTV); recorders; telephones and answering machines; timers; magnifiers; lamps; mobility aids; canes; health aids; glasses; security devices; kitchen aids; recreation aids; and toys and games.

Contact:

LS&S Group, Inc.
P.O. Box 673
Northbrook, IL 60065
708-498-9777 or 1-800-468-4789 (ph)
847-498-1482 (fax)
www.lssgroup.com

lupus Lupus or lupus erythematosus (LE) is the name for a series of chronic autoimmune diseases in which the body's immune system attacks its own tissues. The Lupus Foundation of America estimates that between 500,000 and 1.5 million Americans have been diagnosed with the disease. Lupus occurs more frequently in women than in men, and its more prevalent in people of African-American, Indian, or Asian origin. It is a lifelong illness but is not considered life threatening.

Lupus attacks collagen, the support material for tissue. As a result, it can affect the kidneys, skin, joints, blood, heart, eyes, and virtually any other organ in the body. Since its symptoms of skin rash, painful swelling of the joints, fever, headache, and exhaustion mirror those of other disorders, lupus can be difficult to detect immediately.

The cause of lupus is unknown, but heredity, viruses, exposure to ultraviolet or sunlight, extreme stress, and various drugs may play a role. There is no cure for lupus, but treatment can control and relieve symptoms and often result in a remission.

Since collagen is found in every part of the eye, many eye disorders can result as a complication of lupus or its treatment. Hypertension associated with lupus can swell the blood vessels of the OPTIC NERVE, causing hemorrhaging. When this occurs, the blood vessels of the brain and eye become protectively constrictive, shutting off necessary oxygen to the eye and causing permanent damage.

Vasculitis, swelling of the blood vessels, can center in the eye, causing blockage of the eye's main artery. Sudden, severe vision loss may occur.

Optic neuritis, swelling of the optic nerve, can cause retinitis and an accompanying vision loss. Cortisone treatment may reverse the damage caused by optic neuritis.

UVEITIS, an infection in the eye's IRIS, can be caused by lupus. It is treated with cortisone drugs.

Unfortunately, the drug therapy of lupus patients may contribute to their eye disorders. Many lupus patients are treated with cortisone and other steroids, which may cause cataracts or GLAUCOMA in those predisposed to glaucoma.

Plaquinil, an antimalarial drug used in the treatment of lupus, can cause glaucomalike symptoms, such as the loss of peripheral vision. This drug may also be damaging to the eye's macula.

lutein A nutrient in the carotenoid family that is thought by some people to reduce the risk of developing age-related macular degeneration. While most researchers and doctors agree that good nutrition is important to overall eye health, there is little scientific evidence to support the theory that lutein can prevent macular degeneration, despite recent publicity to the contrary. The National Eye Institute (NEI) in March 2000 issued a statement concerning the value of taking lutein supplements. The NEI advised that claims concerning lutein and eye health should be regarded cautiously and stated that the possible benefits of lutein are uncertain.

Foods that are rich in carotenoids include green, leafy vegetables such as kale and cabbage. While the NEI recognizes that these lutein-rich foods are beneficial to overall health, it questions that direct relationship between lutein and eye health.

Lyme disease An infection caused by *Borrelia burgdorferi,* a spirochete bacteria spread by the bite of an infected tick carried by deer, mice, birds, raccoons, chipmunks, and domestic animals. Lyme disease has a worldwide prevalence and has been recorded in six continents, 20 countries and 48 of the United States. More than 100,000 U.S. cases have been reported to the Centers for Disease Control and Prevention. States most affected by Lyme disease are New York, Connecticut, Pennsylvania, and New Jersey.

Symptoms of Lyme disease include a circular or oblong rash, headache, stiff neck, fever, muscle aches, fatigue, and other flulike discomforts. The symptoms usually subside, only to reappear later or give way to more serious problems such as infections of the eye, muscles and joints, brain, heart, skin, liver and lung, skin tumors, gastrointestinal disorders, birth defects, and loss of nerve conduction.

Early stages of Lyme disease are manifested in the eyes as conjunctivitis, episcleritis, and photophobia. Later, cranial nerve palsies may result and cause exposure keratitis and corneal abrasion. Lyme disease may cause papilledema, optic neuritis, and loss of vision. Ocular disorders may be transmitted from an infected mother to the unborn fetus.

Diagnosis of the disease is problematic. A blood test can measure the immune system response to the infecting spirochete but is not completely reliable. Those who test negative to the disease may be infected.

Lyme disease is treated with oral antibiotics in the early stages and with intravenous antibiotic treatments in later stages. The antibiotic treatment is not a cure. Although some individuals remain symptom free, others experience recurrences and require long-term antibiotic treatment. There is a vaccine against Lyme disease called Lymerix, but it is not always effective. Scientists and doctors are working to improve the vaccine.

macula The macula is the central section of the RETINA responsible for clear central vision. It is located in direct line of sight with the PUPIL.

The retina, which contains the macula, is filled with RODS AND CONES. These light-sensitive cells supply information to the eye about the image seen. The rods react to faint light, movement, and shape. The cones distinguish color and detail but require higher light levels to be effective. The macula contains the greatest number of cones.

Within the macula is an indentation called the FOVEA. The fovea contains the greatest concentration of cones and is the site of sharpest vision. Because the cones require light to work, incoming light is focused by the eye onto the macula, centering on the fovea.

The macula is subject to degeneration. Macular disease may be caused by heredity, other diseases such as arteriosclerosis, or aging. ARM, or age-related maculopathy is the most common type of degeneration. It is a disease in which the macula deteriorates, causing a loss of central vision. The disease may involve hemorrhaging from fragile blood vessels beneath the retina. ARM is a progressive disease that may worsen over time. It may effect one or both eyes. The disease is seldom responsible for total blindness since the patient usually retains some peripheral vision.

macular disease Macular disease is the leading cause of new cases of blindness. The Macular Degeneration Foundation, an educational and research organization founded in 1989, estimates that more than 1.2 million American are affected by this disease and that a new case of adult macular disease is diagnosed every three minutes in the United States.

Macular diseases of the eye that cause deterioration to the macula, or central part of the RETINA. This results in a loss of vision in the central field. The macula is centered in the retina, a light-sensitive layer in the back of the eye. Light reflected off an object is focused onto an indentation of the macula, called the FOVEA. The fovea is the point of clearest sight.

Cones in the fovea interpret the light into information about the object. This information is encoded into electrical impulses by the retina and sent to the brain via the OPTIC NERVE. The brain translates the impulses into an image.

There are two major types of macular disease. The first, inherited macular dystrophies, usually occur before the age of 20. These inherited diseases are rare and usually incurable.

The more common form of macular disorder is called age-related maculopathy, or ARM. It is most common in people who are over 60, but can appear as early as age 40.

It is thought that the disorder is caused by a breakdown in the blood supply to the retina. It may also develop due to an infection, ocular trauma or injury, drugs, other diseases such as diabetes, or heredity.

ARM may fall into one of two categories: wet type or maculopathy. The wet type occurs when new delicate blood vessels form in the CHOROID, a vascular layer of tissue beneath the retina. When these abnormal vessels break or leak into the macula, healthy cells are destroyed and vision loss occurs in that central area. Maculopathy does not involve fluid leakage.

ARM is a progressive disease that may worsen rapidly or slowly over time. The onset usually takes place in one eye first, to be followed by an occurrence in the other eye, two or three years later. The condition may first present itself as a blurring of vision. Printed type may look blurred, vertical lines may look wavy, and central vision may appear blocked or distorted.

Age-related maculopathy can be detected during the normal ophthalmological examination. Those over 50 years of age are routinely screened for the disease. During the exam, the ophthalmologist looks for changes within the retina and choroid. The presence of new blood vessels beneath the retina may be signs of possible degeneration development. The presence of drusen, small whitish spots of waste material scattered on the posterior pole may indicate a propensity for development of the disease.

The patient may also be tested for age-related maculopathy with the Amsler grid. This is a grid with a dot in the middle of two intersecting lines. With one eye covered, the patient looks at the dot. If the patient is unable to see some of the lines or if some lines appear wavy or kinked, ARM may have occurred.

Fluorescein angiography may be performed to view the retinal blood vessels. This is a test in which a fluorescent vegetable dye is injected into a vein in the arm. As the dye travels throughout the body and into the retina, a series of photographs are taken. The photographs point out any irregularities within the retinal vascular system.

Doctors and scientists have been working hard to learn more about ARM. A new drug, Visudyne, was recently approved for treatment of the wet form of ARM. Physicians are hopeful that this drug will begin a series of advancements in the treatment of this disease. But since the peripheral field of vision remains unaffected, it is possible to learn to use the remaining vision to the best advantage. Special viewing techniques and optical aids such as telescopic lenses may be prescribed.

In approximately 10 percent of cases, laser photocoagulation treatments can improve the condition. These treatments use LASERS to cauterize and seal the abnormal leaky vessels of wet type ARM. It is usually a painless procedure, performed on an out-patient basis.

Early diagnosis is critical to the treatment of macular degeneration. If the disorder is caused by drugs or infection, the drugs can be discontinued or the infection treated before further damage can occur. Photocoagulation is most successful in the early stages, since it becomes impossible once the vessels develop near the center of the macula or once the infusion of blood conceals the vessels.

macular edema   A condition of the macula stemming from retinal edema. The macula is an indentation of the retina that contains an abundance of cones, light-sensitive cells that are responsible for discerning color and detail. Light is focused directly on the macula by the eye, making it the center of sharpest sight.

Retinal edema occurs when the capillaries of the retina bleed, filling the spaces between retinal cells with fluid. Retinal edema may be present throughout the retina and involve the macula, or it may contained in a general area that spares the macula. If the macula is spared, vision may be relatively unaffected at first. However, the macula tends to accumulate the fluid. In this case, macular edema occurs. The condition is characterized by inflammation of the macula and blurred or impaired vision. If untreated, macular fluid collects in small pockets of space and forms cysts, a condition called cystic macular edema. The condition leads to degeneration of the macula in which central vision may be permanently lost.

Macular edema is caused by diabetic retinopathy, hypertension, retinal vein obstruction, traction of the vitreous, inflammations such as UVEITIS and RETINITIS, and CATARACT surgery. It is diagnosed with fluorescein angiography, a procedure in which fluorescein dye is injected into a vein in the arm and monitored as it passes through the veins of the retina. Macular edema may right itself spontaneously or persist. Treatment of the condition varies according to the cause. Cases due to inflammation are treated with corticosteroids.

Those conditions of edema caused by vascular problems and diabetes may be treated with photocoagulation, a treatment that uses a laser to seal leaking blood vessels. There is no treatment for edema due to traction or cataract surgery.

magnifiers   Magnifiers and other optical aids are used to increase the size of an image. Magnifiers improve close vision for reading and writing tasks. These LOW-VISION AIDS range from the inexpensive dime-store magnifying glass to sophisticated, expensive video equipment.

Placement-type, hand-held, and stand magnifiers are available in a wide range of sizes and strengths and come with or without built-in illumination. Bar magnifiers are plastic bars that are placed on one line of print to double the original size. Page magnifiers are sheets of plastic placed over a page to magnify the print. Both are available without prescription.

Hand-held magnifiers range from 3X to 10X magnification. Some are modeled after a flashlight and include illumination. These are used for near-vision tasks such as short-term reading. Hand-held magnifiers are not suitable for long periods of reading and writing due to unsteadiness of the hand.

Stand magnifiers are available in 3X to 10X magnification and are mounted on a stand that is placed over the document to be read. The stand places the magnifier the proper distance from the material and frees the hands. Stand magnifiers are generally used with reading glasses.

A loupe, or spectacle magnifier, is a convex lens that clips onto an eyeglass frame. The lens is attached to the frame by a thin, metal arm and swings down into position just in front of the eyeglass lens. Two or more loupes can be simultaneously mounted on the frame to accommodate work or reading done at different distances.

Electronic magnifying systems are more complex and expensive. Video magnifiers, such as closed-circuit television or CCTV, enlarge an original print image up to 60 times. The image is displayed on a large viewing screen. These devices can change the dark letters on a white field of the original to white letters on a dark field to increase contrast and visibility. Many users can use the CCTV to write, type and operate a computer.

High-powered, portable magnifying devices are rapidly becoming available. Small and lightweight, these aids are powered by rechargeable battery packs. They scan print information with a camera mounted on rollers and magnify the image four to 64 times the original size. The image is projected onto a display monitor in either orange print on a black background or the reverse.

Telescopes are commonly used optical aids. They may be hand held, fused into spectacle frames, incorporated into prescription lenses, or worn on a headband. Binocular hand-held telescopes are used for distance magnification and are available in various magnifications. Hand-held binocular telescopes are adjustable and may be used with one or both eyes. They are used with both eyes for viewing sports events, television, and street signs. When used with one eye, binoculars produce a smaller field of view and are used for near and intermediate distance viewing in tasks such as reading or writing.

Binocular telescopes may be fused into spectacle frames for convenience of use. These are used for distance viewing of sports events, television, stage productions, etc. They produce a small field of view and are available in 3X magnification. Binocular spectacles are available without a prescription but cannot be used if a prescriptive correction is necessary.

Hand-held monocular telescopes are available for use with one eye in magnifications up to 10X. They are used for distance of viewing sports or television or in school but are not recommended for walking. Variations of the hand-held monocular telescope may be attached or fused onto prescriptive lenses. Attached versions are available in magnifications up to 3X, and fused versions up to 4X magnification.

Bioptics are optical aids that consist of small telescopes fused onto the upper portion of spectacles, on one or both lenses. The bottom portion of the spectacles contains the individual's corrective prescription. The bioptics involving both eyes enables the user to view distances when walking or driving or to view closer objects or material if magnification is needed. The bioptics that involve one eye only are used for near and intermediate distance viewing for reading material. Bioptics are prescribed by an ophthalmologist or low-vision expert and must be properly centered to the eyes of the wearer. Magnification may extend to six times normal size when used for distance viewing. Wide-angle and zoom lenses may be incorporated into the device.

Near telescopes are fused onto the lower portion of the spectacle frames, with the prescriptive lenses in the upper portion of the frame. They are available up to 8X magnification and are effective for five to 40 inches. The telescopes are angled to be used by both eyes and are used for intermediate distance tasks such as reading or typing.

Headband telescopes are attached to a headband and free the hands for work. They can be worn over prescriptive lenses and are used for near viewing up to one foot or less. They afford a wide field of vision and are most effective for those with equal sight in both eyes.

Some new systems combine the camera and display screen in a hand-held housing. A vacuum-fluorescent display makes a magnified image appear as the camera is moved across the reading material. There also are some new systems that use head-mounted displays, providing portability and a new way of viewing. More information and reviews of various CCTV systems are available by contacting the National Technology Program:

212-502-7642 (ph)
212-502-7773 (fax)
techctr@afb.net

mailing privileges   Materials may be mailed free of postage by legally blind individuals or those unable to read or use conventionally printed materials as a result of a physical disability. The program is entitled "Free Matter for the Blind or Handicapped."

In order to become eligible, the individual must present written certification by a competent authority to the post office where mailings will be sent and received. An authority may include a licensed doctor, ophthalmologist, optometrist, registered nurse, or professional staff member of a hospital or other agency or institution.

Material eligible for mailing includes books, magazines, musical scores, braille material, 14-point Sightsaving Type, records, or cassette tapes. Equipment and parts of equipment used for writing or educational purposes, sound play-back equipment for use by the visually impaired, and equipment designed or adapted for use by visually impaired persons, such as braille watches and white canes are also eligible.

The material must be free of advertising and must be specifically designed for and used by visu-

ally or physically disabled individuals. The mail is subject to inspection by the Postal Service.

Noncommercial agencies or organizations, individuals, and libraries serving eligible persons may mail the material to an eligible person or organization free of charge. The eligible person may exchange or return material postage free to other eligible persons or organizations. Commercial producers of this material may mail it free of postage to an eligible individual or organization so long as the fee, charge, or rental does not exceed the cost of the material.

Eligible persons may send letters in braille, large print, or recorded form. Handwritten or typed letters are subject to postage when mailed to or from an eligible person. Letters must remain unsealed to allow inspection by the Postal Service. All mailed material must be stamped, printed, or handwritten with the words. "Free Matter for the Blind or Handicapped" in the space reserved for postage. Free international delivery of some materials also is included. Special services, however, such as Express Mail or Certified Mail, are not included.

mainstreaming   A term used to describe the practice of educating disabled students, including those with visual impairments, in a standard, public classroom for non-disabled children.

Federal law requires that all disabled children be given a free, appropriate public education in the least restrictive environment. This environment has often been equated with mainstreaming.

The mainstreaming movement grew out of a need for the education of a large population of visually impaired children who were blinded by retrolental fibroplasia during the early 1950s. At that time, the most popular form of education, residential schooling, was unable to immediately provide for the influx of students.

Parents organized to insist that their children be allowed into public schools and that special education be provided according to their needs. Today, although residential schools still provide vital education and training services, the American Foundation for the Blind estimates that nearly 90 percent of disabled students receive all or part of their education in local public schools.

Students may be mainstreamed into a public school program through several models of delivery, including the itinerant-teacher model, and the teacher-consultant model, and the resource-room model.

The ITINERANT TEACHER is one who travels every two or three days to each public school in the district to provide special education modifications to mainstreamed visually impaired children. The teacher provides special equipment, training, and materials adapted to the student's learning needs and consultation services to the regular classroom teacher.

The TEACHER-CONSULTANT is a special educator who advises regular classroom teachers, teacher aides, administrators, and other school personnel in methods that will meet visually impaired students' needs. The greatest proportion of the work is consultative, rather than instructive.

The RESOURCE ROOM is a specially equipped room staffed with special education personnel trained to work with disabled students, including those with blindness or visual impairments. The students live at home and attend public school in regular classrooms taught by teachers who provide general curriculum instruction. Students visit the resource room at regularly scheduled intervals or when needed.

Students may be technically mainstreamed into a public school system through a school's SELF-CONTAINED CLASSROOM for the disabled. This is a classroom in a public school that is specially equipped and staffed with special education teachers for the disabled. All the students in the class have visual impairments or other disabilities.

Many children, often those with low vision or other disabilities that do not interfere with educational progress, attend their local public schools without special-education support.

Scholl, Geraldine, ed. *Foundations of Education for Blind and Visually Handicapped Children and Youth.* New York: American Foundation for the Blind Inc., 1986.

Scott, Eileen P. *Your Visually Impaired Student.* Baltimore: University Park Press, 1982.

malignant melanoma A tumor of the eye that grows from melanin-laden cells in the CHOROID, IRIS, or CILIARY BODY. Also called an intraocular melanoma. According to the U.S. Department of Health and Human Services, malignant melanomas account for up to 80 percent of all eye malignancies, making them the most common primary (originating in the eye) inner-eye tumor. The tumor may develop from a mole or spontaneously and is usually slow to grow and spread. It generally affects one eye only (unilateral), may appear at any age and is more common in whites than blacks. Symptoms include redness of the eye, inflammation, vision loss, and the presence or development of GLAUCOMA. Melanomas of the iris may distort the shape of PUPIL.

A melanoma can be detected in the ophthalmologic examination. It may first appear to be a choroidal hemorrhage, but can be identified further by FLUORESCEIN ANGIOGRAPHY or ULTRASONOGRAPHY.

Three types of treatment are commonly used for intraocular melanomas. They are: surgery, radiation therapy, and photocoagulation. Surgery is the most common treatment. It can involve removing a portion of the diseased eye, or enucleation, which is the removal of the entire eye. Radiation uses X rays and other high-energy rays to kill cancer cells and shrink tumors. It can be used by itself, or in combination with surgery. Photocoagulation treats the melanoma by destroying blood vessels with a tiny beam of light, usually from a laser. Destroying the blood vessels kills the tumor.

Clinical trials to test other treatment methods are ongoing. More information about the trials can be obtained by calling (toll free) the National Cancer Institute's Cancer Information Service at 800-422-6237. If the diagnosis is uncertain, a period of observation may be prescribed, possibly including chemotherapy or radiation treatments.

Little is known concerning the cause of malignant melanomas. Unlike skin or conjunctiva melanomas, sunlight exposure is not related to these tumors. Limited data exists concerning metastatic rates (growth or spread of tumor) and spontaneous regression rates

National Cancer Institute. "What is Intraocular Melanoma?" NCI website: www.cancernet.nci.nih.gov, 2000.

Marfan's syndrome　Marfan's syndrome (arach-nodactyly) is a rare genetic disease. It is characterized by long, thin bones, elongated limbs, especially of the extremities, tall slender figure, lack of subcutaneous fat, nonelastic ligaments, congenital heart disorders, high infant-mortality rate, malformations of the spine, joints, and ears, and ocular disorders.

Ocular disorders include dislocation or subluxation of the LENS, serious refractive errors (near-sightedness, far-sightedness, etc.), GLAUCOMA, CATARACT, and uveal COLOBOMAS. IRIDONESIS, or a trembling of the iris, also associated with Marfan's syndrome. The most common symptom, subluxated lens, is a condition in which the lens becomes displaced in an up and out direction.

The subluxated lens may increase myopia and cause ASTIGMATISM or cataracts. Often, the displaced lens blocks or narrows the angle of the ANTERIOR CHAMBER and causes secondary glaucoma. If glaucoma cannot be treated successfully with medications or surgical procedures, the lens may be removed. In some cases, aphakic (without lens) patients may experience corrected vision with aphakic spectacles or contact lenses.

For more information contact:

The National Marfan Foundation
382 Main Street
Port Washington, NY 11050
800-8-MARFAN (ph)
516-883-8040 (fax)
www.marfan.org

Maternal and Child Health Services Program

The Maternal and Child Health block-grant program evolved from the original Sheppard-Tower Act of 1921. Also known as the Maternity and Infant Act, it was the first national health services grant program. In 1935, the act was amended and revised by Title V of the Social Security Act to include services for disabled children.

Amendments to Title V in 1963 authorized a grant program to improve health and prenatal care for low-income women. The effort was designed to reduce preventable mental retardation and birth defects. The legislation provided funding for research studies and additional grant funds for states under the Maternal and Child Health program and the Crippled Children's program.

The Social Security Act Amendments of 1965 extended and improved health-care services for mothers and children. Project grants were established to develop maternal and children's health-care programs and comprehensive training services for specialists working with disabled children. Project grants were authorized to support and improve health-care services to low-income school-age and preschool-age children.

In 1967, amendments to the Social Security Act combined the separate Crippled Children's Service grants and Maternal and Child Health Services grants into one authorization. One-half of the funding was allotted to formula grants; the other half was divided 40 percent for project grants and 10 percent for training and research. In 1981, this grant authority was consolidated with those for all the programs established in Title V into one state block-grant authority by the Omnibus Budget Reconciliation Act.

The words "crippled children" were removed from the wording of the Act in 1985 and the words, "children with special health-care needs" was substituted. In 1986 and 1987, appropriations were raised for the Maternal and Child Health program.

Block grants awarded to the states may be used to provide health-care services, and fund development, administration, training, education and evaluation of the programs. According to the Office of Special Education and Rehabilitative Services, the law authorizes the states to use MCH block-grant funds to:

- Assure mothers and children access to quality health services
- Reduce infant mortality, preventable diseases, and disability conditions among children
- Reduce the need for in-patient and long-term care services
- Increase appropriate child immunization
- Increase health assessments and follow-up diagnostic and treatment services for low-income children

- Provide preventative and primary-care services for children and prenatal, delivery, and postpartum services for low-income mothers
- Provide rehabilitation services for blind or disabled children under 16 who receive Supplemental Security Income benefits
- Provide information services regarding diagnosis, hospitalization, and after-care for children who have disabilities or conditions that may lead to disabilities
- Provide for Special Projects of Regional and National Significance (SPRANS), research and training for genetic disease testing, counseling, and information dissemination
- Provide grants relating to hemophilia and sudden infant death syndrome

U.S. Department of Education. *Summary of Existing Legislation Affecting Persons with Disabilities.* Washington, D.C.: USDE, 1988.

Maxi Aids Inc.   Maxi Aids is one of the largest suppliers of adaptive living aids in the United States. Formerly known as Seeing Technologies Inc., the company has an extensive on-line catalog and also offers traditional catalogs of its products.

It offers products including alarm vibrators, adaptive calculators, canes, CCTVs, computer products, games, personal need devices, glasses, kitchen and cooking adaptive devices, mobility devices, magnifiers, radios and recorders, paging devices, sensory products, talking products, and telephones.

Contact:

Maxi Aids
42 Executive Blvd.
Farmingdale, NY 11735
631-752-0521 or 1-800-522-6294 (to place an order)
631-752-0738 (TTY)
631-752-0689 (fax)
www.maxiaids.com

Medicaid legislation   In 1965, amendments to the Social Security Act added Title XIX, a grants program that allowed states to establish medical-assistance systems. Title XIX extended the Kerr-Mills medical-aid program for low-income blind and disabled individuals and dependent children.

The new program became known as Medicaid. Unlike Medicare, it allowed states to offer coverage not only to those who receive public assistance, but also to eligible needy people who did not qualify for welfare or Medicare. The program varies from state to state.

Although the original legislation of 1965 made no specific reference to disabilities, Medicaid has become the main source of medical services funding to severely disabled individuals. In 1992, U.S. federal and state budgets included $118 billion in Medicaid benefits. This may be because later amendments added specific benefits for mentally ill and mentally retarded institutionalized individuals, and because the funding targets low-income groups where the incidence of disability is greater.

Medicaid eligibility is determined by financial need. Recipients generally fall into one or more of the three qualifying categories: categorically needy, medically needy, or qualified severely impaired.

The categorically needy receive AID TO FAMILIES WITH DEPENDENT CHILDREN (AFDC) benefits or SUPPLEMENTAL SECURITY INCOME (SSI) benefits or qualify under specific regulations for their state.

Medically needy persons may have incomes too high to qualify for AFDC or SSI benefits yet cannot afford to pay for necessary medical treatment. States determine a different qualifying income level for those who are medically needy.

Qualified severely impaired individuals are those under 65 who receive federal SSI benefits because of blindness or disability and are able to be employed but do not have incomes that allow them to pay for health-care coverage.

Medicaid provides hospital services, both inpatient and outpatient, as well as laboratory tests or X-ray services. Special nursing facility services and, for those over 21 years old, home health services are also provided.

The benefits cover the recipient's doctor services and diagnostic tests such as those classified as EPSDT, or early periodic screening, diagnosis and treatment services, for those under 21. Additionally, some rural health-clinic care and family-planning services are also provided under the plan.

States must arrange to transport recipients to and from medical services if needed; they must allow the recipient to choose the medical caregivers and must provide health-care services statewide. If adequate medical care is provided, states may limit the quantity, extent, and range of these services.

If listed in the state plan, the state may provide any optional services that are allowed under state law and permitted by the Secretary of Health and Human Services. Since each state designs a program to meet the specific needs of its citizens, coverage differs greatly from state to state.

The optional services may include private nursing, health-clinic, and dental services. Physical and occupational therapy and rehabilitation services may be covered, as well as hearing, speech, and language therapy or treatment.

The plan may include prescriptions such as drugs, eyeglasses, dentures, prosthetics, and prosthetic aids. Other services may include those not covered specifically under federal law in such areas as diagnostic screening, inpatient hospital procedures, nursing or intermediate-care facility services, in-patient psychiatric treatment for those under 21 or over 65, and case-management services for specific categories of eligible people.

U.S. Department of Education. *Summary of Existing Legislation Affecting Persons with Disabilities.* Washington, D.C.: USDE, 1988.

Medicare legislation   Title XVIII of the Social Security Act authorizes the Health Care Financing Administration, a division of the Department of Health and Human Services, to offer Medicare health-insurance benefits to qualified handicapped and elderly individuals. Generally, eligible individuals are those 65 years or older who qualify for Social Security benefits. Disabled individuals may qualify for Medicare after a two-year waiting period if they are:

- No longer able to work and their pre-disability contributions to the Social Security FICA meet the required limit

- People with severe childhood disabilities who are dependents of eligible Social Security recipients who are retired or have died

- People with childhood disabilities who qualify for Social Security benefits

- Disabled widowed persons, 50 years of age or older

- Diagnosed as having an end-stage renal condition

In 2001, nearly 40 million people in America were eligible for some Medicare health coverage. Medicare has two parts: Part A is hospital insurance and Part B is medical insurance. Part A helps pay for necessary in-patient and limited home services including hospital or emergency-room care, nursing facilities, hospice services, and some home-health care.

Part B of the insurance plan helps pay for doctors, services, outpatient hospital care, and other medical treatment not covered by Part A. Services covered by the plan are paid according to reasonable costs and fee schedules. Any eligible individual may register for Part B benefits. Although the individual is required to pay a monthly premium, some states or other agencies may pay the premium for a disabled person.

At the end of March 2001, a bill was pending in Congress that would make orientation and mobility specialists, rehabilitation teachers, and low-vision therapists eligible providers under Medicare.

U.S. Department of Education. *Summary of Existing Legislation Affecting Persons with Disabilities.* Washington, D.C.: USDE, 1988.
Health Care Financing Administration. "Medicare Basics." www.medicare.gov, 2001.

migraine   A migraine is a type of recurrent headache. It differs from the normal tension headache in that it usually affects one side of the head only and is often accompanied by visual disturbances, nausea, and vomiting.

Migraines are thought to be caused by a sudden dilation of the arteries in the brain and scalp following a period of spasm or narrowing. The sudden expansion of the arteries causes the blood to surge against the artery walls and surrounding tissues. The dilation and constriction may occur when the body over-produces serotonin and nor-epinephrine, amines or biological substances that dilate and constrict blood vessels of the body and brain.

Migraine attacks tend to run in families and may be triggered by a variety of causes. It is estimated that between 11 and 18 million Americans suffer from migraines, most of them women. In addition, it is estimated that up to 38 million Americans have the genetic propensity for migraines. The following have been linked to migraine attacks: intense direct, reflected, or flickering lights; rapidly changing images, sudden or persistent noises; reaction to stress; strong odors; allergies; hypertension; hormonal changes; nitroglycerin; anesthetic; drugs; alcohol; cheese; chocolate; cured foods; MSG; poor ventilation; change in barometric pressure; exercise; tight clothing; steam; motion; dental problems; a shock or blow to the head; and too little or too much sleep.

The two major categories of migraine headaches are common and classic. Each is preceded by a pre-headache state, called the prodrome stage, which may last from five minutes to an hour. During this stage, symptoms of the oncoming migraine may be noted. They include nausea, vomiting, weakness or tingling on one side or section of the body, mental confusion, fatigue, irritability, dizziness, pallor, euphoria, water retention, and lack of coordination.

Common migraines are associated with light, noise or odor sensitivity, and vomiting or nausea. Classic migraines may include these symptoms but are further characterized by visual disturbances. Patients may experience blurred vision, TUNNEL VISION, double vision, SCOTOMAS, scintillating scotomas, fortification spectra (angled, shimmering lines), HEMIANOPSIA, or distorted vision.

Blurred vision is common to migraine attacks and may be accompanied by tunnel vision, the loss of peripheral or side vision. Tunnel vision has been described as vision seen when looking through a straw. Double vision, or DIPLOPIA, may result during a migraine if ophthalmoplegia, paralysis of the eye muscles, occurs. When a muscle is paralyzed, one eye moves out of alignment and the brain receives two images instead of one, or double vision.

Scotomas are blind spots in the field of vision of one or both eyes. The vision in the scotoma may be blurred or completely obliterated. Scintillating scotomas are blind spots that shimmer with bright light to block out vision. Scotomas may appear anywhere in the field of vision and may move during the course of the prodrome stage or during the headache stage.

Fortification spectra is a shimmering, glittering pattern of bright or colored lights in the field of vision. The lights form shapes such as auras or semicircles and appear in zigzag formations much like a prism. They may block vision or lie atop it.

Hemianopsia is a decrease or loss of vision in one half of each eye. The entire right or left half of the field of vision may be obliterated or may be blocked by fortification spectra.

Distorted vision may result from migraine. Objects or people may appear elongated or stretched out of shape as by a funhouse mirror. This phenomenon is sometimes called the Alice in Wonderland syndrome in reference to the distorted figures pictured in *Alice's Adventures in Wonderland.* The author, Lewis Carroll, was said to have suffered migraines and collaborated closely with the illustrator to produce illustrations that captured the visual effects he experienced.

The visual effects of the prodrome stage may disappear with the onset of the headache or my overlap. When the visual symptoms occur, but a headache does not follow, the condition is known as a migraine equivalent.

The migraine headache itself is often severe. It usually affects only one side of the head and may include the face, extending as far as the jaw. Patients may experience light sensitivity, head, neck, and scalp sensitivity or tenderness, nausea and vomiting. The headache may last from one to 24 hours. In rare cases, the headache may last for days.

Migraines can occur at any time of life. They may appear in children as recurring attacks of headache and vomiting or as migraine equivalents. The attacks may disappear or return later in middle life. Migraines can occur for the first time in middle age and may decrease in regularity as time goes on. Women are more likely to suffer from migraines, but the problem tends to improve with menopause.

At present, there is no cure for migraines. Analgesics such as aspirin and acetaminophen or either compound with codeine may be taken to ease pain at the first sign of the headache. Severe pain is often treated with vasoconstricting agents such as ergotamine. These drugs constrict the blood vessels of the scalp to reduce the flow of blood. Ergotamine must be taken during the early stages of the headache and cannot be taken in conjunction with drugs for hypertension.

Migraines may recur. Patients may reduce recurrences by avoiding triggering factors and managing stress and tension. Drugs to prevent migraine attacks may be prescribed in cases in which the severity or frequency of migraine attacks has not been affected by the elimination of triggering factors. The drugs, such as Bellergal, Pizotyline, Propranolol, Elavil, and Sansert, have varying degrees of effectiveness, side effects, and safety. New treatments for migraines are being developed and tested.

Migraines can be very upsetting and distressing to those who suffer from them and to their families and friends. Also, there are many misconceptions about migraines, including the theory that a migraine is not a bona fide physical illness.

Joel R. Saper, M.D., director of the Michigan Head-Pain & Neurological Institute, explained the problem of misconception as it relates to migraines. "There is no condition of such magnitude that is shrouded in myth, misinformation, and mistreatment as is this condition, and there are few conditions which are as disabling during the acute attack," Saper said.

There is a support group for migraine sufferers called Migraine Awareness Group: A National Understanding for Migraineurs, or M.A.G.N.U.M.

Contact:

M.A.G.N.U.M., Inc.
113 South Saint Asaph, Suite 300
Alexandria, VA 22314
703-739-9384
www.migraines.org

mobility See ORIENTATION AND MOBILITY.

Mowat Sensor The Mowat Sensor is a mobility aid designed for use by visually impaired persons and developed by HUMANWARE. The device uses high-frequency sound waves to detect objects in the user's path. The sensor vibrates if an object is present and increases the vibration rate as the user nears the object. The sensor has a short range for objects less than one meter away and a longer range for objects up to four meters away.

Approximately the size of a flashlight, the device may be hand held or carried in a pocket or purse. A model for those with poor tactual sensation produces an audible signal heard through an earphone attachment. Other similar devices are manufactured under various names, including the Bliss Passive Detector.

The device is designed to be used with a long cane or dog guide. Several hours of practice and/or training with a qualified instructor are required for proficient use. (See ELECTRONIC TRAVEL AIDS.)

multiple sclerosis (MS) A chronic disease of the central nervous system. According to the National Multiple Sclerosis Society, approximately 333,000 Americans have been diagnosed with MS or MS-related diseases, and approximately 200 new cases are diagnosed each week.

The disease attacks the body's myelin, a fatty substance that coats and insulates nerve fibers of the brain and spinal cord. As the myelin is damaged, sclerosed or hardened tissue, called plaques, form. The plaques interrupt or obstruct the impulses transmitted along the nerves.

Symptoms of MS include tingling in the limbs or extremities, numbness, blurred or double vision, nystagmus, impaired sensation, fatigue, weakness, dizziness, slurred speech, tremor, spasticity, and bladder, bowel, or sexual function problems.

Half of all those who are diagnosed with MS may experience visual disturbances. The three most common disorders are optic neuritis, DIPLOPIA, and NYSTAGMUS.

Optic neuritis, or inflammation of the OPTIC NERVE, often results in a condition termed retrobulbar neuritis. It may first appear as a loss of vision in one eye, blurring of vision, color blindness, or blind spots. The disruption of vision usually first occurs in the central field of vision and progresses to peripheral fields.

Optic neuritis may be treated with steroids or the drug ACTH. Recurrence is possible, but remission of the visual impairment is good. Most cases respond to treatment in three months.

Diplopia, or double vision, may occur if the eyes do not move together to focus on an object. Diplopia occurs when the myelin along nerve fibers controlling coordination of the eye movement is damaged. Diplopia is treated with steroids and ACTH or by patching one eye. The condition usually improves within several weeks but may recur.

Nystagmus is an involuntary, jerky movement of the eyes that makes focusing difficult. It may cause dizziness and blurred vision. The condition is treated with steroids, ACTH, and Meclizine for symptoms of dizziness. Within a few weeks the symptoms may subside, although recurrences are possible.

The symptoms and progression of MS are unique to the individual. Although an initial attack may never be followed by a recurring incident, most people experience periods of exacerbation, in which symptoms of the disease are most pronounced, and remission, symptom-free periods.

The degree of disability varies by individual but two thirds of all those with MS remain ambulatory over their lifetimes. The disease is rarely fatal and studies indicate that life expectancy is only reduced by 15 percent or less.

MS usually first appears between the ages of 20 and 40. Women, whites, and those who live in colder climates are more likely to develop the disease. Twice as many women as men have MS. Studies suggest that where one was born and lived for the first 15 years of life affect the risk of developing the disease more than later places of residence.

The cause of MS is unknown. It is not contagious or inherited, although certain genetic conditions within individuals may make them more receptive to MS. These factors include exogenous (outside the environment) factors such as viruses and endogenous (inside the environment) factors such as body immunity.

Because families tend to share similar exogenous and endogenous factors, susceptibility to the disease may run in families. Four percent of all families with an incidence of MS have an additional case of MS.

Although there is no cure for MS, it may be treated with medications to reduce the symptoms. Muscle relaxants may reduce spasticity and medications may be prescribed to reduce pain, tension, bowel and urinary distress.

The drug ACTH or steroids such as prednisone may shorten the duration and lessen the intensity of exacerbations. ACTH is usually administered by injection and monitored for effects on the body in the hospital. Steroids are given orally or by injection but also require monitoring. Side effects of these medications may include weight increase, fluid retention, mood alteration, and tendency toward the development of ulcers. Since 1993, three new medications to treat relapsing forms of MS have been approved by the Food and Drug Administration. They are: Betaserona, Copaxonea, and Avonexa. These medicines have been shown to lessen the severity and frequency of MS attacks. They also help to reduce accumulations of lesions on the brain and to slow the progression of disability.

Since increasing evidence links MS to disorders within the body's immune system stemming from a viral infection, current areas of research include virology and immunology. Some researchers believe that MS is associated with physical trauma, but that theory is controversial.

Frames, Robin. "Insight into Eyesight." *MS: Facts and Issues.* New York: National Multiple Sclerosis Society, 1985.

National Multiple Sclerosis Society. *Living with MS.* HealthNet Library, CompuServe, 1988.

National Multiple Sclerosis Society. *What Is Multiple Sclerosis?* New York: NMSS, 2001.

myasthenia gravis Myasthenia gravis is an autoimmune disease in which abnormal antibodies in the blood disrupt transmission of impulses from the nerve endings to muscle tissue. This condition results in severe or fatal (in the case of respiratory failure) fatigue of the muscle. It is estimated that there are about 36,000 cases of the disease in the United States, with a prevalence of 14 in every 100,000 people. Women are affected more often and earlier in life than men.

The disease may affect one group of muscles or those of the entire body. Approximately 75 percent of all initial myasthenia cases involve the ocular muscles, and nearly 90 percent develop some ocular involvement over time. Those cases that involve only the ocular muscles for a period of two years will probably be limited to the ocular muscles and not progress systemically. Ocular myasthenia cases account for approximately 20 percent of all cases.

Ocular symptoms of the disease include PTOSIS (drooping eyelid), lid twitch or quiver, and NYSTAGMUS (uncontrollable movement of the eyes). Ptosis may be absent at the start of the day but becomes more pronounced as the day progresses.

Myasthenia gravis is diagnosed with a Tensilon test. The drug Tensilon is injected to stimulate nerve transmission. Muscle strength is measured before and after the injection. Those who show a temporary gain in strength or improvement of symptoms after the injection test positively for myasthenia gravis.

Myasthenia gravis is generally treated by a neurologist. Treatment may consist of oral drugs and corticosteroids. Removal of the thymus gland may produce an improvement in symptoms.

myopia Nearsightedness, occurring when the refractive power of the eyes is too great in relation to the length of the eyes. Myopic eyes are too "long" for their refracting capabilities. Myopic people see close objects more clearly than distant objects. Corrective concave lenses in the form of contacts or eyeglasses are prescribed to correct the problem.

High myopia is a condition in which the eye is extremely long or large, producing extreme nearsightedness. In very large eyes, the structures within them are stretched, causing the retina to become thin and weak. Tears or detachments that impair vision can develop as a result.

Myopia usually occurs from the preteen to teenage years. As the child grows, the myopia may worsen with each growth spurt. Once the child reaches maturity, it generally levels off and stabilizes for many years.

myths Myths about blindness have existed for centuries and grew from ignorance about the condition and nature of blindness. Myths are perpetu-

ated by modern attitudes toward, and stereotypes of, blindness.

Some commonly held myths surrounding blindness include the concept of all forms of blindness as darkness, the concept of blind as dependent, the connection between blindness and punishment as in the Oedipal legend, the belief that the other senses compensate for a loss of sight, and that people who have a vision loss have ESP or musical talent.

Being blind does not necessarily mean seeing nothing, or being in darkness. Of the half million people who are legally blind in the United States, most retain some usable vision. Only a fraction have no light perception or usable vision. Because darkness is so closely associated in society with ignorance, evil, and fear, the concept of blindness as darkness also links it to these negative traits.

The lack of understanding about visual abilities of the blind fosters the perception of blind persons as dependent. Throughout history, blind persons have been seen as liabilities to the social group, wards of society, or beggars. This myth disregards the abilities of blind individuals to work and be self-supporting and exists today in the unwillingness of employers to hire blind persons.

The evil-eye myth stems from ancient times when blindness was perceived as a sign of evil or a punishment from God for some evil-doing or sin. Those with the evil eye were thought to be able to kill with it, and were therefore shunned.

The Oedipal legend supports the myth that blindness is equated with evil. Oedipus blinded himself as a punishment for wrong-doing. The legend supports blindness as a just punishment for sins and suggests that blind persons may have brought the condition on themselves.

A commonly held myth about blindness concerns the compensation of senses. It is falsely believed that once eyesight is gone, nature heightens the other senses to compensate for the lack of sight. In reality, the blind person may learn to use the other senses in more efficient ways to gather information, but the senses remain unchanged.

Blind persons are often believed to have extraordinary abilities or talents, as well. It is commonly held that blind individuals develop extrasensory powers, or ESP, as a compensation for the sight loss. Perhaps because of some popular blind performers, the myth exists that blind persons are innately musically talented.

Curiously, the reverse situation is also widely believed. It is held that blind persons lose sense abilities, especially hearing, with the loss of sight. This myth prompts people to shout questions to a blind person with normal hearing.

As blind and visually impaired persons become more widely integrated into social, vocational, and education situations, myths may dissipate. Through personal experiences, society can discover that blind persons are not condemned or blessed as a group, but rather, are individual members of society who happen to lack some degree of sight. (See ATTITUDES, EMPLOYMENT.)

Carroll, Thomas J. *Blindness, What It Is, What It Does, and How to Live With It.* Boston: Little, Brown, 1961.

Goldberg, Maxwell H., and John R. Swinton. *Blindness Research: The Expanding Frontiers.* University Park: Pennsylvania State University Press, 1969.

Haskins, James. *Who Are the Handicapped?* New York: Doubleday, 1978.

Jernigan, Kenneth. *Disability and Visibility: Uncle Tom, Blind Tom, and Tiny Tim.* Baltimore: National Federation of the Blind, 1970.

Mitchell, Joyce Slayton. *See Me More Clearly.* New York: Harcourt, Brace, Jovanovich, 1980.

National Alliance for Eye and Vision Research (NAEVR)

A nonprofit advocacy organization made up of a coalition of professional, consumer, and industry organizations involved in research in eye and vision disorders. The organization works to provide the best vision possible for all Americans through education, advocacy, and vision research. Its goals are supported by the National Institutes of Health, the National Eye Institute, and other federal research organizations.

NAEVR was founded in 1997 as an affiliated organization of the ALLIANCE FOR EYE AND VISION RESEARCH. Its purpose is to carry out the advocacy activities of that coalition. It is particularly concerned about maintaining federal funding for the NATIONAL EYE INSTITUTE to allow the NEI to carry out its extensive research programs. NAEVR actively lobbies for NEI funding. It also is working to raise government awareness of the connections between tobacco use and eye disease, and the devastating effects of macular degeneration on many elderly people. NAEVR hopes to convince Congress of the need for intensive, focused research in these areas.

Contact:

National Alliance for Eye and Vision Research
426 C Street, NE
Washington, DC 20002
202-544-1880 (ph)
202-543-2565 (fax)
www.eyeresearch.org

National Association for Parents of the Visually Impaired (NAPVI)

An association that serves as a source of support, information, and service to families of the visually impaired. Founded in 1980, the association membership consists of parents and families of the visually impaired, agencies and community groups, and individuals interested or affected by visual impairment.

The organization offers encouragement and emotional support to families and provides information to parents on care, treatment, education, and services available to visually impaired children. NAPVI communicates its expectations to service agencies at the local, state, and federal levels to obtain and ensure quality services to visually impaired and blind children.

NAPVI awards the annual Outstanding Contribution Award to a Professional Working in the Field of Blindness. It publishes a quarterly newsletter called *Awareness* that provides resource information for parents.

The organization disburses fact sheets, brochures, and a publications list and holds a biennial National Parent Conference.

Contact:

National Association for Parents of the Visually
  Impaired
P.O. Box 317
Watertown, MA 02471
800-562-6265 (ph)
617-972-7441 (fax)
www.spedex.com/NAPVI

National Association for Visually Handicapped (NAVH)

A nonprofit, national voluntary health agency. It serves the partially sighted, those not completely blind but who lack adequate vision even with the best possible corrective lenses. Founded in 1954, the organization was formerly known as Aid to the Visually Handicapped or National Aid to the Visually Handicapped.

NAVH produces and distributes large-print books, texts and reading materials free on request to partially sighted persons. It serves as a large-print consultant to commercial publishers and maintains a free, large-print lending library.

The organization offers counseling and advice services to young adults, seniors, and families of the partially sighted. It cooperates with senior citizen centers, hospitals, and institutions and offers adult discussion groups and teenage cultural, social, and educational group activities.

NAVH maintains public and professional education programs addressing the needs of the partially sighted. It serves as a public clearinghouse on services for the partially sighted and disseminates information on available commercial aids. It cooperates with commercial manufacturers of aids in field testing. It offers a large variety of visual aids for sale. Visual-aid counseling is offered to all clients who visit a facility.

Publications include *In Focus,* an annual children's newsletter, *Update,* a large-print, quarterly newsletter, *Seeing Clearly,* an annual newsletter for adults, the *Program Report Annual Bulletin,* the biennial *Catalog of Large Type Publications,* and pamphlets, brochures, and manuals. NAVH holds an annual convention in New York City.

Contact:

National Association for Visually Handicapped
22 W. 21st Street
New York, NY 10010
212-889-3141 (ph)
212-727-2931 (fax)

Or, contact the San Francisco site of NAVH at:

3201 Balboa Street
San Francisco, CA 94121
415-221-3201 (ph)
415-221-8754 (fax)
www.navh.org

National Braille Association (NBA) The National Braille Association (NBA), founded in 1945, is an organization that produces and distributes braille, large print, and taped reading materials for the visually impaired. The NBA offers transcription workshops and collects and studies improvements to transcription techniques.

The membership numbers over 2,500 and includes volunteers and professionals who produce the materials, blind and visually impaired people, teachers, librarians, educators, publishers, professional workers and volunteers for the blind, and parents of the blind or visually impaired.

The organization maintains request registries for those seeking texts in braille, large print, or on tape. The Reader-Transcriber Registry receives requests for nontextbook or nontechnical material transcription. The Braille Textbook Assignment Service accepts requests for college textbooks and other technical materials.

In 1963, the NBA established the Braille Book Bank (BBB) in Rochester, New York. The BBB is a nonprofit organization maintained by volunteers and is partially underwritten by donations. The Braille Book Bank is a major source of textbooks and career materials in braille for visually impaired college students. It maintains over 1,800 titles in master copies for immediate thermoform duplication. Each year, more than 36,000 volumes of paper braille are added to the collection as books are transcribed by request. The Braille Book Bank offers three catalogs for ordering material under the titles *The Textbook Catalog, The Music Catalog* and *The General Interest Catalog.* The catalogs are free on request to the Braille Book Bank, 422 South Clinton Avenue, Rochester, New York 14620.

The NBA established the first volunteer electronic library in the United States. Volunteers transcribe materials with computers. The finished transcriptions are sent on diskettes to the NBA Braille Book Bank for storage or reproduction onto embossed paper braille or as paperless cassette braille. The transcriptions are available by request to individuals, schools, agencies or businesses. Electronic methods reduce costs allow the NBA to provide materials in braille comparable to the print cost. The NBA publishes the journal *Bulletin* four times a year. It holds a biennial national conference.

Contact:

National Braille Association
3 Townline Circle
Rochester, NY 14623
716-427-8260
716-427-0263 (fax)
www.nationalbraille.org

National Eye Institute (NEI) The National Eye Institute (NEI) was established by Congress in 1968 as a part of the federal government's National Institutes of Health. Funded by Congressional appropriations, the NEI funds approximately 80 percent of all vision research supported by the federal government agencies and national private philanthropic organizations.

The goal of the NEI is to conduct and support research relating to ocular disease and disorder treatments and cures, training concerning blinding eye diseases and disorders, research and training in health concerns and requirements of the blind, and clinical sciences regarding the mechanisms of visual function and sight preservation.

The NEI funds grants for research concerning the prevention, diagnosis, and treatment of blinding and visually disabling disorders and diseases. All research is classified under one of five major programs: retinal and choroidal diseases; corneal diseases; cataract, glaucoma, and strabismus; amblyopia; and visual processing. Special consideration is given to projects relating to visual impairment and the rehabilitation process that can be related to the major programs.

The NEI distributes its plan, which outlines the major needs and opportunities within the vision research field, to members of the vision research community, scientists, government officials, and the public. It encourages coordination among private and governmental agencies that support vision research.

The NEI works with individual investigators to encourage submission of grant applications in targeted priority areas, presents plan recommendations to scientific meetings, organizes workshops and symposia on plan-identified topics, and establishes research resources, such as animal colonies.

In January 2001, Dr. Paul A. Sieving was named director of the NEI, replacing acting director Dr. Ruth L. Kirschstein. Sieving was with the Kellogg Eye Center of the University of Michigan before joining the NEI.

The NEI compiles and publishes research results in the National Advisory Eye Council Report, entitled *Vision Research.*

It also offers a variety of free brochures, posters, Spanish-language materials, and a school program publication. These and other publications can be ordered on-line at www.nei.nih.gov/publications.

Contact:

National Eye Institute
National Institute of Health
2020 Vision Place
Bethesda, MD 20892
301-496-5248
www.nei.nih.gov

National Federation of the Blind (NFB) The National Federation of the Blind (NFB), founded in 1940, is the largest organization of the blind in the United States. Membership includes more than 10 percent of the nation's blind persons. The organization is dedicated to the complete, equal integration of blind persons into society.

The NFB serves as a public clearinghouse on information concerning blindness, directs and conducts research, produces and disseminates information to blind persons, and researches and monitors legislation concerning the blind.

It advises and refers blind individuals to services, provides assistance to blind persons with discrimination concerns, consults with congressional committees and state legislatures, serves as an advocate for the rights of blind individuals, and evaluates and promotes new technology. NFB offers over 26 scholarships to blind students and grants an award for the greatest contribution to welfare of the blind.

With the United States Department of Labor, NFB developed Job Opportunities for the Blind (JOB), a program that matches qualified blind workers with employers. JOB directs seminars on career planning for unemployed blind people and educational seminars concerning blindness for employers.

In 1990, the NFB opened the International Braille and Technology Center at the National Center for the Blind in Baltimore, Maryland. The center is a comprehensive facility, offering training, evaluation, and demonstration of various technology.

Staff at the International Braille and Technology Center is available to answer any kind of question about assistive technology for the blind. The center can be accessed through the NFB's phone number, which is listed below.

Publications include *The Braille Monitor,* a monthly journal, *Future Reflections,* a bimonthly magazine and numerous pamphlets, brochures and materials in print, braille, and on records and cassettes. NFB holds an annual conference.

Contact:

National Federation of the Blind
1800 Johnson Street
Baltimore, MD 21230
410-659-9314 (ph)
410-685-5653 (fax)
www.nfb.org

National Industries for the Blind (NIB) A private, nonprofit organization that develops industrial employment for blind and multihandicapped blind Americans. It includes 108 associated industries in 36 states, Puerto Rico and the District of Columbia.

NIB allocates federal government orders and offers grant programs, management training programs, technical expertise in new product and service development, industrial engineering, contract administration, purchasing, quality assurance, and production maintenance to its associated industries.

The organization was developed in 1938 following the passage of the Wagner-O'Day Act, which mandated that federal agencies purchase products from workshops for the blind meeting specific qualifications. In 1971, the Wagner-O'Day Act was renamed the Javits-Wagner-O'Day Act and amended to include severely disabled workers and services as well as products. The products for sale to the federal government are approved by the Committee for Purchase from the Blind and other Severely Handicapped, a presidentially appointed committee.

The first products included mops and brooms but have since expanded to include 1,300 quality blind-made products such as components for the Army's Kevlar helmet, tracheotomy kits, and various kitchen gadgets stocked in commissaries for sale to military families worldwide.

Contact:

National Industries for the Blind
1901 N. Beauregard Street, Suite 200
Alexandria, VA 22311
703-998-0770 (ph)
703-998-8268 (fax)
www.nib.org

National Keratoconus Foundation (NKCF) A nonprofit agency founded in 1986 to increase awareness and understanding about KERATOCONUS and support research concerning the disorder. The organization began with a grant from Jane Neely and her husband, Norman, who had keratoconus and was frustrated by how little information was available.

The mission of NKCF is to provide information and support about the condition to patients, their families, and eye care professionals, and to encourage research and new technology for treatment of the disorder.

NKCF provides educational materials, support groups and programs, a newsletter, links to other keratoconus-related sites, a patient registry, an outreach program, a referral service, and patient education seminars. It also oversees a research program and a corneal tissue collection program.

Contact:

National Keratoconus Foundation
8733 Beverly Boulevard, Suite 201
Los Angeles, CA 90048
800-521-2524
www.nkcf.org

National Library Service for the Blind and Physically Handicapped This act was originally legislated in 1904 by Congress to permit free braille books to be mailed to blind adults. The Pratt-Smoot Act of 1931, and further amendments in 1934, authorized the Library of Congress to establish a national library service that provided free braille and talking books to blind adults.

In 1952, an amendment to the act deleted the word "adult," thus allowing the service to expand and include visually impaired children. Further amendments in 1962 extended the program to include braille musical scores, textbooks, and

1966,
rsically
or the
talysis,
coordi-

rs free
for the
length
ecords,
ough a
Books,
ind re-

2000 it
egional
9 more
d mag-
) read-
e 2000

is who
aterials
visual

hysi-

1291 Taylor Street NW
Washington, DC 20542
202-707-5100 (ph)
202-707-0712 (fax)
202-707-0744 (TDD)
nls@loc.gov (e-mail)
www.loc.gov/nls

National School Lunch Act   As amended, the National School Lunch Act of 1946 offers assistance to public and private institutions, schools, camps, and day-care centers, including those that serve handicapped or mentally retarded students, to provide meals to eligible children. The assistance outlined in the act includes grants, reimbursements, and commodity donations.

The School Lunch Program, as authorized under Section 4 of the act, provides institutions with the funding and food donations necessary to serve free or reduced fee lunches to eligible children. Children qualify according to their family income and the number of children participating in the program.

The participating schools, child-care centers, and residential-care centers are reimbursed for the lunches that must meet nutritional guidelines determined by the Department of Agriculture. The rate of reimbursement is set by the states according to figures in the Consumer Price Index.

The Commodity Distribution Program, as outlined in Section 6 of the act, allows donations of food bought by the federal government under price-support or surplus-removal programs. Formula grants to state agencies are used to distribute the food to eligible schools, institutions, child and elderly nutrition programs, nonprofit summer camps, families, and individuals.

Section 13 of the act provides for the Summer Food Service Program, a nonprofit summer meal program for children in summer camps or institutions, including those that serve the disabled. The program awards formula grants to states that introduce, support, or extend the program and pay according to the number of meals served. The meals must meet nutritional criteria set by the Department of Agriculture.

The Child-Care Food Program, Section 17 of the Act, provides grants-in-aid to states maintaining nonprofit meal programs for children in nonresidential day care. The programs serve meals, including breakfast, lunch, snack, and dinner, to eligible children. Qualified nondisabled children under 12 years of age or disabled children of any age are entitled to two meals and one snack per day under the program. The meals must meet the Department of Agriculture's nutritional requirements.

The states distribute the funds to facilities such as public or private nonprofit institutions or organizations, day-care and recreation centers, and other day-care services. Grants are awarded according to how many meals are served based on reimbursement rates set by the federal government.

U.S. Department of Education. *Summary of Existing Legislation Affecting Persons with Disabilities.* Washington, D.C.: USDE, 1988.

night blindness The inability to see clearly at night or in low light. The condition results from damage or defect in the rods of the RETINA.

The retina receives reflected light from an object. Light-sensitive cells called RODS AND CONES translate the light into electrical impulses that the retina sends to the brain through the OPTIC NERVE. The brain changes the impulses into an image.

The cones, packed into the center (or macular section) of the retina, discern detail and color and require bright light to work effectively. The rods function in dim light and are responsible for detecting movement and shape. Any dysfunction of the rods may cause damage to night vision. Any peripheral vision loss that restricts the field to 5 degrees central vision results in night blindness because the usable foveal area contains no rods.

Damage to the rods may occur as a result of nutritional deficiency or disease. Vitamin-A deficiency may cause night blindness since the presence of vitamin A is necessary for proper rod functioning. Vision impairment due to vitamin-A deficiency is common in developing countries. A resulting disease, XEROPHTHALMIA, is the second major cause of blindness in the world.

Xerophthalmia causes changes in the CORNEA, CONJUNCTIVA and anterior segments of the eye. In acute cases, the cornea can perforate, the IRIS may adhere to the cornea, and the eyeball may be destroyed. A common and early symptom of xerophthalmia is night blindness. The condition can be detected with an electroretinogram or a thorough corneal examination. The condition is treated with megadoses of vitamin A given orally.

Night blindness is also a first symptom of RETINITIS PIGMENTOSA (RP), a degenerative disease of the rods and cones. RP first affects the rods, decreasing vision in the peripheral fields and causing night blindness. RP is a hereditary condition for which there is no cure or treatment.

NoIR Medical Technologies A company that produces plano medical sunglasses, which chemically absorb ultraviolet (200–400nm) and near infrared (800–1400) rays. The glasses may be prescribed in cases of preoperative CATARACT, postoperative CATARACT, RETINITIS PIGMENTOSA, MACULAR DISEASE, ALBINISM, RADIAL KERATOTOMY patients, contact lens wearers, and monochromatic persons.

Preoperative cataract patients may wear glasses with light-amber colored lenses and a 40 percent total light transmission (TLT) rate to provide glare protection and increased visual acuity. Postoperative cataract patients may wear 10 percent TLT amber lenses or 18 percent TLT gray-green lenses. These lenses absorb ultraviolet and infrared rays that were formerly absorbed by the eye's natural lens, removed in cataract surgery.

Individuals with retinitis pigmentosa may wear 2 percent TLT dark-amber or 10 percent TLT amber lenses. These enhance vision and protect the eyes from a maximum amount of visible light.

Patients with macular disease may wear 40 percent TLT light-amber lenses to provide a high quality of visible light, and those with albinism may wear 1 percent TLT dark grey-green lenses to provide maximum protection from light.

Individuals undergoing radial keratotomy surgery may wear 10 percent TLT amber lenses or 18 percent TLT grey-green lenses. Contact-lens wearers may use 10 percent TLT amber or 18 percent TLT grey-green lenses, and monochromatic or color-blind persons may wear 90 percent TLC red lenses.

Contact:

NoIR Medical Technologies
P.O. Box 159
South Lyon, MI 48178
734-769-5565 or 800-521-9746 (ph)
734-769-1708 (fax)
www.noir-medical.com

nondiscrimination laws Congress has enacted legislation that entitles individuals with disabilities, including blindness and vision impairment, to freedom from discrimination on the basis of disability. The laws guarantee the right to a free, appropriate education, the right to medical treatment for infants born with disabilities, the right to protection from harm in institutions, the right to protection from discrimination in federally conducted programs, the right to access to federally supported or operated facilities and programs, and the right to access to advocacy and protection programs or services for developmentally disabled or mentally ill individuals.

Eight major bills were passed during the 1970s and 1980s that aimed to ensure these rights. They include the Rehabilitation Act of 1973, the Education of the Handicapped Act, the Architectural Barriers Act, the Civil Rights of Institutionalized Persons Act, the Child Abuse Prevention and Treatment and Adoption Reform Act, The Civil Rights Commission Act Amendments of 1978, the Developmental Disabilities Assistance and Bill of Rights Act, and the Protection and Advocacy of Mentally Ill Individuals Act.

The *Rehabilitation Act of 1973* provides assurances that disabled individuals are protected from discrimination in acceptance to, or benefits from, federally funded or operated programs. Sections of the act protect against employment discrimination by federal agencies or contractors. The act authorizes grants to states to establish systems for protection and advocacy for disabled rights.

The Individuals with Disabilities Education Act, formerly known as the *Education of the Handicapped Act,* ensures the right of all disabled children to a free and appropriate public education. It supplies assistance to states to support this education and offers grants to states that provide appropriate educational programs to disabled students.

The *Architectural Barriers Act of 1968* required all buildings constructed or altered with federal funds after 1969 to be accessible to persons with disabilities, in compliance with accessibility guidelines issued in 1969. The act was amended to include public buildings and government-leased buildings intended for public use.

The *Civil Rights of Institutionalized Persons Act of 1980* granted the right of the U.S. Department of Justice to sue states for violation of rights of institutionalized persons.

The *Child Abuse Prevention and Treatment and Adoption Reform Act of 1978* includes a section prohibiting the withholding of medically indicated therapy or treatment to physically or mentally disabled infants.

The *Civil Rights Commission Act Amendments of 1978* expanded the jurisdiction of the Civil Rights Commission to include protection from discrimination to disabled persons on the basis of disability.

The *Developmental Disabilities Assistance and Bill of Rights Act* ensures the rights of appropriate services, treatment, and rehabilitation to those with developmental disabilities.

The *Protection and Advocacy for Mentally Ill Individuals Act of 1986* establishes a formula-grant program to states to provide mental-health advocacy programs and services. The Fair Housing Act, as amended in 1988, prohibits housing discrimination on the basis of a variety of factors, including disability.

In the spring of 1990, a landmark disability rights bill called the *Americans with Disabilities Act* passed in the United States Senate and House of Representatives. The bill bars employment discrimination for qualified applicants with disabilities and calls for changes in the workplace if needed to accommodate the worker. It requires accessibility to all new businesses, trains, and buses, and requires telephone companies to provide operators to relay messages from deaf to hearing individuals.

The National Voter Registration Act of 1993 is intended to increase the number of registrations of people with disabilities and of minorities. Both groups have historically had very low registration rates.

The Rehabilitation Act prohibits discrimination on the basis of disability in programs conducted by federal agencies or supported by public funds. It also applies to employment in federal jobs and to the employment practices of federal contractors. The standards pertaining to employment discrimination are the same as those used in the Americans with Disabilities Act.

The Rehabilitation Act also sets requirements for electronic and information technology that is developed, maintained, owned, or used by the federal governments. All technology that falls into those categories must be accessible to people with disabilities, whether they are federal employees or members of the public. To be considered accessible, an information technology system must be operable in a variety of ways and not be dependent on a single sense or ability of the user.

The Architectural Barriers Act requires that buildings and facilities that are built with federal money or leased by a federal agency comply with federal accessibility standards. These standards apply to new buildings, and those that have been remodeled or altered. U.S. post offices are included in this act.

U.S. Department of Education. *Summary of Existing Legislation Affecting Persons with Disabilities.* Washington, D.C.: USDE, 1988.

US Department of Justice. *A Guide to Disability Rights Laws.* www.usdoj.gov, 2000.

nonoptical aids   Nonoptical aids or environmental aids change, improve, or maximize residual vision by improving conditions in the environment. Nonoptical aids include illumination, light transmission, reflection control, and contrast.

Illumination is improved through use of brighter or dimmer room lighting, as needed according to the cause of disability. Ideal lighting provides maximum illumination and minimum glare. Lighting may consist of standard lamps to small lamps that attach to spectacle frames.

Light transmission is improved through lenses, filters, and absorptive lenses that reduce glare and highlight contrast. These are especially helpful for individuals with conditions such as albinism, CATARACTS, GLAUCOMA, and MACULAR DISEASE, which result in light sensitivity, or photophobia. Lenses, filters, and absorptive lenses are available in a wide range of degrees of protection, from simple filters that reduce glare to photochromic lenses that use gray, green, and amber filters to block all ultraviolet light.

Reflection is controlled by visors, side shields, specially treated lenses, and typoscopes. Visors may be supplied by the brim of a hat or can be a filtering visor lens attached to the spectacle frame. Sideshields are filters that attach to the sides of spectacle lenses to control the light on the sides of the eyes. A typoscope is a slit-reading device that isolates one line of type at a time, thus reducing glare from the light reflected from the page. Typoscopes are especially helpful for those with cataracts.

Contrast is enhanced by using highly contrasting colors near one another such as black ink on white or yellow paper, or fluorescent strips on stair risers. Contrast for reading pale or bluish print may be improved by using pale-yellow tinted lenses or by placing a clear yellow or amber sheet over the page.

nonverbal communication   Nonverbal communication involves ideas or emotions expressed by the face and body. Components of nonverbal communication include eye contact; facial expressions; head nodding or listing; shrugs; body posture; hand, arm, and foot gestures; touching; and regard for personal space.

A review of literature on communication skills of the blind indicates that blind individuals present different behaviors than sighted individuals. Individuals who become blind after birth (adventitiously) tend to exhibit more standard types of behaviors than do congenitally blind individuals (Bonfanti, 1979).

Nonverbal communication is generally learned through observation. Because blind or severely impaired persons do not have the opportunity to observe these gestures, they often do not form a pattern of appropriate gestures. This lack of knowledge can result in inappropriate behavior or a lack of nonverbal feedback to the other party. The resulting awkwardness or confusion can impede communication with sighted individuals.

Blind people may show a lack of facial expression, inappropriate voluntary or involuntary facial expressions, distracting or unattractive physical behaviors such as rocking or eye rubbing, excessive blinking, lack of eye contact, overuse or underuse of hand or arm gestures, and more intense touching techniques.

Blind individuals can be trained in nonverbal communication skills. The individual is made aware that such gestures or signals are received, translated, and acted on by the receiving party. Instruction includes methods to improve eye contact, form appropriate voluntary facial expressions, improve posture and appearance, develop appropriate, light touching behaviors, and correctly judge personal space or territory.

The training usually involves tactile props and techniques. It may include instruction in the workings of the eye and explanations of clues received visually as opposed to tactually. Although results vary with the individual, training usually results in some improvement of nonverbal skills.

Bonfanti, Barbara H. "Effects of Training on Nonverbal and Verbal Behaviors of Congenially Blind Adults." *Journal of Visual Impairment and Blindness* (January 1979), pp. 1–7.
Scholl, Geraldine, ed. *Foundations of Education for Blind and Visually Handicapped Children and Youth.* New York: American Foundation for the Blind Inc., 1986.

nutritional amblyopia   See TOXIC AMBLYOPIA.

nystagmus   The term for an involuntary movement of the eyes. The eyes may move vertically, horizontally, in circles, or some combination of the three. The condition causes focusing problems and blurred vision. Nystagmus may be congenital or acquired as a result of another disorder.

Jerking nystagmus is the most common form of the disorder. The eyes move faster in one direction than the other. It may be caused by lesions or changes in the brain stem, cerebellum, or vascular system; overstimulation of the systems within the inner ear; hypertension; stroke; multiple sclerosis; Ménière's disease; labyrinthitis; drug or alcohol toxicity; or brain inflammations, including meningitis and encephalitis.

Pendular nystagmus is the less common form of the disorder. The eyes move horizontally and equally quickly in both directions. Pendular nystagmus may be caused congenitally as in congenital CATARACT or disorder of the OPTIC DISC. It may be acquired after birth as the result of ASTIGMATISM, albinism, OPTIC ATROPHY, or corneal opacification or cataracts.

The underlying cause of nystagmus is treated to alleviate the symptom. If the cause is astigmatism, prescription eyeglasses may be helpful. When the cause is a disease or disorder that can be treated, control of the disease usually results in control of the nystagmus. In unmanageable conditions the patient may learn to hold the head or body in accommodating positions or learn to focus with one eye only. A nonprofit agency to serve people affected by nystagmus was formed in 1999. The American Nystagmus Network offers on-line support and discussion groups and provides information concerning the condition.

It does not, however, offer medical advice.

Contact:

American Nystagmus Network
P.O. Box 45
Jenison, MI 49429-0045
www.nystagmus.org

object of regard   The object of regard is the object on which the eyes are focused.

oculist   See OPHTHALMOLOGIST.

Ocusert   The trade name of a medication used in the treatment of GLAUCOMA, a condition in which intraocular pressure builds within the eye. Manufactured by the Alza Corporation, which merged with Johnson & Johnson in the second half of 2001, Ocusert is a thin membrane worn in the eye like a contact lens. The membrane rests in the conjunctival cul-de-sac and continually dispenses pilocarpine into the eye.

Pilocarpine is a parasympathomimetic drug that constricts the PUPIL and facilitates an increased aqueous humor outflow from the eye, decreasing intraocular pressure. It also is available in drop and gel form.

Ocusert may be prescribed in one of two strengths: Ocusert Pilo-20, which releases 20 micrograms of the drug per hour, or Ocusert Pilo-40, which releases 40 micrograms of the drug per hour. The Ocusert is effective for one week, at the end of which time it must be replaced.

Ocusert may induce MYOPIA (nearsightedness) within the first few hours of insertion because it stimulates the CILIARY BODY. Ocusert should not be used by those with a history of acute inflammatory disease of the anterior segment of the eye because pupil constriction will occur and may exacerbate the problem. It is also contraindicated for those with glaucoma who have had an extracapsular CATARACT extraction because posterior SYNECHIAE (adherence of the iris to the lens) may occur.

The Ocusert membrane may be placed in the eye by the patient. Recommended insertion time is just before retiring since the myopia induced by the drug will have stabilized by morning. The system must be stored in a refrigerator.

Office of Disability Employment Policy   (ODEP)
An office formed in 2001 within the U.S. Department Labor that attempts to increase employment of persons with disabilities. This office was formerly known as the President's Committee on Employment of People with Disabilities. Programs and staff of the former President's Committee on Employment of People with Disabilities were integrated in the new office.

The mission of ODEP is to improve and increase employment of persons with disabilities through policy analysis, technical assistance, and development of best practices. It also stresses outreach, education, and constituent services, and promotes hiring of disabled persons.

The President's Council on Employment of People with Disabilities was founded in 1947 by President Harry Truman to encourage business and industry to offer employment opportunities to returning disabled veterans of World War II. Among its goals and duties were to serve as an adviser to the president; attempt to improve public attitudes toward disabled workers through education and awareness programs; and serve as an advocate for policies and practices for disabled employment rights. It also advised disabled workers, sponsored a national resource and consultation service, compiled and disseminated public information and technical materials, and contributed to standardizing guidelines and practices governing the employment of disabled persons. The President's Council on Employment of People with Disabilities also served as a public relations channel with the media.

The President's Council worked in close alliance with an organization of volunteers in each state to conduct programs and activities that it initiated and developed. It also awarded prestigious prizes to disabled persons who demonstrated outstanding achievement, and sponsored scholarships.

ODEP has undertaken a cultural-diversity initiative aimed at increasing job opportunities for minority disabled people. It also is working to create a better understanding among the public of, as well as job opportunities for, people with cognitive disabilities.

Contact:

Office of Disability Employment Policy
1331 F Street, NW, Suite 300
Washington, D.C. 20004
202-376-6200 (ph)
202-376-6205 (TTD)
202-376-6219 (fax)
www.dol.gov/pcepd/index.htm

onchocerciasis One of four major causes of blindness in the world including TRACHOMA, XEROPHTHALMIA and CATARACT. The disease occurs primarily in developing countries and is found mainly in West Equatorial Africa, Central America, and South America. According to Helen Keller International, it may have infected over 30 million people and blinded an estimated 1.5 million people. It is projected that 20 percent of all those infected will become visually impaired. In Africa, approximately 40,000 people become blind each year due to this disease.

Onchocerciasis, also known as river blindness due to association of the infection with vector breeding sites, is a systemic disease caused by the filarial worm *Onchocerca volvulus*, a parasite transmitted by the blackfly. Humans become infected with the disease when the worm infests the body through tainted water or direct contact. The worm may live up to 15 years within the human skin, kidneys, blood, or cerebrospinal fluid. The disease causes corneal inflammation or KERATITIS, corneal scarring, and vision loss. It may be seen in conjunction with chronic IRIDOCYCLITIS and GLAUCOMA.

A drug called Stromectol, manufactured by Merck & Co., Inc., was approved by the U.S. Food and Drug Administration in 1997. Stromectol is a very effective antiparasite medicine, and can be used to treat onchocerciasis. It is available under the name Mectizab in many parts of the world, including Africa and Central and South America. However, the treatment is very expensive and may not be affordable to all people.

Prevention of the disease may include insecticides to rid the community of the worms, avoidance of breeding sites such as rivers and open waterways, wearing protective clothing, and excising of skin nodules that contain the worms.

(See WORLD BLINDNESS.)

Bath, Patricia E. "Blindness Prevention Through Programs of Community Ophthalmology in Developing Countries." *Ophthalmology*, vol. 2. K. Shimizu and J. Oosterhuis, eds. Amsterdam: Excerpta Medica, 1979.

Center Watch. "Drugs Approved by the FDA." www.centerwatch.com/patient/drugs, 2000.

Cupak, K. "The Importance of Eye Camps in Underdeveloped Countries." *Ophthalmology*, vol. 2. K. Shimizu and J. Oosterhuis, eds. Amsterdam: Excerpta Medica, 1979.

Helen Keller International. *Facts About Helen Keller International.* New York: HKI, 1988.

Phillips, Calbert I. *Basic Clinical Ophthalmology.* London: Pitman Publishers Limited, 1984.

World Health Organization. *Available Data On Blindness (Update 1987).* New York: WHO, 1987.

opacification A cloudiness or lack of transparency that blocks the transmission of light. This usually refers to a clouding of the eye's lens, which leads to a CATARACT.

Opacities in the lens are very common in aging persons and are not termed cataract until the opaque lens fibers significantly interfere with vision. Opacities often progress so gradually that the patient is unaware of the cataract until it becomes large or crosses the center of vision. Opacities that do develop into cataracts can be removed by surgery. Prognosis is excellent, and satisfactory results are achieved in 90 percent of cases.

ophthalmia neonatorum An inflammation of the eyes of newborn infants. The condition generally affects the CORNEA and CONJUNCTIVA. Once a common cause of blindness arising from unhygienic conditions at birth, the infection is now successfully treated with antibiotics immediately after birth.

The condition is not hereditary but occurs during birth. Bacteria such as gonococcus, staphylococcus, streptococcus, or pneumococcus and viral infections such as chlamydia are present within the maternal birth canal. The inflammation is transferred from the mother to the infant's eyes as the child passes through the birth canal.

A herpes infection is the most common infection transmitted at birth, affecting approximately 1 in 5,000 births, according to the International Herpes Alliance. Gonococcus or staphylococcus germs and other bacteria may cause ophthalmia neonatorum also. Symptoms of the infection are apparent shortly after birth when the cornea, conjunctiva, and eyelids of the infant begin to inflame. The eyes may be treated with local antibiotics such as penicillin, streptomycin, or tetracycline administered at one hour intervals. Systemic antibiotics may be prescribed if the cornea is involved. If not treated, the condition can cause blindness and spread to other parts of the body.

The standard postbirth therapy to prevent ophthalmia neonatorum consists of the administration of silver nitrate, or comparable antibiotics, in eyedrop or ointment form. In order to prevent blindness from ophthalmic neonatorum, all states have passed laws that require the routine application of silver nitrate drops or antibiotic ointment to all newborn infants' eyes.

ophthalmic technician   A skilled assistant who works with an ophthalmologist. Ophthalmic technicians complete patient medical histories, perform simple vision tests, administer eye drops or ointments, change eye dressings, take optical measurements, and assist in surgery. Under the supervision of an ophthalmologist, the ophthalmic technician may also aid patients in fitting contact lenses, instruct patients in lens care, and perform some treatment procedures.

Ophthalmic technicians must have completed high school before entering the accredited training programs offered by medical schools, hospitals, and colleges. The two-year training program is followed by two years of supervised work experience in a clinical setting. Graduates of the program are required to take the certification exam issued by the Joint Commission on Allied Health Personnel in Ophthalmology. Certification is not, however, a requirement for employment in all cases.

ophthalmologist   An ophthalmologist (or oculist, the term used in Europe) is a medical doctor (MD) who has completed college, four years of medical school, a year of internship, and a minimum of three years of specialized residency training concerning diseases and surgery of the eye. Many receive additional training in one or two years to subspecialize in areas such as CORNEA TRANSPLANT surgery, retinal surgery, or low-vision services.

Ophthalmologists test vision, prescribe corrective lenses, diagnose and treat eye diseases and defects, prescribe medications, and perform surgery. They are subject to the licensing practices and requirements outlined by state and professional organizations for physicians. Each state medical board issues a license to an applicant after the physician passes a comprehensive examination covering general medical knowledge. Ophthalmologists may be certified as members of the American Board of Ophthalmology, a national organization formed to ensure optimum ophthalmological care, after passing written and oral examinations according to subspecialty.

ophthalmoscope   An instrument used to magnify and illuminate the inside of the eye. Examination of the eyes with an ophthalmoscope is a routine part of the annual eye exam.

The hand-held instrument shines a bright light on the back of the eye, making it possible to view and evaluate the health of the RETINA, blood vessels, and OPTIC NERVE. The examiner uses the ophthalmoscope to look for abnormalities of these eye parts, as well as indications of diabetes, hardening of the arteries, high blood pressure, and other diseases. Since the blood vessels in the inside of the eye are the only ones in the body able to be viewed in their natural state, they provide a window to the general health of the patient. Routine examinations with an ophthalmoscope often uncover disorders or diseases unsuspected in the patient.

Another version of the ophthalmoscope, a *binocular indirect ophthalmoscope,* is used to evaluate the entire surface of the retina. The light is attached to a headband worn by the examiner. Examination of this kind can determine whether the retina is healthy and functional enough to warrant CATARACT surgery.

Optacon   A reading machine developed by Telesensory Systems Inc. that converts print into tactual letter configurations that are read with the fingertips. The Optacon, which is no longer manufactured but still used by some people, is designed to increase access to print and not to replace braille.

The Optacon user slides a miniature camera across a line of print with the right hand. Simultaneously, the left hand rests on an electronic array consisting of 100 vibrating pins. The Optacon electronically converts each letter of print into a letter configuration formed on the array and read by the tip of the index finger of the left hand. The Optacon can translate a variety of print styles and sizes. Adaptations to the machine include models that adapt to typewriters, computer terminals and electronic calculators.

Individuals must be extensively trained to use the Optacon effectively. The speed of the reading machine is slower than voice synthesized models or sight reading. (See TELESENSORY SYSTEMS INC.)

optical aids   See MAGNIFIERS.

optic atrophy   Optic atrophy is a loss of nerve tissue on the OPTIC DISC, the place where the OPTIC NERVE joins the eye. The optic disc is nonseeing and corresponds to the blind spot in vision. Optic atrophy may cause a loss of visual field. Both central and side vision may be lost, although visual acuity may remain unaffected. It can also cause abnormal color vision or blurred vision. Often called pale disc, optic atrophy is characterized by pallor, or whiteness, of the disc. Because nearsighted eyes and those of children also have disc pallor, the condition may be misdiagnosed or confused with other conditions.

Optic atrophy may be caused by glaucoma, an obstruction of a retinal vein or artery, a disorder of the optic nerve such as optic neuritis, a tumor, PAPILLEDEMA (swelling of the disc due to intracranial pressure), RETINITIS PIGMENTOSA, toxic-related causes, such as tobacco amblyopia, or injury. Treatment of optic atrophy consists of therapy for the underlying cause with medication or surgery or withdrawal of toxic substances.

optic disc   The part of the RETINA where the OPTIC NERVE meets the eye and the blood supply enters the eye. The optic disc contains no light-sensitive rods or cones and is therefore unable to "see." It is responsible for the blind spot in the normal field of vision.

Optic atrophy, a condition in which nerve tissue has been lost from the disc, results in loss of visual field. This condition may be caused by GLAUCOMA, retinal vascular occlusion, PAPILLEDEMA, RETINITIS PIGMENTOSA, or injury.

The optic disc is subject to swelling. Papilledema is a condition that occurs when the optic disc becomes swollen due to an obstruction to the circulation of blood within the eye or by increased pressure within the cranium. Swelling may also be caused by optic neuritis (swelling of the optic nerve), blockage of a central retinal vein due to arterial disease, MULTIPLE SCLEROSIS, DIABETIC RETINOPATHY, and postoperative conditions following intraocular surgery.

optician   An optician dispenses the lenses and low-vision aids prescribed by optometrists and ophthalmologists. Opticians grind and formulate the lenses and fit them to a frame. In many states, opticians also fit and administer contact lenses. They are not trained or licensed to examine the eyes or to prescribe lenses.

optic nerve   A cord of approximately 1 million nerve fibers that connect the brain to the eye and that supply blood to the RETINA. It sends blood from the back of the eye through blood vessels in the retina to cover the entire surface.

The optic nerve is a conduit of information from the retina to the brain. The retina receives reflected light that falls on an object. It evaluates the light messages and transforms them into electrical impulses. The impulses travel through the optic nerve to the brain, where they are translated into an image.

The optic nerve is joined to the eye in the retina at a point called the OPTIC DISC. Since the optic nerve contains no light-sensitive cells, it is "blind" and renders the spot where it connects to the retina, the optic disc, blind as well. This juncture where the nerve joins the retina is known as the blind spot in the normal field of vision.

The optic nerve is subject to several disorders. OPTIC ATROPHY is the deterioration of optic nerve fibers of the optic disc. As a result, both central or side vision may be lost. Optic atrophy may be caused by a blockage of a retinal vein or artery, an injury, a congenital or hereditary condition, GLAUCOMA or RETINITIS PIGMENTOSA, or following a swelling or disease in the optic nerve.

TOXIC AMBLYOPIA is a condition related to optic atrophy in which the optic nerve is damaged due to toxins such as alcohol or tobacco. Poisoning by these substances results in loss of central vision.

Optic neuritis (also called optic neuropathy) or swelling of the optic nerve, may result in conditions such as retrobulbar neuritis. Symptoms of retrobulbar neuritis include painful eye movements and loss of central vision. The condition is sometimes associated with MULTIPLE SCLEROSIS.

Tumors may develop along the optic nerve pathway. They may cause vision loss and bulging of the eyeball.

For more information about condition affecting the optic nerve, contact:

The International Foundation for Optic Nerve
   Disease
P.O. Box 777
Cornwall, NY 12518
845-534-7250
www.ifond.org

optic neuropathy Optic neuropathy or neuritis is a swelling of the OPTIC NERVE. The condition is serious and may result in permanent vision loss.

Optic neuropathy is often associated with MULTIPLE SCLEROSIS. This form of neuritis, called retrobul-

bar neuritis, involves sudden loss of vision in one eye accompanied by pain associated with eye movement. Blind spots, or SCOTOMAS, may appear within the field of vision as well as COLOR BLINDNESS and difficulty seeing in bright light. Vision may be affected in the entire field or may begin in the center of the field and progress to peripheral areas. The condition is treated with steroids, and the prognosis is excellent. The vision loss may be partially or completely recovered after three months.

Optic neuropathy or neuritis unrelated to multiple sclerosis may be caused by collagen disease such as LUPUS; vascular disease such as arteriosclerosis, arteritis, or arterial hypertension; a viral, fungal or bacterial infection; tumors or cysts; and alcohol or tobacco overuse and other toxic causes. There is also a hereditary form of optic neuropathy that is passed through the mother to her children. It affects males more than females, usually occurring in the mid-20s. This type of optic neuropathy is called leberis hereditary optic neuropathy. Symptoms may include loss of vision in one or both eyes. Treatment may consist of medication for the underlying systemic cause and may include corticosteroids. Vision loss produced by neuritis unrelated to multiple sclerosis may be irreversible.

optometrist An optometrist has a degree of optometry (OD), which is awarded after completing college and four years of optometry school. An optometrist screens and diagnoses common eye problems, assesses the efficiency and health of the eyes, provides low-vision care, prescribes corrective eyeglasses, contact lenses, and low-vision aids.

Optometrists are not physicians, and in the case of disease or surgery, optometrists refer patients to a physician or ophthalmologist.

orbit The bony socket lined with fatty tissue that cradles and protects the eye. The globe of the eye is held in place in the orbit by six extrinsic muscles.

The orbit is subject to several conditions. The fatty tissue surrounding the globe may become inflamed due to bacterial infection. The infection may spread to the globe. Tumors may also form within the orbit.

Hemangioma, a common tumor of the orbit most often seen in children, is benign and rarely requires surgery. Dermoid cyst is a growth that appears at the level of the eyebrow in the upper portion of the orbit. The cyst may be removed for cosmetic reasons and for biopsy. Pseudotumor is an inflammatory mass of the orbit without known cause. This tumor is treated with steroids to reduce the inflammation.

Other rare tumors include glioma of the OPTIC NERVE and rhabdomyosarcoma. Glioma of the optic nerve is a slow growing tumor that causes OPTIC ATROPHY. It may be linked with Von Recklinghausen's disease. Rhabdomyosarcoma is a rare tumor of the orbit seen in children. It is highly malignant and rapid growing but may be controlled by radiation therapy if treated in the earliest stages. Tumors originating from diseases of the body may metastasize to the orbit.

Tumors of the orbit often cause DIPLOPIA (double vision) or EXOPHTHALMOS, bulging of the eyes. Exophthalmos, also known as proptosis, is also caused by thyroid dysfunction, muscle palsy, injury, and infection. ENOPHTHALMOS, the appearance of sunken eyeballs, may occur due to an injury that displaces the fatty tissue lining of the orbit.

Injuries to the orbit may result in vision-limiting conditions. A common injury, the blow-out fracture, occurs when the globe is forced back into the orbit. A fracture forms on the orbital floor and bone is forced downward. Such an injury often causes damage to the rectus muscle and infraorbital nerve. The injury may be treated with placement of a plastic implant in the orbital floor and return of the displaced tissue to its correct position.

Fractures of the skull may extend into the orbit and cause cranial nerve palsy or optic nerve damage. A blow to the eye may result in OPTIC DISC atrophy. Such conditions resulting from injuries may affect vision or result in vision loss.

orbital cellulitis   An inflammation of the orbit. The infection is considered an emergency and must be treated promptly. If untreated, the OPTIC NERVE may become damaged and vision permanently lost. If allowed to spread to the brain, the infection could cause meningitis.

Orbital cellulitis may be the result of an infection of the sinuses that spreads to the bony orbit socket. Symptoms include forward displacement of the eye, restricted ocular motility, fever, and red, swollen eyelids. Movement of the eye also may be limited. Treatment involves admission to the hospital where antibiotics are administered in intensive therapy. Surgery may be performed to drain an abscess. If treatment is timely, the prognosis for the eye and vision are excellent.

orientation aids   Maps, scale models, or verbal descriptions of a building or site that enable visually impaired persons to navigate independently. Orientation aids are particularly appropriate to large public facilities, such as airports, train stations, hospitals, hotels, or universities.

Orientation aids may be visual, verbal, or sculptural. Visual types include diagrams or maps and may include raised lines or features. TACTILE MAPS with visual information are beneficial to both visually impaired and sighted users.

Verbal aids are spoken or written descriptions of the site or descriptions of routes to travel the site. Verbal aids may be recorded onto cassette or tape or printed. Many verbal aids are designed to be used en route.

Sculptural aids are three-dimensional models of the environment or site. If made to scale, models give the most information about spatial relationships and concepts.

Orientation aids are recommended for inclusion in standardized locations in all public facilities or sites by the Committee on Architectural and Environmental Concerns of the Visually Impaired, a standing committee of the American Association of Workers for the Blind. (See TRAVEL AIDS.)

orientation and mobility   The term used to describe methods to navigate safely, gracefully, and confidently in an environment. Orientation and mobility skills are taught as a part of the rehabilitation and education program for the blind and visually impaired.

Formal orientation and mobility programs came into existence after World War II. In response to the need for rehabilitation-skills training for blinded veterans, the United States military established rehabilitation programs at four hospitals. Richard E. Hoover, an ophthalmologist working as a director of physical reconditioning, orientation, and recreation at Valley Forge General Hospital in Phoenixville, Pennsylvania, developed a long cane and a set of methods for using the cane that are the basis of today's orientation and mobility programs.

As word of the benefits of Hoover's program grew, a demand for mobility training developed. In 1959, at a conference cosponsored by the American Foundation for the Blind and the Office of Vocational Rehabilitation, guidelines for mobility instructor criteria were outlined. Training programs were established in universities, and by 1960 Boston College established a graduate Peripatology Program, to be followed in 1961 by the establishment of the Center of Orientation and Mobility in Western Michigan University.

Current programs in universities require course work in education, physical and behavioral sciences, sensory training and awareness, preventive and restorative resources, and field training. Qualified orientation and mobility instructors are certified by the American Association of Workers for the Blind.

Orientation and mobility skills instructors individualize the program to the needs and abilities of the user. It is important for blind children to have orientation and mobility training early, in order to develop confidence in their surrounding and their ability to negotiate their environments. Although programs vary, orientation and mobility courses usually include sensory training, concept development, motor skills, orientation to surroundings, self-protection, long-cane skills, and use of a human guide.

Sensory training involves learning to use and sharpen the SENSES, including remaining vision, to their greatest abilities. The senses are used to determine landmarks, orient oneself to surroundings, and maneuver safely within an environment. The training may include development of echo perception or echo location, listening to the echo of self-emitted sounds to determine objects or surfaces in the environment.

Concept development is essential for those congenitally blind and includes learning spatial concepts such as perpendicular and parallel, and understanding fundamental structures such as compass directions, the layout of a building, or the design of a city block.

Motor skills include proper posture and body movement and the maintenance or improvement of coordination. These skills may be enhanced or developed through exercise, such as walking, skipping rope, jumping, or running.

Orientation training may include skills using landmarks and shorelines, squaring off, and trailing. Landmarks are objects in specific areas used to orient oneself in the environment. Shorelines are places where two different surfaces meet, such as where the floor meets the wall or where the floor meets the rug.

Squaring off uses landmarks as guides for determining direction, such as lining up with the edge of the curb to cross the street. Trailing involves lightly trailing the back of the hand to follow a shoreline such as a table edge, a hedge, or a wall. The back of the hand is used to avoid injuring the fingers.

Self-protection includes teaching protective body techniques. Upper-body protective techniques involve using the arm to protect the upper body and face from obstacles. The user carries one arm horizontally in front of the body with the elbow bent at a 90 degree angle. The arm then comes into contact with impeding objects before the body. If the head or face is the area most likely to come into contact with obstacles (such as when horseback riding) the arm is held up vertically to the side of the body with the hand held slightly ahead, protecting the face. The upper- and lower-body protective technique combines the horizontally held arm with the other arm held in front of the body, below the waist, at a 45-degree angle.

Long-cane skills are taught once the preceding skills are mastered. Training involves correct grip, movement of the cane, and use of the cane while walking to identify and circumvent obstacles.

Although use of a human guide is the least independent form of travel, it is sometimes necessary. The training in use of a human guide includes mastery of the SIGHTED GUIDE TECHNIQUE, a method for traveling with a sighted person.

Visually impaired persons receiving orientation and mobility training may be instructed in the use of optical or electronic travel aids prescribed by an optometrist or ophthalmologist. Optical aids include telescopes, magnifiers, and hand-held or spectacle-mounted devices that improve or enhance remaining vision.

Electronic travel aids include the laser cane, the Pathsounder, the Sonicguide, and the Mowat Sensor, all of which require specialized training to use. Electronic travel aids send out light beams or ultrasound waves that come into contact with objects in the path. When the beam or waves hit an object, the device responds by vibrating or emitting a sound. Electronic travel aids are used by approximately 1 percent of visually impaired persons and often cannot be used with a dog guide.

Dog-guide training is not a part of a standard orientation and mobility program. Only approximately 1 percent of visually impaired persons use DOG GUIDES because restrictions of age, health, hearing ability, remaining vision, and temperament limit those who may qualify to receive a dog. Those who do qualify for a dog guide are trained with the dog at the dog-guide school in specifically designed orientation and mobility programs.

American Foundation for the Blind. *How Does a Blind Person Get Around?* New York: American Foundation for the Blind, 1988.

Kelley, Jerry D., ed. *Recreation Programming for Visually Impaired Children and Youth.* New York: American Foundation for the Blind, 1981.

Scott, Eileen P. *Your Visually Impaired Student.* Baltimore: University Park Press, 1982.

Skurzynski, Gloria. *Bionic Parts for People.* New York: Four Winds Press, 1978.

orthokeratology A procedure that uses contact lenses to reshape the CORNEA to reduce MYOPIA. The curvature of the cornea is measured, and hard contact lenses are prescribed at a slightly flatter degree. As the cornea is flattened, new lenses are prescribed at increasingly flatter degrees. The process may take up to three years to complete.

The eyes are regularly measured and the visual acuity tested to determine the degree of correction.

The goal is to reshape the cornea to allow a visual acuity of 20/20 without correction. As this is achieved, the lens-wearing time is gradually reduced.

After the process, the cornea may maintain its new shape for a period of time but eventually reverts to its original shape. Retainer lenses may be prescribed to discourage regression. The retainer lenses may be worn as little as once every month or as much as eight hours a day.

Objective analysis of the procedure has revealed the dangers of permanent damage to the cornea, unimpressive and transient success rates, discomfort during the procedure and expense. Those with mild myopia stand the best chance of success, but those with severe myopia may benefit only in a reduction of strength needed in the lens prescription.

The procedure, although acclaimed by some doctors, is not widely used.

orthoptist A skilled health-care worker who diagnoses and treats people who have fused-vision, eye-muscle, and crossed-eye disorders. Orthoptists work under the supervision of an ophthalmologist to teach patients vision exercises that enable the patient to accurately focus and coordinate the movement of both eyes. They may also be trained in GLAUCOMA and vision-field testing.

Orthoptists must complete a minimum of two years of college or registered nurse's training in addition to the two years orthoptist academic program offered by hospitals, medical schools, or eye clinics. They may be certified by the American Orthoptic Council, although this is not a requirement for employment in every case.

Overbrook School for the Blind A private, not-for-profit school geared toward students with vision impairments and other challenges. It was founded in 1832 by Julius Friedlander, a young teacher who moved to Philadelphia from Germany for the purpose of starting a school for children with impaired vision or blindness. Overbrook is located on a 22-acre campus in West Philadelphia. About 200 students attend the school. Most commute, but there is some student housing available.

Overbrook educates children between the ages of three and 21 who are legally blind. Some have other impairments as well. There is no charge to families of the children who attend the school. State funding and funding from the child's school district covers the cost. The school also provides services to children who do not attend Overbrook and initiated a campaign in 2001 to provide advanced technology in its classrooms. In addition to academics, the school offers life skills classes, a work experience program, and extracurricular activities.

Contact:

Overbrook School for the Blind
6333 Malvern Avenue
Philadelphia, PA 19151
215-877-0313 (ph)
215-877-2709 (fax)
www.obs.org

panophthalmitis A painful condition in which inflammation or infection affects the entire globe of the eye. This may result from the inflammation of posterior UVEITIS or an infection due to surgery or injury.

Panophthalmitis also occurs when an inflammation or infection that affects the posterior chamber and center of the globe, a condition called endophthalmitis, spreads past the center to involve the ANTERIOR CHAMBER and the SCLERA.

The underlying condition is usually not treatable once it has reached the stage of panophthalmitis. Panophthalmitis usually results in complete, permanent loss of vision in the affected eye. The eye may begin to shrink and it may require surgical removal.

paperless braille Cassette braille, an information system that is stored on discs and accessed in braille. The system reduces the storage space normally needed for thick braille texts.

To use paperless braille systems such as VersaBraille, the individual runs his fingers over display cells to read the text. The push of a button accesses the next segment of recorded material. The user can produce, edit, and record braille with the system.

Although it consists of several pieces of equipment, the system is portable. It can be adapted for use with computer terminals, calculators, and typewriters.

papilledema A swelling of the OPTIC DISC due to an increase in intracranial pressure. Intracranial pressure may be the result of cerebral tumor or abscess, hypertension, subdural hematoma, or hydrocephalus, an increase in cerebrospinal fluid within the cranial cavity. It is a symptom of intracranial pressure increase and is often accompanied by vomiting and headache, enlargement of the blind spot, and transient blurring or loss of vision. It almost always is bilateral, and may develop over hours to weeks.

Since papilledema may indicate a tumor, it is a serious condition that requires prompt medical attention. Papilledema may be diagnosed by a visual-field examination, ULTRASONOGRAPHY, computerized TOMOGRAPHY, and FLUORESCEIN ANGIOGRAPHY, a test in which fluorescein dye is injected into the body and observed as it travels through the eye.

Pseudopapilledema is a degeneration or abnormality of the disc that exhibits the same symptoms as those of papilledema. Pseudopapilledema may actually be a misshapen disc or multiple drusen, waste particles of the optic nerve.

Papilledema is treated according to its cause. Hydrocephalus is treated with a shunt to drain the extraneous fluid. Tumors are surgically removed. Medication or surgery may be necessary for hypertension or hematoma.

partially sighted See LOW VISION.

pathsounder One of the ultrasonic ELECTRONIC TRAVEL AIDS designed for use by visually impaired persons. The device is manufactured under several names, including the Russell Pathsounder and the Polaron.

The device consists of a small box that may be hand held or worn at chest height from a strap around the neck. The box sends ultrasonic waves into the path of the user to detect objects up to 16 feet away. The reflected waves are converted into an audible sound to warn the user.

The device is designed to be used in conjunction with a long cane, and some manufacturer's models may be used with a dog guide. Use of the Pathsounder requires training from a qualified instructor.

peripatology   See ORIENTATION AND MOBILITY.

peripheral vision   The side vision of the visual field. It gives information about the area surrounding central vision, where detail is perceived.

Peripheral vision is controlled by the rods, light-sensitive cells of the RETINA. The retina is the inner layer between the CHOROID and the vitreous gel that contains photosensitive RODS AND CONES. The rods and cones provide information about the shape, color, size, and movement of an object in view. The retina processes the information from the rods and cones and encodes it into electrical impulses. The impulses are sent via the optic nerve to the brain where they are translated into an image.

The rods outnumber the cones by an average of five to one and are scattered throughout the retina. They react to faint light, shape, and movement. Because the rods do not require high levels of light to function, they enable the eye to see at night. Because they are scattered throughout the retina, unlike the cones which are concentrated in the center, they are responsible for peripheral vision.

Diseases of the retina and other disorders of the eye may damage cones or destroy peripheral vision. RETINITIS PIGMENTOSA (RP) is a hereditary group of diseases that attack the retina and cause degeneration of the rods and cones. The rods are affected first. As they are destroyed, night vision deteriorates and peripheral vision is lost. As the disease progresses, ever-increasing tunnel vision results. Currently, there is no treatment for RP.

RETINAL DETACHMENT may cause a sudden loss of peripheral vision. A retinal detachment occurs when the retina pulls away from the epithelial layer next to the choroid. This may be caused by holes or tears in the retina, by traction or by leakage of the VITREOUS gel. The tears may result from aging, injury, cataract surgery, or severe myopia (nearsightedness). As the retina detaches, it fails to function in the detached area, and vision is lost. Detached retinas are usually treated surgically.

GLAUCOMA is a disease that attacks and destroys peripheral vision. It is the leading cause of blindness among adults in the United States. It may be caused by heredity, aging or as a result of another eye condition. As the AQUEOUS FLUID in the ANTERIOR CHAMBER of the eye fails to drain normally, the fluid builds within the eye, forcing the vitreous in the *posterior chamber* against the retina and optic nerve. The pressure cuts off the blood supply to nerve cells in the retina and optic nerve, damaging them and destroying vision. Since glaucoma first affects those cells that determine peripheral vision, a loss of peripheral vision is a major symptom of glaucoma. Other symptoms include pain, blurred vision, the presence of halos around lights, and a loss of night vision. Without treatment, glaucoma causes increasing tunnel vision. Vision lost as a result of glaucoma cannot be restored, but once diagnosed, glaucoma may be effectively treated and controlled with medication or a combination of medication, laser treatments and surgery.

Perkins School for the Blind   The Perkins School for the Blind, established in 1829 as the New England Asylum for the Blind, was the first school for the blind in the United States. It was later referred to as the New England Institution for the Blind and then finally renamed The Perkins School for the Blind in honor of an early benefactor, Colonel Thomas Handasyd Perkins. Both HELEN KELLER and ANNE SULLIVAN, her teacher, were students at the Perkins school.

Under the directorship of Dr. Samuel Gridley Howe, the school offered instruction for blind and deaf-blind individuals. A printing department, later named the Howe Memorial Press, was added that produced books and materials in Boston Line Type, a raised and enlarged Roman alphabet, and in braille.

Today the school educates and trains children and adult blind, visually impaired, deaf-blind, and multi-impaired individuals. The Adult Services Program provides community housing options, offering instruction in independent-living skills and rehabilitation programs for those 18 years and older.

The Severe Impaired Program offers individualized instruction and residential care to severely or multi-impaired individuals aged 10 to 22. The Deaf-Blind Program serves individuals aged five to 22 and provides academic education, vocational training, and daily living skills.

The Perkins School offers secondary services to adolescents in high school or special educational programs, a lower-school program of individualized instruction for children in elementary school, and a preschool program and infant-toddler program for assessment and training for children from birth to five years.

The project with industry program explores employment opportunities for blind and visually impaired adults and provides job-placement services, job analysis, adaptive engineering, and training support.

The school operates the Howe Press, which manufactures the Perkins Brailler, a braille typewriting machine. The Howe Press offers the braillers, brailler accessories, brailling slates and accessories, games, maps, mathematical aids, music, and braille paper through its mail-order catalog.

The school also runs the Hilton/Perkins Program, aimed at improving the quality of life for multi-handicapped blind or deaf-blind children around the world by offering increased educational opportunities.

The Perkins School maintains the Samuel P. Hayes Library, the world's largest collection of print material on the nonmedical aspects of blindness and deaf-blindness. The library contains 25,000 volumes in print, braille or on recorded discs or cassettes. The school publishes a biannual newsletter, the *Howe Press Newsletter.*

Contact:

Perkins School for the Blind
175 North Beacon Street
Watertown, MA 02172-9982
617-924-3434 (ph)
617-926-2027 (fax)
www.perkins.pvt.k12.ma.us

phacoemulsification A type of CATARACT extraction invented in 1967 by Dr. Charles Kelman. During the procedure, a small incision (one-tenth of an inch) is made in the eye. An ultrasonic, titanium needle is then inserted into the incision. The surgeon presses a foot pedal to activate the needle. The needle vibrates 40,000 times per second to break down or emulsify the hard nucleus of the cataract. The liquefied cataract is then sucked back up through the needle and removed from the eye. The posterior capsule is left intact, and one suture is placed to close the incision. Recovery from surgery is almost immediate. Patients may often return to work and routine activities the following day.

When phacoemulsification was first introduced, it was associated with a higher complication rate due to the inexperience of the surgeons. As more ophthalmologists gained expertise in the procedure, the complication rate dropped and the method is no longer considered controversial.

phoroptor An instrument used in the ophthalmologic examination. The phoroptor determines the refraction errors, or the degree of inability to properly focus.

It is a large butterflylike apparatus that has two round sections affixed to a vertical base. The patient faces the phoroptor, with one round section centered in front of each eye. The patient places his chin on a chin rest and looks through lenses in each round section to read a wall chart.

The phoroptor holds hundreds of lenses of varying degrees in each round section. The examiner uses a dial to change the lenses in front of each eye. The patient is asked to determine which lenses provide the clearest vision or image of the chart.

From the information provided by the patient in response to the phoroptor lenses, the examiner can prescribe the proper corrective lenses.

photocoagulation A procedure in which light is used to coagulate or congeal hemorrhages. Photocoagulation is used routinely in ophthalmological therapy and as an alternative to surgery.

Light was first used in the 1950s to coagulate retinal detachments. The procedure used a German device that produced a powerful beam of light from a xenon arc. In the 1960s LASERS were introduced and became the instrument of choice for photocoagulation because they generate less heat and can be focused more precisely.

The low energy, finely concentrated light of the laser is directed into the eye where it is absorbed by the tissue. The energy converts to heat, which forms a burn. The burn develops into scar tissue, which congeals the hemorrhage.

Photocoagulation is used to treat DIABETIC RETINOPATHY. An ARGON LASER is directed into the eye where the light is absorbed into the pigmented layer of the RETINA. The surgeon makes several "burns" around each leaking vessel of the retina. The resulting scar tissue stops the leaking. Unhealthy tissue that is generating neovascularization (new, weak vessel growth) is treated with the laser to destroy it and prevent the cycle of new growth.

In much the same manner, photocoagulation is used to treat subretinal neovascularization, a complication of AGE-RELATED MACULOPATHY. A break in the pigment epithelial layer beneath the retina causes the underlying vessels to bleed into the retina and cause scarring. The scarring destroys vision in the macula, the central section of the retina responsible for sharpest sight.

This treatment utilizes a laser, which is absorbed only in the deepest layers of the retina where such damage occurs. The light passes through the upper, unaffected layers and treats only the targeted areas below.

Photocoagulation may be used in some instances to treat GLAUCOMA. A laser may be used to create a series of burns that develop into scars and form openings in the meshwork of drainage channels that allow fluid to flow more easily from the eye.

Photocoagulation is generally a painless procedure, usually performed without anesthesia. The patient sits in front of a slit lamp or biomicroscope in a dimmed room. Topical anesthetic drops, dilating drops or a contact lens may be placed in the eye.

The surgeon administers from 50 to several hundred rapid bursts of energy to the affected areas of the eye. The patient may see flashing lights and may experience slight discomfort or brief, painful moments. The procedure may last from five to 30 minutes, and the patient is usually able to walk or drive home afterward. Follow-up treatments may be necessary.

Although photocoagulation may improve vision in some cases, it is not always a cure. It frequently cannot restore lost vision and may only serve to stop or impede the progression of a disease or disorder.

Berland, Theodore, and Richard A. Perritt. *Living With Your Eye Operation.* New York: St. Martin's Press, 1974.
Eden, John. *The Eye Book.* New York: Penguin Books, 1978.
Krames Communications. *The Retina Book.* Daly City, California: KC, 1987.
Medem Medical Library. How is Diabetic Retinopathy Treated? www.medem.com/search, 1997.
Reynolds, James D. "Lasers in Ophthalmology." Health-Net Library, CompuServe, 1989.
Schweitzer, N. M. J., ed. *Ophthalmology.* Amsterdam: Exerpta Medica, 1982.
Shulman, Jules. *Cataracts.* New York: Simon and Schuster, 1984.

photophobia   Photophobia, or fear of light, is a condition in which the eyes have little tolerance for light. The eyes may experience pain as a result of exposure to light or may involuntarily squint or blink in response to light.

Photophobia is not a disease but, rather, a symptom or result of an ocular disease or disorder. Photophobia is a first sign of congenital GLAUCOMA in infants. It may be caused by or seen in a multitude of disorders including IRITIS, corneal lesions, ALBINISM, CATARACTS, BLEPHARITIS, MIGRAINE, TRACHOMA, UVEITIS, some types of drugs, and SYMPATHETIC OPHTHALMIA. Since photophobia is a result or symptom of disorder, its occurrence should prompt an ocular examination.

photorefractive keratectomy (PRK)   A corneal surgery that can reduce or correct mild to moderate myopia (nearsightedness), with or without mild astigmatism. The surgery, which normally is done on an outpatient basis, involves removing the epithelium, or surface layer, of the cornea. A special laser is then used to precisely reshape the cornea. The actual surgery generally takes only about a minute, although the overall procedure requires more time.

An ophthalmologist programs the PRK laser—an excimer laser—to specifically meet the needs of each patient. The laser produces a highly concentrated beam of light that removes micro-thin layers of tissue from the cornea. This results in a flattening of the cornea's front surface, which generally improves the condition of myopia. Much research has been done to determine exactly how much laser is required to treat a particular amount of myopia.

Most people who undergo PRK report that they no longer have to wear glasses or contacts. Tests show that about two-thirds of patients who undergo PRK can see 20/20 or better without corrective lenses. Nearly all—about 95 percent—can pass a standard driver's license exam that requires 20/40 vision without glasses or contacts.

PRK was first performed in the United States in 1996. The procedure still is used, but the newer LASIK procedure has become more popular. PRK is normally without complications, but, as with all surgeries, there are some risks involved. These include the possibility of infection or drug reaction, which, in extreme cases, could result in loss of vision. Some people find they need reading glasses at an earlier age than average (about 40) after PRK, even though they did not wear glasses before the procedure. Some PRK patients have experienced problems with night vision, and a small percentage of patients realize a decrease in best corrected vision.

People who have uncontrolled autoimmune or vascular disease, are pregnant or nursing, have KERATOCONUS, or have previously had a RADIAL KERATOTOMY normally are not advised to consider PRK.

pinguecula See CONJUNCTIVA.

Plaquinil See LUPUS.

pleoptics Pleoptics or pleoptic methods are part of orthoptic training, the use of exercises to correct or improve vision disorders. Pleoptic methods use flashing devices to improve macular and foveal orientation and fixation in cases of AMBLYOPIA, a condition of blindness in one eye due to disuse.

The treatment consists of producing an afterimage on which the patient is taught to focus. The macular region of the RETINA is stimulated with a bright or dazzling light. When the light is turned off, the patient fixates on the macula's after-image, encouraging the individual to use the MACULA.

Pleoptic treatment may last several weeks to several years. Results of pleoptic treatment have been disappointing in light of early expectations, and the methods are now more widely used in Europe than in the United States.

pneumatic retinopexy A fairly new procedure used to repair a RETINAL DETACHMENT. A retinal detachment occurs when the retina becomes separated from the back of the eye. Some detachments are caused by retinal holes or tears, which must be surgically repaired.

With pneumatic retinopexy, freezing treatment is placed around the retinal tear, after which an expanding gas bubble is injected into the eye. The gas pushes against the area of the retinal tear and closes it, eliminating the need for a SCLERAL BUCKLE.

The procedure requires only local anesthetic and often can be done in a doctor's office. It does not, however, work for all types of retinal detachments. Pneumatic retinopexy was first introduced in the United States in 1985.

posterior chamber The posterior chamber of the eye is the area between the IRIS and the LENS. It is the counterpart to the ANTERIOR CHAMBER located between the CORNEA and the iris. Both chambers are filled with AQUEOUS FLUID, the clear liquid that nourishes the CORNEA and lens and carries away waste.

The aqueous is produced by the CILIARY BODY epithelium. The ciliary body also has a muscle group that bends the lens of the eye to focus properly. The aqueous flows from the ciliary body into the posterior chamber to bring nutrients to the lens. It then flows through the PUPIL of the eye into the anterior chamber to reach the back of the cornea. After the fluid has circulated, it leaves the eye through the Schlemm's canal, a drainage point at the junction of the cornea and the iris.

The posterior chamber is the site of surgery for posterior intraocular lens implantations. As a part of CATARACT surgery, a plastic lens is often placed either in front of, or behind, the iris to replace the portion of natural lens lost to surgery. Posterior lens implantation places the artificial lens behind the iris.

Posterior is also a term used to describe the back portion of the eye behind the lens. This area is filled with the vitreous, a clear gel-like material that makes up 80 percent of the volume of the eye. The vitreous gives volume to the eye and supports the other organs within the globe.

The expanded definition or boundaries of the posterior area may include the RETINA, OPTIC NERVE, and portions of the CHOROID and SCLERA, which are positioned in the back of the eye. This area may be injected with antibiotics or other medications in the treatment of disease or infection. It may be the site of surgery as in RETINAL DETACHMENT operations, or vitrectomies. In retinal detachment surgery, the retina is reattached to the epithelial layer next to the choroid. During vitrectomy, the chamber behind the lens is drained of diseased vitreous gel and filled with a sterile saline solution.

The posterior section behind the lens may be subject to floaters, bits of debris or blood in the vitreous. Light passing through the vitreous casts shadows of the debris onto the retina, causing images of the debris to float through the field of vision. Floaters appear in normal vision and are not considered as a symptom of disease unless they appear suddenly or in large numbers.

potential acuity meter (PAM)   A slit-lamp attachment used to assess the potential, usable vision of those with cataractous lenses or corneal opacities.

The PAM uses a prism system and self-illumination to project a small SNELLEN CHART through a clear section of the cornea or lens and onto the retina of the person being examined. In by-passing the opacities, the examiner can efficiently use the Snellen chart to measure visual acuity.

presbyopia   Aging of the eyes. As the eye ages, the lens deteriorates and loses the ability to focus near objects. The first symptoms usually arise after 40 years of age and include difficulty in reading or doing close work.

Prescriptive convex lenses in reading glasses or bifocals may correct the problem. In addition, a Texas-based company called Presby Corp. has developed and is marketing a surgical technique called Surgical Reversal of Presbyopia. The procedure uses a tiny device called a scleral expansion band to expand the diameter of the sclera. This causes the distance between the scleral and the lens to increase, restoring the effective working distance of the muscle, as in a younger eye. The company is conducting investigational clinical trials at six universities to test the procedure.

President's Committee on Employment of People with Disabilities   See OFFICE OF DISABILITY EMPLOYMENT POLICY.

Prevent Blindness America   The oldest national voluntary health organization working to prevent blindness. Founded in 1908, it has been formerly known as the National Committee for the Prevention of Blindness, the National Society for the Prevention of Blindness, and the National Society to Prevent Blindness. The goal of the organization is to preserve sight and prevent blindness through community-service programs, public and professional education, and research.

Prevent Blindness America activities include preschool vision testing, distributing a family home eye test called "How's Your Vision?," local glaucoma screening and educational programs, and promoting industrial and recreational eye-safety programs. The organization also promotes cooperative public and educational programs with governmental and voluntary health and social-service agencies, and sponsors the National Center for Sight, a toll-free number for eye health and safety information. The line is open from 8:30 A.M. to 5 P.M. Central time, and can be reached at 800-331-2020. Prevent Blindness America also maintains a website with extensive information and links to other eye care–related sites. In addition, it sponsors research projects to find the causes and treatments for eye diseases and disorders.

Publications include *Insight,* an annual report, and a wide range of pamphlets and brochures dealing with eye safety, home-vision screening, eye health, and industrial and recreational eye safety. The organization also publishes *Prevent Blindness News,* a 12-page newsletter printed three times a year.

Contact:

Prevent Blindness America
500 E. Remington Road
Schaumburg, IL 60173
800-331-2020
www.preventblindness.org

prevention of blindness According to the Prevent Blindness America there are currently more than half a million legally blind people in the United States, and more than 50,000 people become blind each year. Prevent Blindness America estimates that 50 percent of blindness can be prevented with current medical knowledge and techniques and that 90 percent of all accidental eye damage can be averted with proper eye-safety practices and appropriate eyewear.

The leading causes of blindness in the United States are GLAUCOMA, MACULAR DISEASE, CATARACT, OPTIC NERVE ATROPHY, DIABETIC RETINOPATHY, and RETINITIS PIGMENTOSA. These causes represent an estimated 51 percent of blindness cases. The leading causes of new cases of blindness are macular degeneration, glaucoma, diabetic retinopathy, and cataract.

There are approximately 11.4 million visually impaired persons in the United States, those who have serious vision problems but who cannot be classified as legally blind. Of this group, 1.4 million have severe vision impairments that hinder them from reading ordinary newsprint even with the aid of corrective lenses.

The most common causes of vision impairment are cataract, INJURIES, glaucoma, and CONGENITAL DISORDERS. Cataract is responsible for up to one-third of all new cases of vision impairment. Injury-related vision impairments number close to nearly 1 million, with an estimated 40,000 new cases caused by injury each year.

The best defense against blindness or vision impairment due to disease or disorder is an annual or biannual eye examination after the age of 35. Many diseases are easiest to control and have the best success records when diagnosed and treated in the early stages.

Injury-related vision impairments may be prevented by wearing protective eye wear and improving eye-safety practices, such as improving contact-lens hygiene and overwear time and wearing seat belts while traveling in the car. The materials and products most commonly associated with injuries to the eyes are metal fragments, contact lenses, motor vehicles, and chemicals.

Work-related accidents account for at least 61,000 eye injuries each year. Prevention of blindness due to occupational hazards or injuries is closely monitored by the Occupational Safety and Health Administration (OSHA), which enforces occupational health and safety standards, and the American National Standards Institute, which specifies manufacturing standards for protective eyewear.

Work-related injuries may be prevented by the consistent use of appropriate eye-protection gear. A recent survey by the Bureau of Labor Statistics showed that three out of five workers who suffered an eye injury wore no eye protection. Of those who did, 40 percent wore the wrong kind. Protective eye-safety wear includes safety goggles or glasses, side shields, eye-cup side shields, ventilated goggles, face shields, and helmets. Safety glasses or goggles are made of impact-resistant glass, plastic, or polycarbonate prescription or non-prescription lenses. The glasses frames are reinforced more strongly than normal types and are heat resistant.

Side shields that attach to, or that are part of, the safety goggle frame protect the eyes from flying particles or objects from the front and sides of the wearer. Eye-cup side shields protect the wearer from flying objects from the front, side, top, and bottom.

Goggles fitted with regular or indirect ventilation protect the wearer from chemical splashes, dust, sparks, and flying particles. Face shields protect from splashes, heat, glare, and flying objects and must be worn over safety goggles or glasses. Welding helmets with appropriate filter plates or lenses protect the wearer from splashes of molten metal, sparks and the intense heat and light of welding. The helmets are worn over safety glasses or goggles.

Sports-related injuries account for more than 40,000 emergency room eye treatments annually. Sports with the highest injury frequencies are baseball, basketball, racquet sports, and football. More than 90 percent of all eye injuries and resulting vision impairments may be prevented in sport-related activities by wearing safety eyeguards or industrial-quality safety glasses.

Over 420,000 persons in the United States have lost some sight due to home eye injuries, nearly 45 percent of all injuries. Home injuries are usually product related and are due generally to home structure or construction materials such as nails and lumber, home-maintenance products such as glues and bleaches, personal-use products including contact lenses and sun lamps, and home shop equipment such as batteries and manual tools. Household products cause more than 32,000 serious injuries each year.

Home eye injuries can be prevented by wearing eye protection such as safety glasses (ANSI Z-87) when using hazardous materials or working with tools. Safety goggles should be worn as a protection against battery fragments or acid when jump-starting a car.

Ultraviolet absorbing sunglasses should be worn in sunlight, due to evidence that UV rays can damage the eyes and contribute to the development of various disorders, including macular degeneration and cataracts.

Public education programs organized by non-profit associations, state departments of education, public health-care providers, and civic and service groups serve to prevent blindness by alerting and educating the public about eye care, eye safety, and eye diseases. Many such organizations perform free eye examinations, provide training and education programs for professionals in the eye-care field, support research into eye diseases, and work for legislation to enforce and extend existing laws for eye protection and safety. (See VITAMINS, WORLD BLINDNESS.)

Krames Communications. *A Guide to Eye Safety.* Daly City, California: KC, 1987.
Prevent Blindness America. "Safety." www.preventblind-ness.org, 2000.
Prevent Blindness America. "Facts and Figures." www.preventblindness.org, 2000.

prisms   Prisms are inexpensive optical additions to prescriptive lenses that maximize use of remaining vision. They are used to improve ocular conditions such as NYSTAGMUS, DIPLOPIA, macular disease, or peripheral-field defects.

Prisms are horizontally incorporated into frames for prescriptive lenses or noncorrective spectacles to treat nystagmus, an uncontrollable jerking of the eyes that impairs focusing on an object. The prisms may relieve symptomatic headache and improve acuity and stabilization of vision.

Vertically applied prisms are used to treat diplopia, or double vision, due to retinal surgery. The prisms compensate for the impaired abilities of the extraocular muscles.

Those with macular disease may be helped by prisms. If the MACULA, or central section of sight, is impaired or destroyed, prisms can be placed to move the image from the FOVEA (central macular region) to an area outside the fovea that is usable.

Prisms such as the Fresnel prism are used for peripheral-field (side vision) defects. They are incorporated into prescription lenses or pressed onto noncorrective spectacles in sections above and below or to the sides of the usable central visual field. By moving the eyes or the head slightly, the user can see through the prisms into the restricted field.

progressive addition lenses   Seamless, multifocal lenses that allow the wearer a smooth transition from the distance portion of the lens into the reading portion. No line is visible, either to the wearer or anyone else. The power of a progressive addition lens gradually increases as the wearer looks from the distance portion to the reading portion, creating an appropriate lens power for every distance. A disadvantage of these lenses is that the sides tend to become distorted, making side vision appear to be wavy. Technology for creating these lenses, which first appeared in the late 1970s, continues to improve, however, and wearers find the distortion to be less troublesome as they get accustomed to the lenses.

proliferative retinopathy A retinal disorder that occurs as a complication of DIABETES. It is a serious disease that can result in permanent vision impairment or blindness.

Proliferative retinopathy is one of three types of DIABETIC RETINOPATHY, which also include exudative, or background retinopathy, and preproliferative retinopathy. Diabetic retinopathy is a circulatory disorder that causes the blood vessels that nourish the RETINA, a light-sensitive inner lining in the back layer of the eye, to weaken, disintegrate or become blocked. The vessels may leak fluid, bleed, grow unnaturally, bulge, or stop functioning completely.

Exudative retinopathy is a first stage of diabetic retinopathy in which small hemorrhages occur from the retinal vessels. Hard exudates form rings around the damaged vessels. This condition rarely affects vision and may last indefinitely or progress to a more serious stage. The preproliferative stage is marked by an increasing number of hemorrhages, dilation of the retinal vein, and the occurrence of soft exudates. Preproliferative retinopathy is a serious condition that may rapidly progress to the proliferative stage.

Proliferative retinopathy involves neovascularization or development of abnormal blood vessels within the retina and VITREOUS. The vessels develop as a result of ischemia, tissue anemia due to an obstruction to the flow of blood. The new, weak vessels grow between the vitreous and the retina, near the OPTIC DISC. They leak and cause retinal and vitreal hemorrhages. The vitreous may shrink and pull the vessels with it, causing hemorrhaging, fibrous-tissue development, retinal tears, retinal detachment, and secondary glaucoma. At first, a person with proliferative retinopathy may notice few symptoms of the disorder. As the condition progresses, floaters may be seen, and vision may become blurred or lost.

Proliferative retinopathy is diagnosed by an eye examination. FLUORESCEIN ANGIOGRAPHY may be used to aid diagnosis and locate areas of greatest proliferation. During this procedure, fluorescein dye is injected into a vein in the arm and monitored as it flows through the retina. B-SCAN ultrasonography, or sonar vision, may be applied if the

transparent tissues have become opaque due to hemorrhage.

Treatment consists of photocoagulation or laser therapy. Originally, the treatment involved areas of the retina in which the neovascularization had occurred. Now, the photocoagulation is applied extensively in the retina in a method called panretinal photocoagulation (PRP). During this treatment, over 1,000 laser burns are placed on the retina, excluding the macular area. These areas are destroyed, allowing the limited blood supply to reach and nourish the MACULA, or area of sharpest sight.

Vitrectomy may be necessary in cases of extreme vitreal hemorrhage or traction detachment. A specialized instrument is inserted into the vitreous where it breaks down blood deposits and scar tissue. It then removes the matter and the diseased vitreous fluid by suction. Simultaneously, a sterile saline fluid is injected to replace the vitreous fluid. Approximately two thirds of those who undergo vitrectomy gain improved vision.

Proliferative retinopathy may regress spontaneously. In cases of progressive proliferative retinopathy, early treatment of the ocular condition and the underlying diabetes may prevent or limit vision loss.

Galloway, N. R. *Common Eye Diseases and Their Management.* Berlin: Springer-Verlag, 1985.
Rhoade, Stephen J., and Stephen P. Ginsberg. *Ophthalmic Technology.* New York: Raven Press, 1987.
Vaughn, Daniel, and Taylor Asbury. *General Ophthalmology.* Los Altos, California: Lange Medical Publications, 1977.

proptosis See EXOPHTHALMOS.

prosthesis A prosthetic or artificial eye is used to replace an eye that has been enucleated, or surgically removed. Prosthetic eyes have been in existence for centuries. Ancient Egyptian cultures fashioned wax, plaster- or precious-stone eyes to adorn their dead.

Roman surgeon priests made artificial eyes for the living out of wood, shells, bone, ivory, stone, and precious metals. In the 16th century, Venetians developed the first glass eyes, but the precursor of the modern type of prosthetic was developed in the 17th century by French surgeons.

Before World War II, most prosthetic eyes were manufactured of glass in Germany and exported to other countries. After the war, plastic prosthetics were invented and manufactured throughout the world. Modern prosthetic eyes are made from glass or plastic by ocularists. They are custom shaped to match the eye socket of the individual and the coloring of the natural eye. Prosthetic eyes are generally nondistinguishable from natural eyes.

Two or more days after enucleation the eye socket is fitted with a plastic shell that will cradle the prosthesis. Three or four weeks later, the prosthetic eye is fitted. The eye is attached to the remaining extrinsic muscles in the orbit to ensure natural movement.

The prosthetic eye is worn constantly to prevent contraction of the eye socket. It is cleansed daily and may be lubricated with drops for this purpose. A slight mucous discharge is a normal characteristic of prosthesis wearers, but profuse discharge could indicate an infection.

Infection often stems from roughening of the prosthesis. The prosthesis should be polished once or twice a year to buff out scratches and reduce irritation, and should be checked for wear by a specialist at regular intervals. Most plastic prosthetic eyes last five years on average.

pterygium   See CONJUNCTIVA.

ptosis   A sagging of the upper eyelid. It may be congenital or acquired and can affect one or both eyes. The disorder may appear congenitally in children or in adults due to aging, nerve palsy, inflammation, styes, tumors, cysts, MYASTHENIA GRAVIS, oculomotor palsy, Horner's syndrome, or use of guanethidine eyedrops.

Mild ptosis that does not affect vision may require no treatment. Severe forms of the condition may affect vision by obstructing the pupil or may be cosmetically unattractive. After careful diagnosis as to the cause, ptosis may be corrected surgically in some congenital, nerve palsy, or age-related cases.

Surgery may be performed on children of three or four years of age or younger if the ptosis is uni-

lateral and causing AMBLYOPIA. The surgery may be performed under local anesthetic for adults and general anesthetic for children. The type of surgical procedure used depends on the severity and underlying cause of each case.

Three surgical procedures are most commonly used. The *Fansanella-Servat* involves the removal of a portion of the lid from the inside. The outer skin is not incised. The shortened lid is lifted off the eye. This procedure is used to treat mild cases of ptosis. The *levator resection* is used to treat moderate cases. During this procedure several incisions are made in the lid. A sling is placed inside the lid to permanently lift it. The *frontalis suspension* is reserved for severe cases of ptosis. A section of the muscle that raises the eyelid is removed. The surface skin of the eyelid is usually involved in the incision. The shortened muscle keeps the lid elevated. Complications from eyelid surgery may include infection, bleeding, scarring, and corneal drying. Over- and undercorrections may occur.

Treatment of other forms of ptosis involves treating the underlying cause. Neostigmine may be prescribed in cases of myasthenia gravis. When surgery is contraindicated, special spectacles with an attached crutch to raise the eyelid may be prescribed.

pupil   The small opening centered in the IRIS of the eye. It allows light to pass into the eye. The pupil can change size to accommodate different light extremes. The iris, or colored part of the eye, regulates the size of the pupil by using adjacent dilator and sphincter muscles to open and close it. In bright light, the pupil constricts to screen out excess light. In low light, it opens up to allow the maximum amount of light to enter the eye.

The pupil may open wider in response to a stimulus other than light. Emotions of fear, excitement and delight, and loud noises may dilate the pupil. Drugs may artificially dilate or constrict the pupil. Cycloplegic drops dilate the pupil. Different types such as tropicamide, cyclopentolate, or atropine are effective from three hours to seven days. The pupil is dilated to examine the back of the eye and to treat conditions such as IRITIS and CYCLITIS. Occasionally, dilation of the pupils can bring about an attack of GLAUCOMA in eyes with narrow ANTERIOR CHAMBERS.

Meiotic drops constrict the pupil. Pilocarpine, ecothiopate, or phospholine iodide may constrict the pupil from 4 to 12 hours. The pupils are constricted to reduce intraocular pressure.

The pupil is black because the inside of the eye showing through it is dark. Any change in the color or shape of the pupil may indicate a disorder within the eye or the body. A light-colored pupil, called leukokoria, may indicate the presence of a tumor.

A constricted or misshapen pupil may be evidence of iritis. An enlarged pupil may indicate glaucoma or increased intracranial pressure. Pupils of unequal size may also be the result of anisocoria, a congenital defect.

radial keratotomy (RK) A type of CORNEA surgery developed in the Soviet Union by Dr. Syvatoslav Fyodorov. The surgery is designed to improve myopia (nearsightedness). The ultimate goal of the surgery is to restore the patient's vision to 20/20 without the use of contact lenses or eyeglasses. The words *radial keratotomy* refer to the radial cuts or incisions made on the cornea during surgery.

Those with mild myopia can expect the best results from radial keratotomy. Possible candidates must require glasses or contact lenses to correct their vision. The best results are for those with a refraction between -2.00 to -4.00 diopters and a visual acuity level of 20/80 to 20/200. Those with high myopia (-5.00 or greater) will not achieve the same results.

Although prospective RK patients must be mildly myopic, people with very slight myopia are discouraged from undergoing surgery for such minimal correction. Those with corneal disorders, GLAUCOMA or pre-glaucomatous conditions, lenticular astigmatism, or other eye disorders are also often not considered good candidates for this surgery.

The presurgical examination involves an external examination of the eye, a vision acuity test, and a refraction test. Additional tests may include corneascope photographs, a slit-lamp examination, intraocular-pressure testing, motility studies, and cornea measurement and depth testing.

Approximately one hour before surgery, the patient is treated with two or more sets of eye drops to dilate and anesthetize the eye. Many surgeons also administer an antibiotic such as gentamicin sulfate.

In the operating room, the surgeon takes a number of exact readings and measurements of the eye to determine the surgical plan. The cornea is stamped with a trephine, a cookie-cutter-like instrument that marks an incision pattern that the surgeon uses as a guide. The pattern includes a center circular clear zone and a variable number of incision lines radiating out from the clear zone. The surgeon uses a diamond blade to cut from the clear zone circle outward. The procedure flattens or shortens the cornea, to produce better refraction and improved vision.

The surgery is done on an outpatient basis (without overnight hospitalization) and generally requires 30 minutes per eye. The eye is covered with a patch for 24 hours, and eye drops such as pilocarpine hydrochloride are used for a week.

After surgery the patient may experience pain, sensitivity to light, tearing, decrease or fluctuation of visual acuity, over- or undercorrection, and astigmatism. Patients may achieve from 20/20 vision to 20/200 vision, or experience no improvement at all.

Studies indicate that radial keratotomy improves vision in the majority of cases. However, the procedure remains a controversial one and the prospective candidate for RK is encouraged to research the procedure, its risks and benefits and the surgeon involved to develop a reasonable expectation.

Waring, A. O., et al. "Results of the Prospective Evaluation of Radial Keratotomy (PERK) Study on Year After Surgery." *Ophthalmology,* vol. 92, no. 2 (February 1985): 177.

radiation burns Burns caused by light. Ocular radiation burns can be caused by ultraviolet rays, infrared rays, X rays, microwaves, laser beams, and gamma rays.

Burns due to ultraviolet rays include SNOW BLINDNESS, welders' flash, and sun-lamp injuries. Ultraviolet waves do not penetrate the globe and therefore deliver a burn to the CORNEA, or clear, outermost covering of the eye. Symptoms of these burns are usually delayed two to nine hours and include extreme pain, a sensation of sand in the eyes, and severe light sensitivity. The burns heal themselves within two to three days but antibiotics or steroid drops may be prescribed. Ultraviolet burns can be prevented by wearing protective eyeglasses or goggles.

Eclipse blindness is an ultraviolet burn caused by watching the sun during an eclipse. Although the ultraviolet rays of the sun do not enter the globe, the heat generated within the eye during prolonged exposure to these rays produces a burn to the MACULA. The macula is the area of clearest sight within the RETINA, the light-sensitive layer at the back of the eye. The damage to the macula from an eclipse burn is irreversible and causes loss of central vision. An eclipse cannot be safely viewed directly. Sunglasses, photographic film, or film negatives afford no protection to the eyes. An eclipse may be safely viewed indirectly by observing the image of the sun projected onto a flat surface through a small hole in a piece of paper.

Infrared rays can penetrate the eye and may cause CATARACTS. In the past, ocular infrared burns were found among steel workers and glass blowers. The adoption of safety goggles and eyeshields has virtually eliminated the problem.

X rays may produce cataracts in threshold doses of approximately 1,000 rad but may vary with exposure times. Simple dental or diagnostic X rays will not endanger the eyes. X rays that are used therapeutically to treat lesions near the eyes should be given only when the eyes are appropriately shielded.

Microwaves may cause cataracts but only when the eye is in the direct line of the beam. According to current knowledge, microwave ovens constitute no threat to vision.

LASERS are intense beams of light that can enter the globe of the eye. They are used therapeutically in ophthalmology to heal hemorrhages in the retina. The beam is focused directly onto the point of therapy that is exposed to the light for a specific amount of time. Industrial lasers can produce retinal burns when viewed directly or by reflection off other objects.

Gamma rays can produce cataracts and loss of vision. The rays released by atomic bomb explosions resulted in mass amounts of cataract cases following the bombings of Hiroshima and Nagasaki during World War II.

radio information services   Radio channels and programs that provide news and information on community events. Many services read sections or complete issues of local newspapers and offer information of interest to visually impaired listeners.

Radio services may be broadcast on open, freely accessible channels or on closed channels that require a reception box available to the user through the broadcasting station. State radio information services are often titled Radio Reading Service, Radio Talking Book, or Radio Information Service. (See Appendix for listing by state.) Local cable television stations may provide similar services.

Television descriptive services such as Descriptive Video Service (DVS) and Washington Ear provide narration describing various visual features of dramatic television programs. During the program, the narrator supplies details of the costuming, lighting and physical actions taking place. The service uses a separate channel accessible through an adapter that is compatible with standard television and video cassette recorders with stereo capabilities.

Contact:

Descriptive Video Service, WGBH-TV
125 Western Avenue
Boston, MA 02134
617-300-5400 (ph)
617-300-1026 (fax)
http:\\main.wgbh.org

The Metropolitan Washington Ear, Inc.
35 University Boulevard East
Silver Spring, MD 20901
301-681-6636 (ph)
301-681-5227 (fax)
www.washear.org

Rail Passenger Service Act The Rail Passenger Service Act, as amended by the Amtrak Improvement Act of 1973, founded the National Railroad Passenger corporation. The corporation must ensure that no elderly or disabled person is denied transit on any intercity passenger train operated in connection with the corporation.

The corporation was instructed to renovate existing facilities and equipment to make them accessible to elderly or disabled persons, to ensure that new facilities or equipment comply with accessibility standards, to provide special employee training dealing with traveling needs or concerns of the elderly and disabled, and to assist elderly and disabled passengers in the terminal and as they board and alight the trains.

Amtrak was instructed in 1990 to make access improvements at some stations that it shared with a commuter authority. Those instructions were a result of the Americans with Disabilities Act of 1990. They were noted in Amtrak's 1997 Reform and Accountability Act.

U.S. Department of Education. *Summary of Existing Legislation Affecting Persons with Disabilities.* Washington, D.C.: USDE, 1988.
Amtrak Reform Council. "The Amtrak Reform and Accountability Act of 1997." www.amtrakreform-council.gov, 1997.

Raised Dot Computing (RDC) See DUXBURY SYSTEMS, INC.

raised-line drawing kit A tactual aid used to make pictures or graphs. It consists of a board covered with a soft underlay of rubber. The user places a sheet of acetate over the board and draws on it, creating raised lines and an embossed picture.

Randolph-Sheppard Act The Randolph-Sheppard Act of 1938 established an employment-opportunities program in which blind individuals could operate vending facilities on federal property. Amendments to the act, legislated in 1974, extended its scope to include federal property operated by all federal agencies or departments and added operational guidelines to be authorized by state licensing agencies.

The act amendments outlined procedures and regulations to ensure fair treatment between blind vendors, the licensing agencies, and the federal government, and established greater control and participation by the Rehabilitation Services Administration. In cases in which vending machines directly compete with blind vendors, the amendments allowed the income from the machines to accrue to the vendor or to be used by the state licensing agency as a sick fund or vacation/retirement fund. (See BUSINESS ENTERPRISE PROGRAM.)

U.S. Department of Education. *Summary of Existing Legislation Affecting Persons with Disabilities.* Washington, D.C.: USDE, 1988.

reading machines Machines that "read" printed material aloud via a voice synthesizer. They are used by visually impaired and blind persons who are unable to read with magnification.

Most reading machines, such as the Kurzweil Reading Machine, employ a computer-controlled camera that scans the lines of print and recognizes words from its programmed computer memory. These machines can read textbooks, articles, and tests, as well as a user's own written work. The voice synthesizer says each word aloud. The user puts the text on the glass plate of the scanner and pushes buttons on a control panel to activate the voice synthesizer. On several models, the user can control the speed, volume, and pitch of voice and can direct the machine to repeat material or to read punctuation marks.

The Optacon is an optical-to-tactual converting reading machine. It translates print into letter configurations that are read with the fingertips. The user slides a camera across a line of print with the right hand. Simultaneously, the left hand feels the letter configuration formed on an array of vibrating pins. The user must be extensively trained to use the machine.

Recording for the Blind and Dyslexic   (RFB&D) A non-profit, national service organization that records and lends educational books free of cost to the blind and the physically or perceptually handicapped. Based in New Jersey, the organization maintains 32 recording studios across the United States and circulated 238,543 titles in 2000.

The organization was founded in 1948 by Anne T. MacDonald to provide books to blind World War II veterans completing their education on the GI Bill of Rights. The service has since expanded to make books available to anyone who is print handicapped (i.e., cannot read conventional printed material due to a visual, physical, or perceptual disability). Because an increasing number of people with learning disabilities were using the service, the name of the organization was changed in 1995 to Recording for the Blind and Dyslexic. It formerly was known as Recording for the Blind.

Over 91,000 people of all ages are served by the RFB&D. Although most are students, many are professional people seeking work-related materials; others are pursuing nonvocational interests or hobbies.

In order to request a text, a borrower must be registered with the RFB&D. Registrants complete an application that includes verification of a visual, physical or perceptual impairment by a medical or educational authority. The registered borrower may then request a text by telephone or mail. If the text has already been recorded, it is copied onto cassettes, checked for quality, and shipped to the borrower. If the book has not been recorded, the borrower sends two copies of the book to the RFB&D. The book is recorded and sent in installments as it is completed. When finished, the master tapes remain in the RFB&D library.

The RFB&D maintains a Master Library of over 83,000 educational manuscripts ranging from elementary to postgraduate levels. In 2000, 4,300 new titles were added, most as a result of borrowers' requests. Librarians also provide reference services and bibliographic searches drawing from a computerized data bank containing information from the Master Library and the National Library Service for the Blind and Physically Handicapped.

RFB&D has more than 5,700 volunteers. It is working to introduce digital audio technology to its members. Members will soon be able to access information on CD-ROM or on the Internet.

The RFB&D honors outstanding blind college seniors with annual Scholastic Achievement Awards. The awards are presented to those chosen for exceptional character and scholarship.

Contact:

RFB&D
20 Roszel Road
Princeton, NJ 08540
609-452-0606
www.rfbd.org

reduced rates   Reduced rates for telephone and transportation fares are frequently available to legally blind individuals. Legal blindness is a term describing visual conditions of either visual acuity of 20/200 or less in the better eye, after correction, or a visual field of 20 degrees or less in the better eye, regardless of visual acuity.

Verification of legal blindness by a doctor or ophthalmologist may in some cases be used to obtain reduced monthly service rates for touch-tone dialing and speed calling. Telebraille devices may be offered to those who are deaf/blind and can read braille. Those with low vision may be eligible to receive free 411 information or large-number overlays for the telephone dial.

Interstate bus lines and Amtrak offer reduced fares to legally blind individuals as do many city public transportation systems. Identification cards may be necessary to obtain the reduced fare and are often issued by the individual transportation agency. An identification card verifying legal blindness can also be obtained from the American Foundation for the Blind. (See FINANCIAL AID.)

refraction   A term used to describe the bending of light. The eye must refract light efficiently in order to see clearly.

When light falls on an object it is reflected to the eye. The light enters through the eye's CORNEA, a thin, transparent covering. The cornea bends or refracts the light and focuses it toward the inner sections of the eye.

The refracted light enters the PUPIL, a tiny hole in the center of the IRIS, the colored part of the eye. The light is then further refracted by the CRYSTALLINE LENS of the eye. The lens focuses the light onto the RETINA, a light-sensitive layer in the back of the eye. The retina transforms the light into electrical impulses or information about the light received. The impulses are sent to the brain by the OPTIC NERVE. The brain translates the impulses into an image. If there is any problem with the refracting or focusing of the light throughout this process, a distortion or blurring of the image will result.

refractive error   Refractive error, or ametropia, is an inability of the eye to focus properly. The CORNEA and the LENS of the eye focus light on the RETINA, which transforms the light into electrical impulses. The impulses are sent to the brain, where they are interpreted and presented as an image. If the cornea and the lens are unable to effectively focus the light onto the retina, a refractive error is present and blurred vision results.

The four most common refractive errors are MYOPIA (nearsightedness), HYPEROPIA (farsightedness), ASTIGMATISM (distorted image), and PRESBYOPIA (aging eyes). Refractive error is often caused by the length of the eye. An average eye is approximately 24 millimeters long. The lens and cornea are designed to work best with an eye this length. An eye that is longer or shorter than this length creates focusing problems. A longer-than-average eye is myopic, or nearsighted. A shorter-than-average eye is hyperopic, or farsighted.

An eye that is too curved or flat presents a distorted image and is termed *astigmatic.* The irregular shape causes the light to focus onto two different points, rather than the one focusing point of normal vision. Astigmatism may be present in myopic, hyperopic, or presbyopic eyes. A presbyopic eye is one in which the lens has lost its natural elasticity due to aging. The lens is unable to change shape to focus on near objects.

Refractive errors are easily detected in the routine eye examination. Contact lenses or eyeglasses may be prescribed to correct the error and allow the eyes to see clearly, or refractive surgery may be recommended. Although early diagnosis and treatment are encouraged because they produce clear vision, refraction errors are not worsened or improved by the use of corrective lenses or glasses.

refractive keratology   The first type of refractive surgery to reshape the cornea, refractive keratology has been widely replaced by photorefractive kera-

tectomy (PRK) and laser in situ keratomileusis (LASIK) surgeries.

Refractive keratology was developed mainly in Russia. During the procedure, doctors use a special scalpel to score the surface of the cornea in order to reshape it. This type of surgery is most successful for mild cases of astigmatism and nearsightedness. Treating more severe cases sometimes resulted in fluctuating vision, a persistent glare and starbursts.

REHABDATA   A bibliographic database of disability and rehabilitation literature produced by The National Rehabilitation Information Center (NARIC). It includes citations to research reports, scholarly papers, journal articles, audiovisual materials, and reference documents.

Each of the more than 50,000 entries in the computerized listing is described by one to five descriptor headings to assist the user in the information search. Each entry contains an abstract and 10 information fields describing the entry.

REHABDATA may be accessed through NARIC. NARIC accepts search requests by telephone, mail, TDD (telecommunication device for the deaf), electronic bulletin board, or in person. Search requests are usually processed within two working days. Or, the Internet can be used to reach NARIC's Instant Disability Information Center. That site contains five databases to facilitate your search. It can be accessed at www.naric.com/search.

Contact:

REHABDATA—NARIC
1010 Wayne Avenue, Suite 800
Silver Spring, MD 20910
800-346-2742 (ph)
301-495-5626 (TDD)
301-562-2401 (fax)
www.naric.com

rehabilitation   Rehabilitation services are programs that provide training or support to disabled individuals from federal, state, or private agencies. Rehabilitation may be offered through a public or private residential school, within a program of special education in a public school (through an organization for the blind), by a private rehabilitation facility (through correspondence courses) or by state rehabilitation agencies.

All 50 states administer programs of VOCATIONAL REHABILITATION and DAILY LIVING SKILLS for the purpose of enabling disabled individuals to become independent, employed, integrated members of society. These agencies are listed under various names, such as Department of Rehabilitation, Commission for the Visually Handicapped, State Services for the Blind and Visually Impaired, and the Bureau of the Blind.

Each state program varies according to the range of services and training available and the amount of financial assistance provided. Services may include medical and vocational diagnostic services, physical restoration, home-management skills training, orientation and mobility instruction, braille instruction, communication-skills training, personal-management skills instruction, books and training supplies, transportation allowance, reader services for the blind, vocational rehabilitation, job-placement services, postemployment services, procurement of job-related equipment and occupational licenses, adaptive aids evaluation and selection, counseling, and family-member services.

Legally blind individuals may qualify for state rehabilitation services if they can provide certification of disability and if the state has a reasonable expectation that such individuals will benefit from receiving the services. Vocational rehabilitation services are provided if the disability results in a substantial handicap to employment and if the state has a reasonable expectation that the recipient will get or hold a job as a result of vocational training.

Rehabilitation services are available at little or no cost to the individual. Some aspects of the rehabilitation program may require financial contribution by the individual. In some states, services such as psychological counseling, equipment purchase, and transportation to school or school tuition may be financed by the state or a combination of the state, the individual, and grants or loans.

In all state programs, each individual's case is carefully evaluated by a rehabilitation counselor for the blind and/or a vocational rehabilitation counselor for the blind with input from the disabled person. Everyone eligible is given an individualized written plan that outlines the rehabilitation goals, the individual's skills and needs, and the process by which those needs will be met.

The plan may provide for a medical examination to ascertain the extent and limitations of the disability in order to assess suitable employment possibilities. Medical treatment or equipment, including surgery, psychiatric counseling, hospital services, prostheses, and eyeglasses, may be provided to reduce or alleviate the disability and improve productivity on the job.

Guidance counseling may be suggested to assess the individual's potential for rehabilitation, independent living, and appropriate employment. Job training may be provided at home, rehabilitation centers, trade schools, or on-the-job settings. Educational tuition and expenses may be supplied if college is necessary to the vocational rehabilitation. The plan may furnish financial assistance during the rehabilitation process.

Rehabilitation services may be provided by social workers, occupational therapists, therapeutic recreation workers, vocational rehabilitation counselors, rehabilitation counselors, or orientation and mobility teachers.

Rehabilitation counselors or teachers are college-trained specialists who provide daily living skills training as well as communication-skills, recreational-skills, and low-vision aids training.

Daily living skills, also known as independent-living skills, concern personal and home management and are frequently taught in the home or in a rehabilitation facility. They include methods for grooming and self-care, dressing, eating, precane mobility, handling and identifying money, personal recordkeeping, labeling food and clothing, cooking, laundering, safety skills, household cleaning, sewing, and home repair.

Communication skills may include listening skills, handwriting, typing, telephoning, braille, procurement of large-print or recorded materials, and personal communication or nonverbal-communication skills instruction.

Recreational-skills training includes instruction in leisure activities and exposure to adaptive games, crafts, and hobbies. The availability of support groups, sports groups, and other social activities may be explored.

Low-vision evaluation is provided by an oph-thalmologist or optometrist who recommends specific aids and often provides training. Rehabilitation teachers can provide training in the use of other nonprescriptive adaptive low-vision aids and appliances such as bold-line writing paper, talking clocks, or glare-free lighting.

Orientation and mobility teachers are college-trained specialists who provide instruction that allows the visually impaired individual to move safely and efficiently in the environment. Skills provided in the instruction include auditory skills, tactual skills, olfactory skills, kinesthetic awareness, perpendicular and parallel alignment, search patterns, recovery skills, use of reference points, soliciting assistance, time and distance estimation, sighted-guide technique, protective techniques, trailing, and use of the long cane and electronic travel aids.

Vocational rehabilitation enables the visually impaired individual to continue employment or train for new work. Vocational training may be offered by the state rehabilitation agency, a rehabilitation facility, a residential or public school, an organization for the blind, or a sheltered workshop.

College-trained vocational rehabilitation specialists work with individual to evaluate existing skills and aptitudes, evaluate and recommend occupations, outline needed skills, provide vocational skills training and education, and recommend and provide training of vocational aids or devices.

Vocational-rehabilitation training may result in employment in the mainstream of industry, employment in a business enterprise program (BEP), a vending, short order, or cafeteria-style stand business program supported by the federal funds, or employment in a sheltered workshop. The individual may also be employed at home as a homemaker and family-care provider.

The success of rehabilitation training varies by individual. The extent of the visual loss, the time in life when the loss occurred and the abilities and aptitude of the individual all affect the outcome. The length of time for rehabilitation services also differs and may continue six months or longer.

American Foundation for the Blind. *Rehabilitation Services.* New York: AFB, 1988.

California Department of Rehabilitation. *Client Information Booklet.* Sacramento, California: CDR, 1987.

California Department of Rehabilitation. *Rehabilitation is Here to Help.* Sacramento, California: CDR, 1986.

Lions Clubs International. *Rehabilitation of the Blind.* Oak Brook, Illinois: LCI, 1984.

National Association for Visually Handicapped. *The Adult Partially Seeing.* New York: NAVH, 1984.

Rehabilitation Act   The Rehabilitation Act was created in 1954 to replace the outdated National Vocational Rehabilitation Act of 1920, which first established the national system of state vocational-rehabilitation agencies. The act was rewritten in 1973 to include emphasis on service to individuals with severe disabilities. It was amended in 1992 in order to revise and extend the programs approved in 1973, and again in 1998.

The 1973 amendments prohibited discrimination on the basis of physical or mental disability in all areas of life affected by the federal government. They stated that no otherwise qualified disabled person could be discriminated against, or excluded from participating in or gaining benefits from any activity or program that receives federal financial support.

The 1973 law established federal funding of nearly $1.5 billion to support training and placing individuals with mental and physical disabilities into full- or part-time employment in the competitive labor market. The act put into effect a variety of services, demonstration programs, training and research grant programs, and a federal-state grant-in-aid program.

The act provides basic federal-state vocational grants that support state vocational-rehabilitation agencies, client-assistant programs (CAP) to inform and advise rehabilitation clients and other disabled persons, innovation and expansion grants that expand state vocational-rehabilitation services to those with severe disabilities, American Indian vocational-rehabilitation services, research and training grants, construction loans and grants for rehabilitation facilities, and grants to public and nonprofit organizations for vocational training services for disabled persons.

The act further supports special projects and supplementary services including severely disabled projects, disabled youth job-training programs and reader and interpreter services. The act establishes the National Council of the Handicapped, which reviews all federal statutes pertaining to those with disabilities and recommends legislative proposals to Congress and the president.

Employment opportunities projects are supported by the act through programs such as Projects with Industry and other public/private ventures that offer training or employment services to disabled individuals.

The act provides formula grants for vocational-rehabilitation agencies to support independent-living services and centers for independent living. It supplies independent-living services for visually impaired persons who are over age 55 and unemployable.

The Rehabilitation Act specifically addresses the hiring and employment of the disabled. Section 501 of the act prohibits discrimination in employment of qualified disabled persons by federal agencies. It instructs federal agencies to establish goals for hiring employees with severe disabilities, to recruit such individuals, and to encourage equal opportunity in career development and advancement.

Disabled federal employees and those applying for federal jobs are protected from arbitrary dismissal and other actions based on disability. The section states that disabled employees may qualify for reasonable accommodation, including aids and personnel that will enable them to perform their jobs.

Section 503 of the act mandates affirmative action by private organizations that do contract work for federal agencies and further supports reasonable accommodations.

Section 504 of the act requires federal agencies and private and public organizations that receive federal funds to make facilities, programs, and activities accessible to disabled employees. Company rest rooms, libraries, cafeterias, and other public areas must be accessible.

Among the changes to the act in 1992 was the addition of the electronic and information technology accessibility guidelines, which are meant to assure that people with disabilities will have equal access to electronic and information technology within federal agencies. The 1998 amendments require each state to establish a state rehabilitation council in order to receive federal funding in this area.

A state that sets up an agency to handle funding for vocational rehabilitation services provided for blind people may still, under the 1998 amendments, establish a separate state rehabilitation council. The latest amendments also strengthen the electronic and information technology guidelines that were approved in 1992.

U.S. Department of Education. *Summary of Existing Legislation Affecting Persons with Disabilities.* Washington, D.C.: USDE, 1988.

rehabilitation center A facility that provides rehabilitation services to persons with disabilities. Rehabilitation services may include medical, psychological, social, and vocational services. The program is designed to offer reeducation and restoration of the disabled individual to the greatest physical, social and economic level possible. Rehabilitation centers may be supported through federal, state, local, or private funding.

Programs offered may include testing, fitting, or training in the use of prosthetic and orthotic devices; prevocational or recreational therapy; physical and occupational therapy; speech and hearing therapy; psychological and social services; personal and work-adjustment counseling; vocational training; evaluation for control of a specific disability; orientation and mobility services for the blind; additional adjustment services for the blind; and employment for those with disabilities who cannot be readily absorbed into the competitive labor market.

rehabilitation engineering center Rehabilitation engineering centers were first established in 1972 as facilities to develop ways to apply advanced technology in medical, scientific, psychological, and social areas for solving rehabilitation and environmental problems of disabled persons.

There are 15 rehabilitation engineering centers in the United States. Each works within a core area of research specialty.

The Smith-Kettlewell Institute of Visual Sciences, located in San Francisco, is the center devoted to the visual sciences. The center designs and modifies sensory aids for the blind and offers rehabilitation engineering services through collaboration with the Pacific Presbyterian Medical Center's low-vision services. (See SMITH-KETTLEWELL EYE RESEARCH INSTITUTE.)

residential schools   The residential-school model is one of five major educational models or plans for instruction of visually impaired students. The others are the TEACHER-CONSULTANT model, ITINERANT-TEACHER model, SELF-CONTAINED CLASSROOM model, and RESOURCE ROOM model.

Residential schools are those in which visually impaired students live and receive educational instruction. It is the oldest form of education for the visually impaired and is offered in nearly every state. Many residential schools for the visually impaired share a campus or facilities with schools for the deaf and are referred to as "dual" schools.

Residential schools may be either state operated or private. State-operated residential schools are funded by state legislatures and provide free tuition, room, board, and transportation. Private residential schools charge fees that may be paid by the public school district of the student.

The campuses, schoolrooms, and educational programs of residential schools are designed and equipped to meet the needs of visually impaired students. The educational materials and curricula can be designed, or the students may be grouped, to meet an individual's instructional requirements.

Trained staff, including houseparents, are on duty 24 hours a day to provide general curriculum instruction, academic remediation, compensatory-learning-skills instruction, personal management and independence-skills training, and information counseling.

The residential-school model is superior to many other models in its attempts to meet all levels of student educational needs as they arise. However, because students may return home only weekly or monthly, some students may suffer from a lack of familial contact or interaction with sighted peers.

Barraga, Natalie C. *Visual Handicaps and Learning.* Belmont, California: Wadsworth Publishing Company, Inc., 1976.

Scholl, Geraldine, ed. *Foundations of Education for Blind and Visually Handicapped Children and Youth.* New York: American Foundation for the Blind, 1986.

resource room   The resource-room model is one of five educational models or plans for the instruction of visually impaired students. The others are the ITINERANT-TEACHER model, TEACHER-CONSULTANT model, SELF-CONTAINED CLASSROOM model, and the RESIDENTIAL SCHOOL MODEL.

The resource room is a specially equipped room staffed with special education personnel trained to work with blind or visually impaired students. The students live at home and attend public school in regular classrooms taught by teachers who provide general curriculum instruction. Students visit the resource room at regularly scheduled intervals or when needed.

The resource-room teacher provides specialized skills instruction and information counseling relating to vision loss and academic remediation. Special instruction may take place individually or in small groups.

The resource room model has an advantage over the teacher-consultant and itinerant-teacher models in that it provides instruction or assistance immediately and according to the needs of the student. However, because of its availability, it may foster dependence and restrict growth toward independent working within a self-contained classroom.

Barraga, Natalie C. *Visual Handicaps and Learning.* Belmont, California: Wadsworth Publishing Company, Inc., 1976.

Scholl, Geraldine, ed. *Foundations of Education for Blind and Visually Handicapped Children and Youth.* New York: American Foundation for the Blind, 1986.

retina   The light-sensitive nerve layer in the back of the eye that lies between the VITREOUS and the CHOROID. It is an information-gathering and processing portion of the eye and is necessary for sight.

As light is reflected from an object, it passes through the LENS and is focused on the retina. Light-sensitive RODS AND CONES collect this light information. The cones, which are responsible for central vision and color, are found throughout the retina but are most concentrated in a depression called the MACULA, the place of sharpest vision. Within the macula is the FOVEA, a central indentation packed with cones. The rods, which are responsible for night vision, are scattered throughout the retina.

The retina transforms the information gathered by the rods and cones into electrical impulses, which it sends through the OPTIC NERVE to the brain. The brain translates the impulses into an image.

The retina is subject to many serious conditions that cause *retinopathy,* any change in the retina due to a disease or inflammation. RETINITIS is any condition in which the retina becomes inflamed. Retinitis is often linked to the choroid, the layer that underlies the retina and that provides blood to the eye. Any inflammation of the choroid may spread to the retina to become CHORIORETINITIS.

Chorioretinitis may be caused by toxoplasmosis, a parasitic infection carried by cats, toxocariasis, an infection in dog feces, congenital syphilis, or other systemic diseases. The condition results in inflammatory lesions. Lesions near the macula result in central-vision loss.

Since the optic nerve joins the eye at the retina, conditions of the optic nerve often affect the retina. PAPILLEDEMA is a swelling of the OPTIC DISC, the place where the optic nerve and the retina meet. The condition may block ocular venous circulation and can result from a rise of intracranial pressure.

Retinal degeneration is any condition in which the retina is reduced to a lesser state of effectiveness. Macular degenerative disease may be caused by heredity, systemic disease, drugs, infections, and aging. Age-related maculopathy (ARM) is a condition of senility in which the Bruch's membrane tends to thicken, neovascularization takes place and central vision is lost.

Angioid streaks are dark brown streaks on the retina near the optic disc. They are caused by changes in the Bruch's membrane and are associated with degeneration of the elastic tissue. Myopic individuals may experience myopic chorioretinal degeneration.

RETINITIS PIGMENTOSA is a misnomer for a degenerative disease that involves no inflammation. The inherited condition involves the progressive degeneration of the retina's rods and cones. The rods are first affected, producing the symptoms of night blindness and limited peripheral field. In later years, the central field may be affected.

Often, progressive loss of vision due to vascular disorders of aging are termed retinal degeneration, as well. Vascular disorders include ARTERIOSCLEROSIS, a narrowing or blocking of the arteries associated with hypertension and heart disease. Arteriosclerosis may block retinal arteries and impair venous return, which may trigger neovascularization (formation of new, weak blood vessels), hemorrhaging and result in vision loss.

Hypertensive retinopathy is related to, and includes, arteriosclerosis, and also contains conditions of edema, exudates, and hemorrhaging. Severe damage may cause loss of vision.

DIABETIC RETINOPATHY, a leading cause of vision loss, is a condition of diabetes in that the retinal blood vessels form aneurysms which swell and hemorrhage. Neovascularization, hemorrhaging, and scarring occur, which may cause retinal detachment and loss of vision.

ARTERIAL OCCLUSIONS are obstructions of the central retinal artery that block blood from reaching the retina. Retinal tissue is damaged due to lack of oxygen, and sight is lost. Obstructions to retinal veins cause hemorrhaging, retinal edema, and vision loss.

SICKLE CELL RETINOPATHY is an inherited disease in which sickle-shaped hemoglobin cells replace rounded red hemoglobin cells. The sickle-shaped cells block the flow of blood, which leads to oxygen deprivation and vascular occlusions of the retina.

RETINOPATHY OF PREMATURITY is a disease of premature infants in which the proliferation of retinal vessels may lead to hemorrhage. The resulting scar tissue causes a vision loss due to RETINAL DETACHMENT, a condition difficult to repair.

Retinal dystrophy is any condition or disease that destroys or damages the tissue of the retina. Common dystrophies include juvenile retinoschisis, a dystrophy of the fovea, Stargardt's disease, a hereditary disease of the central retina, Best's disease, a condition characterized by elevated macular regions, and cone dystrophy, in which color and central vision are progressively destroyed.

Retinal detachments occur when the retina becomes separated from its underlying epithelium and choroid. They may be caused by holes or tears, fluid leakage, or traction. These conditions are caused by injuries, infections, other ocular conditions or disorders, and systemic diseases.

Retinal detachments cause sudden loss of sight that is often permanent. Some detachments can be prevented and corrected by cryotherapy, a surgical procedure performed using a super-cooled cryoprobe.

TUMORS of the retina may be malignant or benign and include retinoblastoma, a hereditary tumor of childhood. This serious growth spreads quickly and may metastasize along the optic nerve to the brain. Tumors may necessitate removal of the affected eye or cause retinal detachments.

retinal degeneration   See RETINA.

retinal detachment   A retinal detachment occurs whenever the RETINA is disconnected from the back layers of the eye. It is a serious condition that may require immediate medical treatment.

The retina is the light-sensitive portion of the back of the eye that receives and encodes information about an object into electrical impulses. It sends the impulses through the OPTIC NERVE to the brain. The brain then translates the impulses into an image.

The retina, the pigment epithelium and the CHOROID are located between the VITREOUS gel and the outer SCLERA of the eye. The retina normally adheres closely to the pigment epithelium and is supported by the vitreous gel. When the retina detaches or separates from the epithelial layer, a retinal detachment occurs.

Retinal detachments are caused by tears or holes in the retina, fluid leakage, or traction. When the retina becomes disturbed, as from a tear or hole resulting from an injury, space may open up between the retina and the epithelium. Fluid from the vitreous may leak into the space, causing a further retraction or a detachment.

The vitreous may experience hemorrhaging from vessels damaged by diabetes or injury. Inflammation may develop and vitreous membranes may form as a result of the hemorrhaging. As the vitreous membranes contract, they may cause detachment of the retina. This contraction is known as traction.

Vitreous detachment can cause retinal holes or tears. In this condition, the vitreous leaves its normal position against the retina and falls to the anterior cavity of the eye. A hole or tear may form as the vitreous collapses from its position.

Rhegmatogenous detachments, or those associated with holes, are most often related to eye injuries, trauma to the eye or head, aging, nearsightedness, degenerative eye conditions, retinal degeneration, and vitreous detachment. Some people are prone to retinal detachment due to hereditary conditions such as Stickler's syndrome and Wagner's disease.

Additionally, CATARACT surgery may be a leading factor in rhegmatogenous detachments. According to the National Institute of Health, detachments ensue in one of every 50 cataract operations. Non-rhegmatogenous detachments are associated with diabetes, diabetic retinopathy, and retinopathy of prematurity.

The most common symptom of retinal detachment is a sudden loss of sight in either the central or peripheral field. It is often described as a curtain or shadow cast on the field of vision. Symptoms may also include flashes of light or the appearance of floaters, spots that seem to float across the visual field. Floaters are bits of debris or blood in the vitreous that cast shadows on the retina. These shadows appear as the floating spots.

Treatment of retinal detachments may be preventative or reactive. Prevention involves the correction of tears and holes that have not yet caused a detachment, or the treatment of an area of the retina that has degenerated. This type of treatment may be considered before cataract surgery. Since holes or tears do not always result in retinal detachments, this procedure is considered controversial. Each case is decided individually, according to the risk of possible future detachment.

Surgery is needed to treat existing detachments. In most cases, the surgeon forms a scar on the hole or tear by thermal or cryotherapy (freezing treatments) methods. The thermal method, called surgical diathermy, utilizes a needle transmitting high-frequency electrical current. The needle is touched to the sclera and the resulting heat stimulates scar tissue formation.

In cryotherapy or CRYOSURGERY, a cryoprobe, an instrument with a tip cooled to between 30 and 70 degrees below freezing, is touched to the sclera. The sclera remains unaffected, but the retina and underlying choroid are frozen and stimulated to form adhering scar tissue. After the scar tissue has been stimulated, a hypodermic needle is then inserted through the sclera to drain any accumulated fluid under the retina. The surgeon may then make an indentation in the back of the eye and place a silicone buckle or belt around the eye to indent the sclera inward and help reattach the retina.

The surgery requires an incision but is performed underneath the membrane that covers the sclera. The inside of the eye is seldom breached. The buckle remains permanently in the eye but is not seen or felt.

The surgery is performed in the hospital or occasionally in an outpatient setting. It may last from one to several hours and may require a brief stay of up to six days in the hospital. Postsurgical eye drops may be prescribed, and the patient is advised to avoid heavy lifting and strenuous activity.

Surgery to correct retinal detachment is highly successful. According to the National Institute of Health, the success rate varies from 85 percent to 90 percent.

retinal dystrophy   See RETINA.

retinal edema   A condition in which the capillaries of the RETINA bleed, filling the spaces between retinal cells with fluid. Retinal edema may be present throughout the retina or it may be contained in a general area.

If the MACULA, the central indentation of the retina and section of sharpest sight, is spared, vision may be relatively unaffected at first. However, the macula tends to accumulate the fluid. In this case, MACULAR EDEMA occurs. The condition is characterized by inflammation of the macula and blurred or impaired vision. If untreated, macular edema may develop into cystoid degeneration, and central vision may be permanently lost.

Retinal edema is caused by DIABETES, hypertension, retinal vein obstruction, traction of the vitreous, inflammations such as UVEITIS and RETINITIS and CATARACT surgery.

Retinal edema is diagnosed with FLUORESCEIN ANGIOGRAPHY, a procedure in which fluorescein dye is injected into a vein in the arm and monitored as it passes through the veins of the retina.

Retinal edema may resolve spontaneously or persist. Persistent cases may cause permanent vision loss. Treatment of the condition varies according to the cause. Cases due to inflammation are treated with corticosteroids. Those conditions of edema caused by vascular problems and diabetes may be treated with photocoagulation, a treatment that uses a laser to seal leaking blood vessels. There is no treatment for edema due to traction or cataract surgery.

retinitis   See RETINA.

retinitis pigmentosa   (RP)   A group of inherited diseases that causes degeneration of the eye's retina. The disease affects 100,000 Americans, and approximately one in 80 persons carries the recessive gene for RP. There are approximately 1,560 new cases of RP diagnosed each year, or an average incidence of 6/1,000,000. RP and related retinal degenerative diseases, including USHER'S SYNDROME and other rare syndromes, affect 400,000 Americans and 4 million people worldwide.

Although the disease name includes "itis," no infection or inflammation is associated with these diseases. Retinitis pigmentosa is characterized by a degeneration of the RODS AND CONES of the retina.

The retina of the eye receives the reflected light from an object. The light-sensitive rods and cones translate the light into electrical impulses that the retina sends to the brain through the OPTIC NERVE. The brain changes the impulses into an image. The rods of the retina function in dim light. They are responsible for detecting movement and shape. Scattered throughout the retina, they are accountable for peripheral vision. The cones, which discern detail and color, require brighter light to work effectively. They are packed into the central part of the retina, the MACULA, and are responsible for central vision.

Retinitis pigmentosa first affects the rods. As the rods are destroyed, vision in low light is decreased, and peripheral vision constricts. As the disease progresses, the cones are affected, and central vision is lost.

Retinitis pigmentosa is hereditary but rarely may accompany other diseases. When accompanied by a serious hearing loss, the disorder is termed Usher's syndrome. There are several types of RP. They include:

- Congenital RP, or Leber's congenital amaurosis, is apparent at birth or in infancy. This rare disease causes a steady, progressive loss of sight.

- Recessive RP is passed to the child of two individuals who carry the gene for RP but who may not have RP. There is a 25 percent chance that a child (male or female) of two carriers will have RP.

- Dominant RP is passed to the child of one affected parent and one unaffected parent. With each pregnancy, there is a 50 percent chance that each child (both male and female) will inherit the disease. Unaffected children usually will not pass on the disease to their children. Three genes thought to cause dominant RP have been discovered.

- Sex-linked RP is passed to a child by the mother, who is the carrier. Sons of a female carrier of sex-linked RP and an unaffected male have a 50 percent chance of having RP. Daughters of such a pairing have a 50 percent chance of being carriers but will not inherit the disease.

The genetic cause and inheritance pattern for sporadic RP is unknown. Research is being conducted to investigate new mutations as they appear with each new generation.

The most common symptom of RP is night blindness or difficulty seeing in dim light. There may be a progressive loss of peripheral or side vision, which results in tunnel vision. As the disease progresses, the individual may experience a loss of central vision. Many individuals may develop CATARACTS, or opaque sections on the LENS of the eye. Some individuals may experience complete blindness as a result of RP, although most will retain some limited vision.

In most types of RP, the onset is during childhood or early adolescence. Congenital, recessive and disease-related types of the disease tend to be more severe than dominant RP. Sporadic RP varies in severity with the individual.

Retinitis pigmentosa is not easily diagnosed. Often during the ophthalmologic exam, a change in the appearance of the retina may indicate RP. However, other tests, such as an electroretinogram, may be necessary to confirm the diagnosis.

An electroretinogram, or ERG, measures the electrical activity of the retina when exposed to light stimulus. Drops are first placed in the eyes to dilate the PUPILS. Anesthetic drops are administered to the eye just before a contact lens attached to electrodes is placed on the CORNEA of the eye. The electrodes record the responses of the retina as lights are flashed in both dark and light environmental conditions.

There is no cure or treatment for retinitis pigmentosa. Vitamin-A therapy, topical treatment with DMSO, and light deprivation have been investigated as cures with disappointing results. Research is continuing in the areas of retinal cell transplantation, gene therapy, pharmaceutical therapy, and nutritional therapy. These areas of research are thought to be very promising for victims of RP.

Low-vision aids such as the NIGHT VISION AID, prescriptive glasses, telescopes, large print, or closed circuit television may be helpful. Genetic counseling may alert families to some types of hereditary RP.

Finkelstein, Daniel. "Blindness and Disorders of the Eye." *The Braille Monitor* (December 1988): 578–579.

The Foundation for Fighting Blindness. "Frequently Asked Questions Regarding Retinitis Pigmentosa." www.blindness.org, 2000.

Pagon, Roberta A. "Retinitis Pigmentosa." *Survey of Ophthalmology*, 33, no. 3 (November–December 1988): 137–168.

Reynolds, James D. "Retinitis Pigmentosa," HealthNet Library. Columbus: CompuServe, 1989.

retinoblastoma   A malignant eye tumor that originates in the retina. It is the most common childhood ocular tumor and may be the most common congenital tumor of any kind.

Retinoblastoma may be either hereditary or sporadic. According to the U.S. Department of Health and Human Services, up to 40 percent of cases are hereditary. The hereditary type is usually present at birth and most frequently appears at approximately one year of age. It often affects both eyes. Children of families with a history of retinoblastoma should be examined regularly for tumors. Even without prior family history of retinoblastoma, all bilateral retinoblastoma tumors should be considered hereditary and capable of being passed to future generations.

The more common sporadic type of retinoblastoma is not hereditary. It usually affects one eye only and appears at approximately two years of age. All forms of the disease are evident by age five in almost all cases.

Symptoms of retinoblastoma may include redness, pain, and inflammation in the early stages. Once the tumor has grown larger, the eyes may cross or the PUPIL may change from black to white or gray. This change in pupil color, called leukokoria, is the actual appearance of the tumor itself, visible through the hole of the pupil.

Once the tumor has been diagnosed, treatment must be given immediately. Both types of retinoblastoma are life threatening and can grow and spread rapidly up the OPTIC NERVE to the brain.

Sometimes, the affected eye is enucleated, or removed. In the case of bilateral retinoblastoma, the more seriously affected eye may be enucleated and the less affected eye given radiation or chemotherapy treatments.

Retinoblastoma is caused by the absence of paired retinoblastoma genes on the 13th chromosome. This can occur from heredity and/or environmental causes. Although retinoblastoma has one of the highest rates of spontaneous regression among all tumors, the cause of regression is unknown.

retinopathy of prematurity (ROP)   A condition that appears soon after birth, generally in premature infants, in which abnormal blood vessels develop in the retina. This condition may progress to a retinal detachment that may cause blindness.

Although the precise cause of ROP is unknown, it is a result of prematurity, with very low birth weight (less than 1,000 grams) as the major factor. These premature infants may develop an overabundance of blood vessels in the retina. This may resolve spontaneously or may result in hemorrhages and the development of fibrous tissue or scar tissue. High MYOPIA, UVEITIS, GLAUCOMA, AMBLYOPIA, STRABISMUS, and RETINAL DETACHMENT may follow as secondary conditions. Total blindness may result.

In approximately 80 percent of retinopathy of prematurity, the retinal vessels heal themselves within the first year of the child's life. Approximately 15 percent of the remainder of cases progress to mild or modest ROP. The remaining 5 percent of cases develop severe ROP with retinal detachment and other secondary conditions.

Treatment of ROP has recently included CRYOSURGERY, or freezing therapy. In cryosurgery, proliferative retinal vessels are sealed with a cryoprobe, an instrument with a tip cooled to between 30 and 70 degrees below freezing. This therapy has shown good results and, if the ROP is severe, has proven to be the most effective treatment. If retinal detachment occurs, it is difficult to treat, resulting in only 30 percent to 50 percent success rates.

Historically, ROP was called RETROLENTAL FIBROPLASIA and thought to be caused by an overabundance of oxygen used in the incubators of premature infants. Modern, well-managed neonatal intensive care units for premature infants monitor oxygen, electrolytes, vitamins, and nutrition, carefully maintaining each at the best level for normal growth and development. Despite these efforts, ROP may be unavoidable for very low birth weight premature infants.

retinoscope   An instrument used during the eye examination for determining the refractive power of the eye. The examiner shines the light of the retinoscope onto the eye from an arm's distance away.

As the light moves across the PUPIL, the speed and direction of the lights and shadows are evaluated and recorded. This data indicates to the examiner the refractive power of the eye and is used to determine nearsightedness, farsightedness, or astigmatism.

retrobulbar neuritis   A form of optic neuritis, or swelling of the OPTIC NERVE associated with MULTIPLE SCLEROSIS. Retrobulbar neuritis is commonly seen among younger patients with multiple sclerosis and is often a first symptom of the disease.

Symptoms of retrobulbar neuritis include sudden loss of vision in one eye accompanied by pain associated with eye movement. Blind spots, or scotomas, may appear within the field of vision as well as color blindness and difficulty seeing in bright light. Vision may be affected in the entire field or may begin in the center of the field and progress to peripheral fields. Retrobulbar neuritis also can be caused by a neurological lesion, and is not necessarily a symptom of multiple sclerosis.

The condition may be treated with the drug ACTH and oral steroids. Although recurrence is possible, the prognosis for remission is good. Patients usually recover partial or full vision within three months.

retrolental fibroplasia (RLF)   The historical term for a disorder responsible for an epidemic of blindness during the 1940s and 1950s. During this period, it was the most common cause of visual impairment in children.

The condition appeared in conjunction with the widespread use of infant incubators. Premature infants or those in respiratory distress were placed into incubators supplied with 100 percent oxygen. The high levels of oxygen caused the retinal arteries and veins of the eyes to constrict. Once the infants were removed from the incubator and breathed normal air, the arteries and veins expanded and proliferated causing hemorrhages and the development of fibrous tissue or scar tissue.

The scar tissue blocked light from reaching the photosensitive RODS AND CONES of the RETINA and resulted in partial or total blindness. Secondary disorders, including RETINAL DETACHMENT, GLAUCOMA, UVEITIS, CATARACT, MYOPIA, and STRABISMUS sometimes followed within months or years.

The epidemic of retrolental fibroplasia reached its peak in 1952, and by 1954 the link between high concentrations of oxygen and retrolental fibroplasia was accepted and medical practices were altered. The blood level of infants is now monitored carefully, and oxygen is used only in amounts sufficient to prevent brain damage or death.

RLF is sometimes confused with RETINOPATHY OF PREMATURITY (ROP), an eye disorder that occurs in premature infants of very low birth weight. Using the terms synonymously is not correct because it implies that ROP is caused by an overabundance of oxygen. In the current epidemic of ROP, oxygen use is not considered to be the cause.

Most of those who developed RLF are now adult and blind. Their condition affected the education system, since the majority of these children entered school during a short span of time. Demands for MAINSTREAMING in education by the parents of RLF children forced public school systems to develop programs that exist today for all disabled children.

river blindness   See ONCHOCERCIASIS.

rods and cones   The photoreceptor cells within the RETINA of the eye. They provide information to the eye about the object in view.

When light falls on an object, the reflected light is focused by the eye's CORNEA and CRYSTALLINE LENS onto the retina, an inner layer in the back of the eye. Rods and cones within the retina provide information about the shape, color, and detail of the object. The retina transforms this information into electric impulses that it sends to the brain via the OPTIC NERVE. The brain translates the impulses into an image.

The retina contains over 125 million rods and cones. The rods outnumber the cones by a margin of nearly five to one. They are scattered throughout the retina and are responsible for peripheral, or side, vision. The rods react to faint light, darkness, shape and movement. Because the rods do not require high levels of light to function, they enable the eye to see at night.

The cones distinguish detail and color. Each cone contains visual pigments that are sensitive to one of the three primary color light wavelengths. One group of cones recognizes green, one red, and one blue. By blending the colors together in different combinations, the eye is able to see a spectrum of hues.

Unlike the rods, the cones require high levels of light to operate. Because of the need for light, they are concentrated into a central area of the retina called the MACULA.

The cornea and lens of the eye focus the incoming light onto the macula. In the center of the macula is an indentation called the FOVEA. The fovea is packed with cones and is the point of clearest, most distinct vision. Because of their location, the cones are responsible for central, or straight-ahead vision.

Diseases or disorders of the retina and hereditary factors may affect or destroy the rods and cones. RETINITIS PIGMENTOSA (RP) is a group of diseases that attack the retina and cause the degeneration of the rods and cones.

RP first affects the rods. As they are destroyed, night vision deteriorates and peripheral vision is lost. As the disease progresses, increasing tunnel vision occurs. Finally, the cones are destroyed, and central vision is affected.

Color blindness affects the cones only. Anopic cones lack the visual pigment that reacts to a certain band of color. Anomalous cones contain faulty visual pigment that fails to react, or reacts incorrectly, to its corresponding color. Both conditions result in the inability to see some color.

rubella   Rubella, or German measles, is known to cause blindness when contracted in utero during the first three months of pregnancy. Although the mother may feel little discomfort, the disease may cause vision impairment, mental retardation, hearing impairment, heart defects, and respiratory problems.

Ocular disturbances may include congenital CATARACT, GLAUCOMA, IRIS, or retinal disorders or defects and undersized eyes. Cataracts may be bilateral or unilateral and may develop slowly or appear severe at birth. Severe cataracts may be removed, but the patient often requires removal of the posterior capsule at a later date. Those with congenital cataracts often develop AMBLYOPIA, dysfunction of one eye due to disuse.

Runyan, Marla   The first legally blind person ever to qualify for the U.S. Olympic team and a finalist in the 1,500 meters event at the 2000 games in Sydney. Runyan also broke the U.S. indoor record in the 5,000 meters category in February 2001.

Legally blind since the age of nine due to STARGARDT'S DISEASE, Runyan played soccer as a child but switched to track and field at age 14. She competed in the high jump by placing reflective tape on the bar, and learned to jump hurdles by counting the number of steps between jumps.

Born in Santa Maria, California, in 1969, Runyan graduated with honors from San Diego State University in 1991 with a degree in education of the deaf. She earned a master's degree in education of deaf-blind children from the same school, and works teaching handicapped children in Eugene, Oregon.

She was quoted as saying, "I think what I represent is achieving what you want in life. It's a matter of attitude. Some people have a negative attitude, and that's their disability." Runyan has been featured on numerous television sports and news shows, as well as in various publications.

sarcoidosis A systemic disease whose symptoms resemble those of tuberculosis. The disease is characterized by nodules in the skin and lymph nodes and fibrosis of the lungs. The disease most often affects young adults and produces ocular disorders in roughly half the cases.

Sarcoidosis causes posterior and anterior UVEITIS, an inflammation of the uveal tract, the pigmented portions of the eye including the CHOROID, the IRIS, and the CILIARY BODY. Prolonged uveitis may lead to secondary GLAUCOMA, CATARACT, MACULAR EDEMA or SCARRING, and loss of vision. Uveitis is treated with local and systemic STEROIDS.

Sarcoidosis, which often produces no symptoms, is diagnosed with a Mantoux test, biopsy of the nodules, X rays, and blood tests. There is no cure for sarcoidosis.

Schirmer's test An ocular test used to determine the amount of moisture or tear production in the eye. The test is often conducted as a part of a routine eye examination or in response to patient complaint of dry eye.

The Schirmer's test is painless and involves the placement of one folded end of a thin strip of filter paper into the lower eyelid. The uninserted end of the strip projects forward, out of the eye. The strip is left in place for one to five minutes during which time the tears of the eye wet the strip.

A measurement is taken of the amount of moisture accumulated in the strip. Normal readings may be 12 millimeters or more, and dry readings may be from 1 to 5 millimeters.

sclera The tough, outer protective layer of the eye. It is seen as the white portion of the eye surrounding the colored iris but it lines the entire globe of the eye. The sclera joins the transparent CORNEA at the front of the eye and circles around to join the OPTIC NERVE at the back of the eye. The sclera lies atop the CHOROID, the vascular layer that supplies blood to the eye.

The sclera may appear red as a result of an infection or disorder of the CONJUNCTIVA, the mucous membrane lining the sclera and the inside of the lids. The sclera is also subject to SCLERITIS, or inflammation of the sclera. Scleritis is closely linked to rheumatoid arthritis, gout, and collagen disease. Symptoms include redness, pain, and erosion of the sclera. The condition is treated with systemic antiinflammatory agents but seldom with steroids, which destroy collagen and exacerbate scleral thinning.

scleral buckling A surgical procedure performed to correct a RETINAL DETACHMENT. A retinal detachment occurs when the retina becomes separated from the back of the eye. Some detachments are caused by retinal holes or tears that must be surgically repaired and that often requires scleral buckling.

The surgery, performed under general anesthetic, first involves producing a scar near the hole with heat, as in surgical diathermy, or with cold, as in cryotherapy. In order to bring the RETINA into position so that the scar will adhere to the retina, a scleral buckle is applied.

A silicon belt or buckle is placed around the eye. This returns the detached retina into contact with the underlying retinal pigment epithelium where it adheres due to the scar tissue. The scleral buckle is permanent and completely unnoticeable by the patient and others.

The surgery takes place underneath the membrane that covers the sclera so that the inner eye need not be breached. The procedure requires a short hospital stay and post-operative eye drops.

scleritis   An inflammation of the SCLERA, the outer protective layer of the eye. Scleritis produces a red, painful eye and sensitivity to light. Scleritis may be linked to rheumatoid arthritis, collagen disease, disorders of menstruation, and gout, but may develop for unknown reasons as well. It is particularly found among young women.

Scleritis leads to thinning of the sclera and may expose the underlying uveal pigment. If untreated, scleritis may lead to necrosis (death of tissue) or perforation of the globe. Scleritis is treated with systemic nonsteroidal antiinflammatory agents. Corticosteroids are usually contraindicated, because they encourage scleral thinning. Treatment generally is directed at the underlying condition.

scotoma   A blind spot or area of blocked vision in the visual field. It may be caused by eye injury, disease, or disorder or migraine headaches.

Each eye contains one scotoma. This is the blind spot in the normal field of vision caused by the OPTIC DISC. The optic disc is the part of the RETINA where the OPTIC NERVE meets the eye. It is here that the blood supply enters the eye. The optic disc contains no photosensitive RODS AND CONES and is therefore unable to "see."

Scotomas may be present in either the central or peripheral field of vision. Macular diseases attack the MACULA, the point of clearest vision in the central field. A scotoma, or blind spot, develops that permanently blocks central vision but that usually leaves peripheral vision intact.

Scotomas caused by RETINITIS PIGMENTOSA and GLAUCOMA block vision in the peripheral or side visual fields. These diseases continue to destroy peripheral vision until tunnel vision results.

Scotomas caused by migraines are temporary. They occur during the preheadache or prodrome stage of migraines and may forewarn of the subsequent headache. Migraine scotomas may appear in any part of the visual field and may move during the course of the prodrome or headache stages. These scotomas may simply block out vision or may be scintillating and shimmer or blink with bright or colored lights. Migraine scotomas usually last from five minutes to an hour. They tend to retreat with the onset of the migraine headache.

screening   Screening examinations are eye examinations that are used to detect the possibility of a visual disorder in individuals. General screenings are routinely performed on the population during patient eye and medical exams, driver's license renewals, and entrance to the armed forces.

Specific screening exams look for particular visual field losses or ocular diseases. Screening exams performed in retirement communities would concentrate on those diseases and disorders associated with aging, such as AGE-RELATED MACULOPATHY, CATARACT, and GLAUCOMA. An exam performed on a patient complaining of lost vision would screen for scotomas (blind spots) or specific field losses.

Often, a screening examination leads to a diagnosis. Evidence of DIABETIC RETINOPATHY found in a routine screening examination detects both the result of the disease and its underlying cause. Diagnostic examinations follow the screening exams. The diagnostic exam is used on those who test positive or who show indications of disease or a disorder on a screening exam. This examination confirms the presence of a disorder and diagnoses the cause. (See EYE EXAMINATION.)

Seeing Eye, Inc.   A nonprofit organization that breeds and trains dog guides for use by qualified blind persons. Incorporated in 1929 by Dorothy Eustis, it was the first dog-guide school in the United States.

The Seeing Eye breeds and trains German shepherds and Labrador retrievers and trains golden retrievers or other working breeds. The school provides a 20- to 27-day in-residence training program for its students. It has placed more than 12,500 trained dogs with nearly 6,000 blind people from the United States and Canada.

Most dog-guide recipients are totally blind or have light perception. Applicants must be physically fit, able to maintain a reasonable amount of walking exercise, able to absorb and apply instructions in the care and use of a dog guide, and show a willingness to be independent. Age limits are usually between 16 and 65 years for new dog-guide candidates.

The Seeing Eye charges a fee of $150 for the first visit and $50 for each subsequent visit. The fee includes the dog guide, in-residence instruction with the dog, the dog's equipment, and round trip economy air fare from any place in the United States and Canada. Payment, which is only a fraction of the cost of the program and intended to impart a sense of ownership to the participant, may be made in installments over a period of years. The fee is not payable by any other individual or organization.

Contact:

The Seeing Eye, Inc.
P.O. Box 375
Morristown, NJ 07963-0375
201-539-4425 (ph)
973-539-0922 (fax)
www.seeingeye.org

Selective Placement Program

The Selective Placement Program was established as an amendment to the Rehabilitation Act of 1973. The amendment allowed the federal government to employ mentally or physically disabled individuals.

Administrators of this program work with state, public and private rehabilitation agencies to refer and place disabled employees. In addition, the program works to reappoint to another suitable position individuals who become unable to perform a job due to a disability.

U.S. Department of Education. *Summary of Existing Legislation Affecting Persons with Disabilities.* Washington, D.C.: USDE, 1988.

self-contained classroom

One of five major educational models or plans for the instruction of visually impaired students. The other models are the RESIDENTIAL SCHOOL, ITINERANT TEACHER, TEACHER-CONSULTANT, and RESOURCE ROOM.

The self-contained classroom is a classroom in a public school that is specially equipped and staffed with special education teachers for the visually impaired. All the students in the class have visual impairments or other disabilities.

The teacher of the class provides general curriculum instruction and special education. The program is designed to fit the unique needs of each individual.

Although one-fifth of all programs for visually impaired students centered on self-contained classrooms in the early 1960s, the model has since lost popularity except in large metropolitan areas serving multihandicapped blind students.

In order to achieve maximum enrollment, self-contained classrooms are centered in one or a few schools within a district. This often necessitates bussing the visually impaired student to a school outside his neighborhood.

Barraga, Natalie C. *Visual Handicaps and Learning.* Belmont, California: Wadsworth Publishing Company Inc., 1976.

Scholl, Geraldine, ed. *Foundations of Education for Blind and Visually Handicapped Children and Youth.* New York: American Foundation for the Blind, 1986.

senses

The body obtains information from all five senses plus the equilibrium and kinesthesis. The tendency is to rely on the sense of sight or to use the other senses to validate sight information when the same information can often be provided by the other senses alone.

When vision is lost or impaired, the affected person must learn to use the other senses in more effective ways. Contrary to the myth, the other senses do not become heightened, nor does ESP develop as compensation for the lost sight. Rather, the visually impaired person integrates the other senses with any remaining vision and uses them more effectively.

Most visually impaired persons have some remaining vision. This vision may range from clear vision within a limited central or peripheral field to being able to determine light. Individual vision may vary from one day to the next due to general health, diet, stress, fatigue, medication side effects, or environmental factors such as glare or artificial light.

Use of the residual vision may require the visually impaired person to adopt new head or body movements, or to use a visual aid such as a magnifier when viewing an object. The remaining vision may allow for information about the size, shape, color, or contrast of the object in view.

The sense of hearing is used for subject identification, direction, distance, size, and structure. Visually impaired people must learn to recognize and discriminate between sounds and to determine the relative distance and direction between the source of the sound and themselves, a concept termed localization. Localization is dependent on adequate binaural hearing, or balanced, relatively equal hearing in both ears.

Hearing may also be used in echolocation, listening for the echo of a sound rising from an object. The person using echolocation makes a sound such as clapping hands, whistling, or snapping fingers and listens for the faint echo that rebounds from the object. The echo's sound changes as the user gets closer to, or farther away from, an object. With practice, echolocation can be useful in determining the distance, size, or existence of an object in the area.

Echolocation users must have adequate binaural hearing and must be able to hear high-frequency sounds. The use of echolocation is more effective in certain environmental conditions. Hard, large surfaces such as walls and cars reflect echoes better than smaller, softer surfaces such as drapes or people. Echolocation is also related to facial vision. Facial vision is the ability to locate nearby obstacles, without touch, by a feeling of pressure on the face. The close objects reflect background noise in a particular manner that can be interpreted to locate objects. Facial vision depends on adequate binaural hearing.

The sense of touch involves every part of the body from the top of the head to the soles of the feet. Touch provides information about the size, weight, density, texture, and temperature of an object or the environment. Touch may be used to compensate for lost vision in specific tasks such as reading braille.

The sense of smell is used to determine location or landmarks, such as the corner bakery, to detect danger such as leaking gas or the presence of smoke, or to confirm information provided by another sense. Smell is closely linked to taste, which is used to identify foods and provide information about the freshness and texture of ingested foods or medications.

Kinesthesis is the body's ability to remember a movement. It is a muscle sense or awareness that allows the body to perform a movement or physical task with little mental concentration. This sense provides information about the tilt in surface or grade, allows one to effectively estimate distances and positions and enables one to touch-type and sign a signature without looking.

The equilibrium is the body's sense of balance. It provides information as to the position of the body and allows for balance in turning or changing position.

sensory aids   Any aids, devices, or systems that enable an individual to overcome, compensate, or alleviate the performance losses caused by an impairment of any of the senses. Sensory aids may either enhance remaining vision or replace the visual information with information in a tactile or auditory form.

Because sensory aids increase independence and are related to job performance, they are often associated with VOCATIONAL AIDS, or aids that enable an individual to perform a job. Such sensory aids include talking computers, electronic devices to enlarge print, reading machines, electronic braille devices, and telephone communication devices. (See ADAPTIVE AIDS.)

shaken baby syndrome   A medical term used to describe a form of child abuse in which a baby or child is shaken violently enough to cause trauma from acceleration forces. Also called shaken infant syndrome, this form of abuse can cause brain damage and bleeding in and on the surface of the brain. It also can result in ocular injuries such as retinal hemorrhages.

The American Academy of Ophthalmology has encouraged parents and caregivers to learn the symptoms of shaken baby syndrome and to make sure a baby who may have been shaken receives an eye exam, which can reveal evidence of shaking. More than 75 percent of all severely shaken babies have retinal hemorrhages, a symptom rarely seen with an accidental head injury.

Babies and toddlers have weak neck muscles, which give them little control over their relatively heavy heads. When shaken, their heads vibrate rapidly back and forth, which can cause devastating damage. It is estimated that 85 percent of children who are violently shaken sustain serious injury, including blindness, hearing loss, learning disabilities, permanent brain damage, paralysis, or even death.

Shaken baby syndrome was first discussed in medical literature in 1972, and public awareness of the syndrome has increased dramatically in recent years. There often are no obvious outward signs of injury to a baby who has been shaken, although the child may appear to be stunned and glassy-eyed or sluggish. Vomiting, difficulty in breathing, inability to lift or turn the head, lack of appetite, and seizures are signs of possible abuse.

The Survivor's Foundation. "Eye M.D.s Urge Parents to Request Eye Exam in Shaken Baby Cases." www.survivors-foundation.org, 2000.

American Humane Association Children's Division. "Shaken Baby Syndrome Fact Sheet." www.csfpa.org/pages/shaken.html, 2001.

sheltered workshops   Any protected work settings for disabled individuals. These work locations may be nonvocational work-activity centers, transitional rehabilitation training and employment centers, or long-term competitive employment centers that provide opportunities for self-support.

The first sheltered workshop was established in the Perkins School in 1840 as a separate work department. The idea was duplicated in other schools for the blind and later became separate workshops administered by voluntary organizations for the adult blind and state agencies.

The Wagner-O'Day Act of 1938 established a program in which federal agencies could purchase selected commodities from qualified workshops for the blind. The act was amended in 1971 as the JAVITS-WAGNER-O'DAY ACT to extend the authority to workshops for all severely disabled persons and to services as well as products.

Early workshops produced handmade objects for household use, including brooms, chair caning, and hand weaving. Modern sheltered workshops are often more industrial in nature and produce such products as military equipment, including the Kevlar helmet, tracheotomy kits, and kitchen gadgets sold to military commissaries.

Many workshops for the blind are associated with the NATIONAL INDUSTRIES FOR THE BLIND (NIB), a private nonprofit organization that develops industrial employment for blind and multihandicapped Americans. The NIB offers technical and management services and allocates federal government orders among its workshops.

sickle-cell disease   A term used to describe any condition that involves inherited sickle-cell hemoglobin of the blood. The disease is most common among those of African descent and those with ancestors from Puerto Rico, Cuba, Haiti, Jamaica, Italy, Sicily, Greece, Cyprus, Turkey, Syria, and South India. Sickle-cell disease affects about 72,000 people in the United States—about one in every 500 Americans of African descent—and the disease trait is present in one of every 10 Americans of African descent.

The disease affects the hemoglobin of the blood, the matter in red cells that enables the blood to carry oxygen to the body. Normal hemoglobin, called hemoglobin A or C, is characterized by round red blood cells which flow easily through the body's vessels. Sickle-cell hemoglobin, hemoglobin S, is contained in sickle-shaped, elongated cells that resist flow and cause obstructions in circulation (microinfarctions), a lack of oxygen to the tissues (hypoxia), and the proliferation of additional sickle cells.

Sickle cells have a shorter life span than normal cells. Their rapid breakdown rate results in a lowered hemoglobin level, or anemia. For this reason, sickle-cell disease is often referred to as sickle-cell anemia.

Sickle-cell disease occurs when hemoglobin A is changed to hemoglobin S by a genetic substitution of one amino acid in the hemoglobin chain. If both parents are carriers of sickle-cell hemoglobin, there is a one in four chance that the child will inherit normal hemoglobin and not carry the trait.

There is a two in four chance that the child will inherit one trait for sickle-cell hemoglobin and one for normal hemoglobin. This child is a carrier of the trait and may develop very mild symptoms of the disease or none at all.

The remaining one in four chance is that the child will inherit both sickle-cell hemoglobin traits. In this case the child will develop sickle-cell disease.

Early symptoms of sickle-cell disease are manifested in infancy and include listlessness, aches in the arms, legs, stomach and back, poor appetite, and pallor. Patients experience "crisis" periods that involve intense bouts of these symptoms. A crisis may last one day to two weeks and is often preceded by an infection, cold, or sore throat. Crises may recur several times a year, but the patient remains quite healthy between occurrences.

In patients with sickle-cell disease, the vision is affected when blood vessels become blocked in the CONJUNCTIVA, CHOROID, or RETINA. In turn, this may cause anterior segment ischemia, PUPIL irregularity, IRIS atrophy, retinal degeneration, and loss of visual field.

A serious condition called sickle-cell retinopathy is a common result of sickle-cell disease. As vessels within the peripheral sections of retina become blocked, the retina becomes starved for oxygen. It develops new vessels that tend to be weak and hemorrhage. The neovascularization may cause leakage into the VITREOUS or RETINAL DETACHMENT. A loss of vision results.

Photocoagulation therapy, laser treatments, are performed once neovascularization has begun. This may stop the hemorrhaging but can cause complications such as vitreal neovascularization. Cryotherapy, freezing treatments, may be performed on the smaller areas of neovascularization.

Scleral buckling may be used to reduce the traction that causes retinal detachment. This normally simple procedure is difficult in cases of sickle-cell disease because there may be overlying bleeding that interferes with localization of the hemorrhage source, and since the procedure may trigger necrosis, localized tissue death, in anterior areas.

It is thought that the sickle-cell trait may have developed as a natural response to malaria, a more serious disease commonly found in descendant countries of those affected by the disease. Those with sickle-cell disease carry a high resistance to malaria. There is no cure for sickle-cell disease, but medical treatment and monitoring may lessen its effects. Doctors recently began using hydroxyurea, a drug often used to treat leukemia, on patients with sickle-cell disease. The drug has been found to reduce the painful crisis periods.

Galloway, N. R. *Common Eye Diseases and Their Management.* Berlin: Springer-Verlag, 1895.

Mayfield, Eleanor. "New Hope for People with Sickle-Cell Anemia." *FDA Consumer,* May 1996, p. 16.

Rhode, Stephen J., and Stephen P. Ginsberg. *Ophthalmic Technology.* New York: Raven Press, 1987.

Schweitzer, N. M. J., ed. *Ophthalmology.* Amsterdam: Excerpta Medica, 1982.

Sickle Cell Anemia Research and Education Inc. *Facts About Sickle Cell Anemia.* Oakland, California: SCARE, 1977.

sighted-guide technique   A method of guiding a visually impaired person. The sighted person holds the disabled person's arm in a relaxed position close to the body. The arm may be straight or bent at a right angle. The visually impaired person grasps the guide's arm just above the elbow. This position allows the sighted guide to walk a step ahead. The visually impaired person can then follow the guide's movements and directions.

The guide may inform the visually impaired person about steps or cracks in the path or overhead obstacles. The guide may pause when reaching the bottom or top landing of a flight of stairs. This alerts the visually impaired person that one last stair remains. When traveling through a narrow passage, the guide moves the guide arm behind himself so that his wrist is behind the small of his back. This alerts the visually impaired person to drop back. The guide then proceeds through the passage, and the visually impaired person follows single-file.

Partially sighted persons may be asked whether they prefer to take a sighted guide's arm in a darkened room. The sighted guide should never force assistance or lend assistance without first asking permission. Rehabilitation classes teach visually impaired persons how to break the grasp of well-meaning but unwanted guides. (See ETIQUETTE; ORIENTATION AND MOBILITY.)

signature guide   An aid that enables the user to sign a signature within a specific space on a page. The guides may be made of plastic or metal and often have a rubber component that holds the guide in place.

Designs vary, but most guides are a template with a rectangular window or opening that conforms to the standard signature area of a check, credit card receipt, etc. The signature guide is placed on the paper with the lower straight edge of the opening centered on the signature line of the document. The individual uses the edge as a guide and signs the signature within the opening.

slate and stylus   The braille slate and stylus are tools used to print braille. The slate is made from two rectangular metal plates hinged together at one end. The upper plate has rows of small, open windows punched out of the metal. Directly underneath each window on the bottom plate is an indentation of a complete braille cell.

The braille cell is made up of six dots, two across and three down. Each dot is numbered. Different configurations or combinations of dots are used to stand for each letter of the alphabet. For instance, dot 1 stands for the letter A, and dots 1 and 2 stand for the letter B.

In order to make a braille letter with the slate and stylus, a card or sheet of braille paper is placed between the two metal plates of the slate. The stylus, a short metal prong fastened to a handle, is held in the palm and used to make the letters. The writer presses the stylus downward onto the paper within an open window. The stylus pushes the paper against the corresponding indentation of the braille cell dot on the bottom plate. A raised dot is formed on the reverse side of the paper. The writer continues to press against the correct dots in the cell until the correct letter is formed. The writing is read when the paper is turned over and the dots are facing upward.

Therefore, in order to write braille, which must be read from left to right, the slate and stylus user must write from right to left and reverse the normal configuration of dots on the braille cell. Rather than learning to picture each letter in reverse, braille writers learn the number configuration of the dots.

slit lamp   See BIOMICROSCOPE.

Smith-Kettlewell Eye Research Institute   A nonprofit, independent medical and scientific institute incorporated in 1963 and dedicated to research on human vision. The 50-person research staff is a blend of laboratory and clinical research scientists with degrees in medicine, ophthalmology, experimental psychology, physiology, engineering, optometry, computer science, and physics.

The institute concentrates on three main areas of interest: clinical studies related to the diagnosis and treatment of eye diseases and disorders, basic research to understand how the eye and brain work as a basis for clinical and rehabilitation programs, and development of devices and vocational programs to aid partially sighted and blind persons.

The development of devices and programs is the main focus of the Rehabilitation Engineering Center. Established in 1975, the nonprofit center is funded by the National Institute on Disabilities and Rehabilitation Research, a division of the federal Department of Education.

The center conducts ongoing research and development programs in the area of sensory aids that are suitable for solving problems in the rehabilitation of blind, low-vision, and deaf-blind individuals. The emphasis is on the design of practical, low-cost aids and efforts to ensure the aids reach the user.

The aids and devices may consist of vocational aids, educational devices, communication aids, and orientation and mobility aids. Major achievements of past years include the Volatile Braille Display, a Universal Job Instrumentation System (Flexi-Meter), the Braille Notetaker, the Auditory Data-Flow Indicator, and the Auditory Arcade. Currently, staff is working to develop medication reminders for blind and blind-deaf consumers, and to expand the usefulness of KnowWare, a system that provides virtual reality maps for blind people.

Contact:

Smith-Kettlewell Eye Research Institute
San Francisco, CA 94115

415 345 2000 (ph)
915-345-8455 (fax)
www.ski.org

Snellen chart   The eye chart routinely used in the EYE EXAMINATION to determine central visual acuity. VISUAL ACUITY is the measurement of the amount of detail an individual sees as compared with the amount of detail a person with normal vision sees. The visual-acuity test involves reading the Snellen chart when positioned 20 feet away. The chart contains nine lines of letters, written in progressively smaller print.

Each line corresponds to a degree of vision. Line one corresponds to 20/200 vision; line two, 20/100; line three, 20/70; line four, 20/50; line five, 20/40; line six, 20/30; line seven, 20/25; line eight, 20/20; and line nine, 20/15. If an individual can read all nine lines, the vision is measured as 20/15, or able to read at 20 feet what a normally sighted person can read at 15 feet. If the person can read only the top line, or big E, that vision is measured as 20/200, or able to read at 20 feet what a normally-sighted person can read at 200 feet. This is classified as legally blind.

The Snellen chart has been criticized for inaccuracy since each line on the chart must cover a wide range of visual ability. Those with borderline vision may fall between two lines of ability and be incorrectly classified.

snow blindness   An eye injury caused by intense light reflected off snow. The bright light in prolonged exposure produces an ultraviolet burn on the CORNEA of the eye. Symptoms of snow blindness appear in both eyes, and include extreme pain, a feeling of sand in the eyes, and severe sensitivity to light. The symptoms are usually delayed two to nine hours after exposure. The burn heals itself within two to three days. Antibiotic or steroid drops may be prescribed to ease discomfort and discourage infection. Snow blindness can be prevented by wearing protective goggles or glasses.

Although the rays that cause snow blindness are the same as those that cause sunburn at the beach, sunbathers rarely get snow blindness. This is because most of the rays at the beach are coming from above and the eyes are afforded some protection by the eyelids, eyelashes, and eyebrows. In cases of snow blindness, the rays are reflected from the snow and enter the eye from below, a relatively unprotected position. (See RADIATION BURNS.)

Social Security Benefits   The Social Security Administration (SSA) operates two programs that provide financial assistance to visually impaired individuals. These programs are called Social Security Disability Insurance (SSDI) benefits and Supplemental Security Income (SSI).

Title II of the Social Security Act provides federal old age, survivors, and disability insurance, also known as OASDI. Disability insurance benefits are paid to people who have paid Social Security taxes but have become disabled before reaching retirement age. A disabled person is described in the act as one who is unable to work due to a physical or mental impairment that is permanent, long-lasting (12 months or more), or may result in death.

Applicants must be unemployed or employed but earning less than a determined amount and must have a qualifying medical disability according to the ruling of the Disability Determination Service. An applicant must also have contributed to the Social Security fund for approximately half of the years since attaining age 21.

Dependents of an eligible disabled person may also qualify for benefits under Section 202 of the Act. Children must be unmarried and under 18 years old, or 19 if a student, or unmarried of any age with a disability that occurred before age 22. Spouses may be eligible if aged 62 or over, or of any age if a child in their care is disabled or under age 16 and receiving Social Security benefits.

A child's benefit is one-half of that received by the eligible living parent collecting Social Security retirement or disability benefits. The payment is three-quarters of the amount when the parent is deceased.

There is a five-month waiting period before becoming eligible for disability insurance. The waiting period is waived if the recipient reapplies for the benefits within five years of discontinuing benefits.

The benefits are paid in cash monthly to eligible people and their dependents. The age of the worker when he became disabled, his earned income and the length of time he was employed determine the amount of the benefit. The amount may be decreased if the worker is a recipient of other state or federal benefits. After receiving disability benefits for 24 months, the recipient is eligible for Medicare health insurance benefits.

Under Section 222 of the act, all recipients and applicants are referred to state vocational rehabilitation agencies to encourage individual productivity and self-sufficiency. After a recipient has been trained and employed for nine months, the vocational rehabilitation agency is reimbursed for its services with Disability Insurance Trust funds.

A trial work period of nine consecutive or nonconsecutive months is allowed to enable recipients to test their vocational suitability without losing benefits. Each month that the recipient earns more than a certain amount is counted as one of the nine.

An extended period of eligibility lasting up to 31 months may be allowed if the recipient retains the disability or if the earned income is below a specified amount. If the individual's earnings exceed the set amount during a month, benefits are not paid during that month. If a recipient never exceeds the set amount, benefits continue indefinitely as long as all other requirements are met.

Supplemental Security Income, or SSI, is a federal program authorized under Title XVI of the Social Security Act to provide a minimum income to low-income elderly and disabled individuals. SSI requires that recipients meet requirements of financial need, and unlike Social Security Disability Insurance, does not base eligibility on the amount of taxes paid into the Social Security Fund.

Needy individuals or couples disabled or aged 65 or older may qualify for SSI benefits if financial needs requirements are met. Disabled children under age 16 are referred to a state agency funded by the Maternal and Child Health Block Grant Program or another appropriate agency. Disabled individuals are described under the program as those who have a physical or mental disability that is permanent, long-term (12 months or longer), or one that may result in death.

Monthly cash benefits are paid directly to recipients. The amount of payment is based on a Consumer Price Index figure. The Social Security Administration considers earned and unearned income, amount of savings and assets, and other factors when determining how much in SSI benefits to allocate to a particular person.

Individuals who live in another household that supplies support or maintenance receive benefits that are reduced by one-third. Those who live in a public or private medical or health-care institution that receives Medicaid or SSI benefits on behalf of the individuals, receive personal allowances each month. Individuals admitted to a medical or psychiatric facility for a projected three months or less may receive full benefits. Those living in a public, nonmedical facility do not qualify for benefits.

Recipients between the ages of 21 and 65 are referred to state vocational rehabilitation agencies to encourage their return to the work force. If it is determined that an individual is eligible and would benefit from these services, the recipient may not refuse them without good cause.

To encourage recipients to work, the program allows individuals to continue to receive SSI benefits and Medicaid coverage if they are able to work but still retain their disabilities. The individual must suffer from the original disability and must continue to meet all the program requirements. Benefits are discontinued when the individual's earnings exceed the amount of benefit, but the individual may still qualify for Medicaid coverage. (See FINANCIAL AID.)

U.S. Department of Education. *Summary of Existing Legislation Affecting Persons with Disabilities.* Washington, D.C.: USDE, 1988.

U.S. Social Security Administration. Part 416—Supplemental Security Income for the Aged, Blind and Disabled. www.ssa.gov/op-Home, 2001.

Social Services Block Grant   The Social Security Act was amended in 1974 to establish, under Title XX, the Social Services Block Grant program. The program allows each state to provide social services to its residents in ways it deems most appropriate and effective. States may use Title XX funds to provide services to disabled persons. Funds may be used to prevent or reduce dependency, attain and maintain self-sufficiency, prevent neglect or abuse of either adults or children, improve or prevent inappropriate institutional care, and obtain institutional care.

Funds may also be used to improve state programs concerning day-care services of either children or adults, protective services, foster-care services, home-care management and maintenance services, transportation and health services, employment services, information and counseling services, and meal-delivery programs. Services must relate to the special needs of children and the elderly, and those who are blind, mentally retarded, emotionally disturbed, physically disabled, or drug or alcohol dependent.

The eligibility of recipients is determined by each state. Allotments to the state are proportionally set according to population. In fiscal year 2001, Congress allocated $1.725 billion for this program.

U.S. Department of Education. *Summary of Existing Legislation Affecting Persons with Disabilities.* Washington, D.C.: USDE, 1988.

Sonicguide   The Sonicguide is an ELECTRONIC TRAVEL AID developed and designed by HUMANWARE INC. for the visually impaired. The device has three components: a pair of spectacles, earphones, and a control box for the electronic components and power supply.

The spectacle-mounted transmitting device sends out ultrasonic waves that bounce off objects in the user's path. The reflected waves are converted into audible tones heard in stereophonic earpieces. The pitch of the tone provides information as to the distance, position, and surface characteristics of the detected object. The device has a range of five meters.

Other similar devices are known by the trade names Kay binaural sensor and Sensory 6. Versions of the device are available for children, wheelchair users, and orientation and mobility instructors. Correct use of all such devices requires training from a qualified instructor.

Sorsby's fundus dystrophy (SFD)   A rare genetic disorder that causes macular degeneration to occur at an early age, usually between the ages of 30 and 40. Researchers are interested in SFD because of its clinical similarity to age-related macular degeneration. Symptoms include retinal edema, hemorrhages, and exudates in the macular area. As the disease progresses, considerable scarring may occur. Symptoms usually occur first in one eye, with the other eye developing symptoms months or even years later. As with age-related macular degeneration, central vision is affected first.

The disorder was first addressed in 1949 in a study of five British families who were afflicted by the disease. It has been identified in patients in Europe, North America, South Africa, Australia, and Japan.

special education   See EDUCATION.

sports and recreation   Sports and recreation activities benefit all persons, both disabled and able-bodied, by developing self-assurance and confidence, competitive spirit and athletic skills, and by providing stress reduction, comradeship, and fun. Local, state, regional, national, and international competitions exist for participation in sports by visually impaired persons as well as persons with other disabilities.

Although some sports or games require some adaptation to allow full participation by visually impaired individuals, many do not. Adaptation is dependent on the participant's eye condition, general health and interests and requirements of the sport.

A visually impaired jogger or runner may run alone on a track with high contrast or distinctive texture to differentiate the path or on a track specially equipped with guide ropes or poles for visually impaired athletes. A visually impaired person may run with a sighted partner while holding onto the guide's elbow, a stick held between the two, or a rubberbandlike tether.

Competitive games in track and field exist for visually impaired athletes. Competitive events include the triple jump, shot put, long jump, javelin throw, discus, and meter races.

Bicycling is possible when the rider rides a tandem bike with a sighted partner in the front, or pilot, position. The visually impaired person sits behind in the stoker position and provides the power base for the pair. Tandem cycling may take the form of leisurely recreation or competitive riding.

Bowling programs and tournaments are offered through blind bowling or athletic associations. Bowling lanes can be adapted with a portable bowling rail that is assembled and placed next to the aisle as a banister guide.

Skiing clubs and programs are available to visually impaired skiers. Many ski areas have staff to teach or accompany blind individuals in either nordic (cross country) or alpine (downhill) skiing.

Nordic skiing is pursued in flat terrain at fairly slow, controllable speeds. Since nordic skiing generally follows tracks made from previous skiers, the sport is only minimally dependent on a sighted guide who calls directions to the visually impaired skier.

Alpine or downhill skiing is a faster sport that relies on excellent communication between the visually impaired skier and the sighted guide. The guide calls out directions to indicate turns and guide the partner around obstacles. Often, visually impaired skiers wear tunics or shirts printed with "Blind Skier" to advise sighted skiers of their presence.

Ice skating, speed skating, or roller skating may be pursued with a sighted guide. The guide may call out directions or may skate in tandem, allowing the partner to hold onto his elbow or a stick held between the two.

Swimming is a popular sport for recreation or competition. A pool with rope lane markers makes swimming laps possible without a sighted guide. Some visually impaired swimmers prefer to use an outside lane that borders the side of the pool and to count the number of strokes required to reach complete a lap.

Competitive blind swimmers are tapped on the head or hand at the end of each lap to indicate the approach of the pool wall. The tapper taps just as the swimmer should start the turn. This enables the visually impaired swimmer to duplicate the turning techniques of nondisabled swimmers in safety.

Boating or canoeing is usually pursued with a sighted guide partner who takes the lead position in the craft. The guide supplies continuous information on obstacles, rapids, or changes in direction. All boaters should wear personal flotation devices.

Horseshoes may be played by adapting the horseshoes by color or texture. The post can be accented with a bright color or by an auditory cue.

Horseback riding is widely available and pursued in the company of a sighted rider who provides information concerning directions and overhead obstacles. Riders may be required to wear a safety helmet.

Exercising and weight lifting programs are available in gyms and fitness centers that provide individualized instruction. Weight lifting or power lifting requires no adaptation for blind participants but may necessitate a "spotter" or guide to monitor the lift.

Judo and wrestling are two sports that need no adaptation for participation by visually impaired individuals. The referee makes verbal calls concerning scoring and penalties.

Gymnastics programs are available through athletic organizations and local gymnasiums. The visually impaired individual may participate in all activities including the uneven bars, balance beam, floor exercise, and vault. A "spotter" or guide may monitor the activity, and an additional layer of floor matting and padding covering all metal parts may be recommended.

Competitive or recreational darts are played on the Audio Dart Game. The dart board talks to control the game. It informs players when it is their turn, the score earned, and the status of the game as it progresses.

Balls of all types including basketballs and children's playground balls are adapted with inner bells or beeps that alert the visually impaired user to the location of the ball. Goal ball is a game played exclusively by the visually impaired. The object is to roll a ball containing bells past the opposing team and into the goal net. Each team consists of three players who alternately roll and defend. The floor is marked with tape to accent the goals and boundaries. See Appendix for sports organizations. (See TOYS AND GAMES.)

squint See STRABISMUS.

Stargardt's disease An inherited disease that causes people to lose central vision, usually in the first or second decade of life. It is sometimes referred to as juvenile macular degeneration. Doctors estimate that between 17,000 and 25,000 people in the United States have Stargardt's disease.

The disease typically starts between the ages of six and 15. Some children lost most of their central vision quickly, while others experience a slow and gradual loss of sight. Researchers in May 1998 identified a gene that causes Stargardt's disease. The gene causes cells to produce a protein that functions only in the retinas of the eyes. Discovery of this gene is significant for several reasons. It will allow doctors to develop a specific test for Stargardt's disease, which frequently is confused with other vision problems, and, it may move researchers closer to finding the cause of age-related macular degeneration.

stereotypes See ATTITUDES.

steroids Drugs used in the treatment of eye diseases and disorders. They are most often used to combat inflammation in the eye. Steroids may be prescribed in pill, ointment, or drop form. They are most often topically applied, because systemic (taken internally) steroids may have more serious side effects.

Steroids increase the eye's susceptibility to infection and may encourage the multiplication of viruses such as HERPES SIMPLEX. Topical steroids may immediately cause a rise in intraocular pressure, which may lead to GLAUCOMA. Over time, systemic steroids may encourage CATARACT development. Thereafter, steroids should be prescribed for a specific disorder and only if other drugs have proven ineffective. They should be taken only as directed and should not be used for extended periods of time.

Stoxil See IDOXURIDINE.

strabismus Strabismus, or squint, is the name for misalignment of the eyes. The terms *cross-eyed, wall-eyed* or *cockeyed* are often used to describe this condition. An eye may move inward, as in convergent strabismus, outward, as in divergent strabismus, or up or down, as in vertical strabismus.

The condition in which eyes tend to turn inward toward each other is termed ESOPHORIA. When one eye turns inward it is called ESOTROPIA. The condition in which the eyes tend to turn outward away from each other is called EXOPHORIA, and when one eye turns outward, it is called *exotropia*. An eye that turns upward is an example of HYPERTROPIA, and an eye which turns downward is an example of HYPOTROPIA.

The eyes may cross consistently, called constant tropia, or occasionally, called intermittent tropia. There is also a type of strabismus in which the deviation of the eyes is hidden much or all of the time. This is called a phoria. The problem is not merely cosmetic, but can cause visual problems. In normal vision, both eyes focus on one object. The brain receives two pictures of one object and translates that information into one three-dimensional image.

In strabismus, one eye views one object while the other views something else. The brain receives pictures of two different objects. Double vision may result, or the brain, in its attempt to reconcile the two pictures, may suppress one, causing a loss of function. This suppression results in a condition called AMBLYOPIA.

Causes of all types of strabismus are not known. Since it is often associated with high amounts of MYOPIA (nearsightedness), HYPEROPIA (farsightedness), or ASTIGMATISM, it is thought that these conditions may contribute to the cause. Strabismus can develop after a major illness or injury, and some forms of strabismus may also be hereditary.

Because many infants under six months of age develop strabismus conditions that they outgrow, a misconception persists that strabismus is self-correcting. Any strabismus that lingers after six months of age, if only occasional, indicates a problem and should be treated by a physician.

Treatment for early stages of strabismus include the prescription of eyedrops and eyeglasses or bifocals. The lenses of the glasses often include a prism to bring the images closer together.

Exercises may be prescribed if amblyopia is present. The exercises train the eyes to stop suppressing one image and to experience stereoscopic vision. Further exercises then train the eyes to bring both images together to form one three-dimensional image. Once the eyes are properly aligned, follow up treatment may include exercises to keep the eyes in place.

If treatment fails, surgery may be necessary. During surgery, one or more of the six muscles attached to each eye are altered to bring the eyes into position or to strengthen or weaken them according to need. Since strabismus is a disorder that affects both eyes, usually both eyes undergo surgery. Some patients may require additional surgery to completely align the eyes.

stroke An interruption of blood flow to the brain. Stroke is the third most common cause of death in the United States after heart attack and cancer. According to the American Heart Association, about 600,000 Americans experience stroke each year.

More than 75 percent of those who suffer strokes each year are over 65. The incidence of stroke increases by more than 100 percent with each decade over 65. Men suffer 30 percent more strokes than women. Blacks suffer 60 percent more strokes than whites, and evidence suggests that people from poor socioeconomic backgrounds are more susceptible than those from affluent circumstances. Strokes tend to run in families, occur more commonly in the southeastern part of the United States, and occur most often during phases of extreme weather temperatures.

A stroke is a type of cardiovascular disease. Blood is brought to the brain via four large arteries. The brain cannot store nutrients, so it needs a constant supply of blood to furnish oxygen and nutrients and carry away carbon dioxide and other waste materials. When the flow of blood is interrupted, a stroke occurs. Any cessation of blood to the brain can cause damage, including paralysis, loss of consciousness, loss of speech, loss of mental functioning, loss of vision, and death.

Strokes are caused by a blockage or bursting of one of the arteries to the brain. These types of strokes, called cerebral thrombosis and cerebral embolism are the most common types of stroke. They account for up to 80 percent of all strokes suffered in the United States.

ARTERIOSCLEROSIS, hardening of the arteries, is the cause of more than half of all strokes. Arteriosclerosis causes fatty plaque to form inside the walls of the arteries, which slows or stops the flow of blood. This causes a stroke called a thrombotic stroke or cerebral thrombosis.

Platelets, blood-clotting cells in the blood, may cling to the arteriosclerotic plaque and form blood clots that can block an artery. Often, such a clot is jarred loose and floats through the blood stream until it becomes lodged in a smaller blood vessel. The blood flow is cut off and a stroke occurs. This type of stroke is called an embolic stroke.

Blood vessels weakened by injury or hypertension (high blood pressure) may break and allow blood to flow into or around the brain and destroy tissue. This causes a stroke known as a cerebral hemorrhage or a subarachnoid hemorrhage. A cerebral hemorrhage is when blood flows into the brain, and a subarachnoid hemorrhage is when a blood vessel on the surface of the brain ruptures and bleeds into the space between the brain and the skull.

Strokes can be categorized by severity into three types: transient ischemic attack, stroke in progress, and completed stroke. Transient ischemic attacks (TIA) precede more severe strokes in about 10 percent of cases. A transient ischemic attack is a blockage of one small blood vessel to the brain. Stroke symptoms such as loss of vision or tingling in the limbs may last from a few minutes to 24 hours, then disappear. TIAs are usually a warning sign of a more serious stroke to follow.

A stroke in progress is a stroke that begins suddenly and steadily worsens during the following few hours or days. The symptoms may include a tingling or numbness of a limb or one side of the body that develops into total paralysis.

A completed stroke is one in which the blood has been interrupted in its flow, and brain damage has occurred. This may result in paralysis to one side of the body, vision loss of one half of the field of vision or one eye, slurred speech, mental confusion, coma, and death.

All three types of stroke may impair vision. Total vision may be lost in one eye, or one-half of the visual field of both eyes may be lost. This condition is called HEMIANOPSIA and is also present, temporarily, in migraine headaches. Loss of vision may be a result of stroke, a symptom of a stroke in progress, or a TIA, a warning sign of a more serious stroke to follow.

Double vision may result from a stroke if the muscles of one eye become paralyzed or damaged. The weakened muscles may not be able to focus the eye properly on an object that the unimpaired eye views. The brain receives images of two different objects, and double vision occurs.

If the stroke damages the brain stem, NYSTAGMUS may occur. Nystagmus is a constant, involuntary movement of the eyes. The condition may impair vision, but the patient can often learn through rehabilitation to work with the condition to see adequately.

Patients suffering from any stroke symptoms require immediate medical attention. The symptoms may be temporary or sustained and include weakness or tingling of face or limbs, difficulty with speaking or understanding speech, hemianopsia, blurring of vision, double vision, total loss of vision in one eye, headache, dizziness, inability to swallow, mental confusion, and loss of memory.

Treatment of stroke may include the use of anticoagulants or blood thinning drugs to reduce the risk of arteriosclerosis. In the case of TIAs, a surgical procedure called carotid endarterectomy may be called for if the stroke was caused by a stenosis or narrowing of the carotid artery. The stenosis is caused by arteriosclerotic plaque that is removed during the procedure.

After a stroke, patients may enter rehabilitative therapy to regain lost abilities. Physical therapy may help restore coordination and use of impaired limbs. Occupational therapy may assist in the recuperation of hand movements and provide alternative methods for performing daily tasks. Speech therapy may improve the ability to communicate. Often, psychiatrists, psychologists, social workers, and vocational rehabilitation counselors may be called on to assist in the rehabilitation process.

Those who survive stroke usually maintain a plateau or a period of no change in condition after the stroke. The plateau may last for hours or days. The recovery period may be rapid or last months and range from complete restoration of abilities to maintenance of long-lasting or permanent impairments. The degree of recovery is dependent on the damage done to the brain, the type of stroke and the condition and age of the patient.

In the last 30 years, death due to stroke has been reduced 30 to 40 percent. In 1950, the death rate due to stroke was 88.8 per 100,000 people. In 1985 the rate was 32.8 per 100,000. The rate continues to fall, and since 1973, the average rate of decline has been 5.5 percent per year. From 1988 to 1998, the stroke death rate dropped 15.5 percent.

This may be because of increased awareness of stroke risk factors. Several conditions are recognized as risk factors for stroke. They are hypertension, heart disease, diabetes, high red-blood-cell count, TIAs, cigarette smoking, and obesity. Treatment or control of these conditions may reduce the risk of stroke.

subluxation of the lens   Subluxation of the CRYSTALLINE LENS occurs when the lens becomes partially displaced due to a break in the fibers of the ZONULES that hold it in place. The condition may be congenital or acquired. It may be caused by a blow to the eye or other injury, MARFAN'S SYNDROME, homocystinuria (a metabolic congenital disorder associated with mental retardation), and aging.

Symptoms of subluxation of the lens include rapid changes in vision and increased myopia (nearsightedness) due to the increased mobility of the lens. On examination, the IRIS may appear wobbly or tremulous, and the lens may be visible in the pupil. The lens may subluxate up and out, as in Marfan's syndrome, down and in, as in homocystinuria, backwards into the VITREOUS, a condition called posterior subluxation, or forward into the ANTERIOR CHAMBER, a condition called anterior subluxation.

Subluxated lenses may develop CATARACTS or may become trapped in the pupil. Aqueous fluid production forces the trapped lens into the anterior chamber, where it may cause a rise in intraocular pressure, or secondary GLAUCOMA.

When the lens has drifted to the anterior chamber, the pupils are dilated and the patient is set in a supine position to encourage the lens to fall back into place behind the iris. If the lens falls into place, the pupils are immediately constricted with miotic drops, although recurrences are common. If the lens fails to move into position, it is surgically removed, or a peripheral iridectomy is performed to allow aqueous flow.

When the lens moves into the POSTERIOR CHAMBER, it may be left untouched if it does not cause UVEITIS or cataract. In such cases, the lens may be removed. If the lens moves from the central pupil area, becomes completely dislocated or detached or is removed, the eye becomes aphakic, or without a lens. Aphakic characteristics such as lack of accommodation, enlarged image, and color distortion can be corrected with prescription contact lenses or spectacles.

Sullivan, Anne Anne Mansfield Sullivan Macy was the teacher and companion to Helen Keller. Born in 1866 in Feeding Hills, Massachusetts, she developed TRACHOMA at age five. The eye disease arose from the poverty and unsanitary conditions of her environment and slowly destroyed her sight.

In 1874, she was sent to a state poorhouse in Tewksbury where she remained off and on for six years. Five unsuccessful operations were performed on her eyes that alleviated the pain but did not improve her sight.

In 1880, Sullivan entered the Perkins Institution for the Blind in Boston. During her time at the Institution, she received two eye operations that improved her vision. Sullivan graduated from Perkins in 1886, as valedictorian of her class.

In 1887, Sullivan was recommended by the Perkins Institution as a teacher for a deaf-blind child named Helen Keller. Sullivan went to live with the Keller family and battled with the unruly child, attempting to teach her the fingerspelling for various objects in the environment. Keller was unable to link the importance of the spelling to the meaning of the object until one day at the well when Sullivan poured water on Keller's hand while fingerspelling W-A-T-E-R into the other hand.

Keller went on to master the manual and braille alphabet under the tutelage of Sullivan on whom Keller bestowed the lifelong title of "Teacher." Keller attended and graduated from Radcliffe in 1904, with the assistance of Sullivan, who attended classes with Keller and translated class lectures and texts.

When Keller began writing articles and her book *The Story of My Life,* John Macy, an editor and Harvard instructor, was recommended to the two women as an editor and writing assistant. Macy and Sullivan married in 1905, and Keller lived with the couple. Sullivan continued to assist Keller in her writing and lecturing career. The marriage grew troubled and Macy sailed alone to Europe in 1913. In 1914, Polly Thomson joined Sullivan and Keller as a companion and assistant.

In 1929, Sullivan's right eye was removed to relieve constant pain. Her vision in the remaining eye and her general health deteriorated rapidly. Sullivan died in 1936. Her ashes reside next to those of Helen Keller and Polly Thomson.

Supplemental Security Income See SOCIAL SECURITY BENEFITS.

surgical procedures Surgery may be required in the treatment of an eye disorder or disease. According to the type of disorder, surgery may be indicated immediately or reserved as a later alternative in cases that do not respond to medication.

CATARACT removal is the most common surgery performed in the United States. There are two main types of cataract surgery: phacoemulsification and extracapsular.

During phacoemulsification, which is the most common method of cataract removal, a small incision is made on the side of the cornea, and a tiny probe is inserted into the eye. The probe produces ultrasound waves that break up the cloudy center of the lens. The lens can then be removed, using suction.

In extracapsular surgery, a slightly longer incision is made on the side of the cornea, and the surgeon removes the hard center of the lens. The remainder of the lens is then removed using suction.

Once the cloudy lens has been removed, it is usually replaced with a clear artificial lens called an intraocular lens (IOL). The IOL becomes a permanent part of the eye and does not require any additional care or attention. The person wearing the IOL does not feel or see it. In some cases, patients cannot have an IOL, due to problems that occur during surgery or another eye problem. In these cases, a soft contact lens or glasses may be used instead.

Certain types and conditions of GLAUCOMA necessitate surgery. Two major forms of surgery are IRIDECTOMY and filtering surgery, called TRABECULECTOMY. An iridectomy is a surgical procedure in which a portion of the iris is removed to eliminate the blockage of angle-closure glaucoma and prevent further attacks. A trabeculectomy bypasses damaged meshwork and creates a new drainage tract to allow the aqueous to flow from the eye.

CORNEAL TRANSPLANT, or keratoplasty, uses a donor CORNEA to replace all or part of a diseased cornea and restore vision. A section of donor cornea is measured to the precise needs of the host and removed from the donor cornea with scissors. A corresponding section of host cornea is measured and removed. The donor cornea is placed into the remaining cavity and sewn into position with small stitches or sutures.

Tear duct surgery is often indicated in cases of WET EYE. Obstructions are cleared surgically by simple probe and irrigation or silicone intubation procedures, or the more serious surgical procedure, a dacryocystorhinostomy.

A TARSORRHAPHY is a surgical procedure in which a section of the eyelids is stitched together at the corner of the eye. The surgery is performed in the treatment of dendritic ulcers, Bell's palsy, thyroid disease, or any disorder in which the eye is in danger of overexposure or drying.

ENUCLEATION is the surgical removal of the eyeball. Enucleation is performed when the eye contains a malignant tumor, when the eye is blind and causes pain, and when the eye is nearly blind and sympathetic ophthalmia (an inflammation that occurs in both eyes as a result of injury to one eye) is a risk.

RADIAL KERATOTOMY (RK) surgery is elective surgery designed to improve MYOPIA (nearsightedness). The surgery uses radial cuts or incisions to reshape the cornea.

sympathetic ophthalmia A rare condition in which one eye becomes inflamed as a result of an injury or trauma to the other eye. The condition is most common among children and occurs following a perforation injury or surgery. It also can occur if a foreign body remains in the eye, causing great irritation.

Sympathetic ophthalmia occurs when the injured eye remains inflamed and infected due to insufficient or delayed cleansing. Over a period of two weeks to several months, an inflammatory response occurs in the UVEA. Examination of the choroid reveals the presence of eosinophils, giant cells and lymphocytes, serious signals that threaten sight in the eye.

After a period of two weeks to several years, the inflammation spreads to the unaffected eye. Symptoms of blurred vision or PHOTOPHOBIA develop. An eye examination with the slit lamp reveals the presence of granulomatous keratic precipitates on the posterior surface of the cornea, a condition that endangers vision.

Sympathetic ophthalmia can be prevented by earnest attention to cleansing and care of the affected eye or by enucleating (surgically removing) the initially injured eye within a two-week period following the injury. Any severely injured eye that remains inflamed or infected up to a two-week period may need to be removed to prevent sympathetic ophthalmia.

If sympathetic ophthalmia occurs after the two-week time period, the condition may be treated with local and systemic steroids. The treatment is often successful, but the condition is inclined to recur.

synechiae A condition in which the IRIS adheres to either the CORNEA or the LENS. The iris/cornea adhesion is termed anterior synechiae and the iris/lens adhesion is termed posterior synechiae. Synechiae of either type may be caused by anterior UVEITIS, an inflammation of the iris and/or ciliary body. Anterior synechiae may be caused by perforation of the cornea or injuries.

Posterior synechiae may cause a blockage of aqueous flow and an iris bombe, in which the iris bows forward unnaturally. This interferes with the flow of AQUEOUS FLUID and causes secondary GLAUCOMA, a disease in which the accumulation of aqueous fluid causes a rise in intraocular pressure.

Symptoms of synechiae include redness, pain, oversensitivity to light, pus in the anterior chamber on examination, constricted pupil, and inability of the pupil to dilate. Synechiae is treated according to its cause. Since the condition generally includes inflammation of the iris, or IRITIS, the treatment usually involves local steroids and mydriatic drops to dilate the pupil. Some injury-induced synechiae may be self-limiting.

synthetic speech Artificial speech created by speech synthesizers. Speech synthesizers convert printed speech into spoken words to put information into, or remove information from, a computer. The first speech synthesizer was invented in 1936 by H. W. Dudley, a scientist at Bell Labs. The machine required an operator with a keyboard and foot pedals to provide the pitch, timing, and intensity of speech. Dudley's machine was called a voice coder, but soon became known as "The Voder."

Many commercially available personal-computer software programs may be used with synthesizers that read material that appears on the computer screen or information sent to it from the computer.

Speech synthesis may be used to access personal electronic mail and general print information as well. Electronic mail or E-mail is a system of receiving and sending personal communications through the personal computer. It is an instant, and with the use of Braille printers or speech synthesis, private form of communication accessible to individuals with visual impairments.

General print information is accessible via speech synthesis through reading machines such as the Kurzweil Reader. Printed material placed on the scanning screen is scanned and read aloud. The voices of synthetic speech read English words and numerals and are available in various forms of male, female, or robotic voice, adult or child voice, voice pitch, speed, and volume. Some synthesizers offer foreign languages, talking calculators, singing, music with several octaves of pitch, musical keyboards, and sound effects.

The voice is projected over an internal speaker, external speaker, earphones, or telephone, depending on the type of hardware. Often, a section of the standard keyboard, a hand or foot switch or a keyboard on a control box is used to control that section of the screen that will be read and how it will be read. Most programs offer options of reading the text letter by letter or word by word and verbalization of the punctuation.

Synthetic speech is a breakthrough in independence for those with visual impairments. The individual can privately transmit and receive personal documents and produce work-related material independently. It allows free access to information at times and in situations convenient to the individual, and not dependent on the assistance of others. Many advances are being made in this area as technology continues to develop.

ABLEDATA. *Speech Synthesizers.* Newington, Connecticut: ABLEDATA, 1989.

Chong, Curtis. "Speech Output for the IBM Personal Computer." *The Braille Monitor* (January 1986): 37–47.

Hagen, Dolores. *Microcomputer Resource Book for Special Education.* Reston, Virginia: Reston Publishing Company Inc., 1984.

Lauer, Harvey, and Leonard Mowinski. *Recommending Computers for the Visually Impaired: A Moving Target or a Losing War?* HealthNet Library. Columbus, Ohio: CompuServe, 1989.

syphilis A venereal disease caused by the spirochete *Treponema pallidum.* The disease may cause ocular disorders both congenitally and after birth.

Approximately 800 cases of congenital syphilis were reported in 1998. Syphilis is transmitted congenitally from the infected mother to the fetus through the womb after the fourth month of pregnancy when the spirochete can pass through the placenta. Congenital syphilis may result in vision loss and ocular impairment, deafness, dental defects, mental retardation, organ damage, and death.

Ocular damage may involve severe KERATITIS, or corneal inflammation, and chorioretinal scarring. Although the infection is present at birth, the keratitis may develop later in life between ages 5 and 25. Severe keratitis may be treated with medication but may result in corneal opacification and PHOTOPHOBIA.

Syphilis contracted after birth can cause chorioretinal scarring, IRITIS (an inflammation of the iris), and OPTIC NERVE atrophy or degeneration. Syphilis can be diagnosed with a Wasserman test, a blood test to determine the presence of the spirochete in the blood. An eye examination may also determine the presence of the disease and is often used to confirm the diagnosis.

Syphilis is treated with ANTIBIOTICS, and ocular disorders are treated with medication. If treated in the early stages, the damage resulting syphilis may be mild. Congenital syphilis can be prevented if the disease of the mother is treated and controlled before the fifth month of pregnancy. Toward this purpose, most states have developed laws that require testing for syphilis at the beginning of each pregnancy. (See VENEREAL DISEASE.)

Centers for Disease Control. "Congenital Syphilis—United States," 1998. www.cdc.gov., 1999.

tactile aids   Tactile aids provide information that visually impaired individuals access through the sense of touch. These may include braille materials, braille-marked tools, or adaptive aids.

Braille materials, printed materials that are read with the fingertips, are reproduced by transcribers, publishers, and printing houses such as the AMERICAN PRINTING HOUSE FOR THE BLIND. Braille markings are found on adaptive aids such as rulers, measuring cups, and clocks in place of printed letters or numbers. A Braillewriter is a six-key typewriter for typing braille. It produces raised dots onto specially designed, heavy braille paper.

The SLATE AND STYLUS are writing tools used to write braille. The user places a sheet of braille paper between the two metal plates of the slate. The stylus, a short metal prong fastened to a handle, is held in the palm and pressed downward onto the paper within an open window. The stylus pushes the paper against the corresponding indentation of the braille cell dot on the bottom plate. A raised dot is formed on the reverse side of the paper. The writing is read when the paper is turned over and the dots are facing upward.

Templates and writing guides are frames used in writing on lines or in specified spaces. Window openings in the templates serve as a guide for signing checks or writing letters. Raised line paper is writing paper with embossed lines to enable the user to follow a straight writing path.

PAPERLESS BRAILLE or cassette braille is an information system that is stored on audio cassette tapes and accessed in braille. The user runs his fingers over display cells to read the text and pushes a button to access the next segment of recorded material. The user can produce, edit, and record braille with the system. It can be adapted for use with computer terminals, calculators, and typewriters.

A raised-line drawing kit is a board covered with a soft underlay of rubber. The user places a sheet of acetate over the board and draws on it, creating raised lines and an embossed picture.

Tactile color is a standardized system of 12 distinctive colors, each assigned a specific texture. This allows visually impaired persons to better participate in creating or enjoying visual artwork. It is also useful in map-making, for labeling, and as an educational resource.

A thermoform machine is a device that heats a sheet of plastic paper so that it may be molded to whatever shape is placed beneath it. Thermoform machines produce copies of braille and can be used to create raised line maps or graphs.

TACTILE MAPS and globes are three-dimensional maps that are used as an orientation aid. They contain raised surfaces, textures, and braille markings and are designed to be read with the fingertips, in a manner similar to braille.

The Cranmer abacus is an abacus that has been adapted to prevent the beads from accidentally sliding. It is used to perform mathematical computations.

The Optacon is a reading machine that converts print into tactual letter configurations. The user scans a small camera over a line of print with the right hand, while resting the left hand on an electronic array. The machine electronically converts each letter into a print letter configuration formed on the array by vibrating pins and read by the left index finger.

See ADAPTIVE AIDS.

tactile maps   Tactile maps or globes are three-dimensional maps that may be used by visually impaired persons as an orientation aid. As opposed to large-print maps that label areas with large print and thick, dark lines on a contrasting light background, tactile maps contain raised surfaces, textures, and braille markings. They are designed to be read with the fingertips, in a manner similar to braille.

Tactile maps may be used to represent countries, states, cities, or site locations. Tactile maps are commonly found in large publicly used facilities such as hospitals, hotels, universities, airports, and train stations to enable visually impaired visitors to navigate independently.

Geographic embossed tactile maps are professionally available, but instructors often produce their own maps for students when commercial maps are not available.

Tactile maps may be produced in a variety of ways. An instructor may trace a map onto paper placed on top of a piece of screening material. The underlying screen forces holes to form in the paper as it is traced. The student traces the line of holes to follow the map lines.

Aluminum foil is also used as a map material. Several layers of cloth or foam padding is placed on a table. A sheet of foil is placed on top and the reverse side of the map is placed on top of the foil. The map is traced in reverse onto the foil, resulting in a raised line map in the foil. Water is differentiated from land by using cross-hatching marks or dots. Similar methods include using dried glue to make raised lines, felt areas pasted onto a cardboard backing, and raised-line drawing kits.

Professional quality maps can be produced with thermoform, the method used to reproduce braille books. Thermoform is a device that heats a sheet of plastic paper so that it may be molded to whatever shape is placed beneath it. Using a thermoform machine, an instructor places a topographical map, including braille lettering, into the device and reproduces it onto a plastic thermoform page.

Tactile maps are approached systematically. The outlines or borders are first traced, and then the inner portions of the map are read. Tactile maps may be larger than standard print maps or may cover a smaller portion of an area in a larger size map in order to accommodate reading by fingertips. (See ORIENTATION AIDS.)

talking books   See NATIONAL LIBRARY SERVICE FOR THE BLIND AND PHYSICALLY HANDICAPPED.

targeted jobs tax credit   See WORK OPPORTUNITY TAX CREDIT.

tarsorrhaphy   A surgical procedure in which a section of the eyelids is stitched together at the corner of the eye. The surgery may be performed in the treatment of dendritic ulcers, Bell's palsy, thyroid disease, or any disorder in which the eye is in danger of overexposure or drying. Tarsorrhaphy is reversible and may be used temporarily.

tax benefits   Additional income tax deductions are available to legally blind individuals. The amount that may be deducted varies depending on marital status and age. A married blind individual, for instance, may deduct an additional $850. Single blind individuals may deduct an additional $1,100. To qualify for the deduction, an individual must be legally blind, which means he or she must have a visual acuity of 20/200 in the better eye, after correction, or a visual field of 20 degrees or less in the better eye after correction. The individual must attach to the tax return a statement from an ophthalmologist confirming legal blindness.

Some medical expenses, such as eyeglasses, necessary home improvements, dog guides, tuition for special education, prosthetic eyes, and, in some cases, attendant care, also may be deducted from income if itemized.

Taylor slate   One of the earliest manipulative/tactile aids for visually impaired students studying mathematics. The slate measures about 11 by 17 inches, with holes running across and up and down in columns. Each hole looks like a plus sign (+) overlying an "X." The one-inch pegs have the same shape as the holes and are stored in a tray on the slate when not in use. At one end of each peg there is a bar, and at the other end there are two conical projections. The angle at which each peg is inserted into the hole determines the numerical value represented. Very popular through the

1930s and into the 1940s, the Taylor slate is no longer used.

teacher-consultant The teacher-consultant model is one of five major education models or plans for the instruction of visually impaired students; the other models are RESIDENTIAL SCHOOL, SELF-CONTAINED CLASSROOM, RESOURCE ROOM, and ITINERANT TEACHER.

The teacher-consultant is a special educator who advises regular classroom teachers, teacher aides, administrators, and other school personnel in methods that will meet the visually impaired student's needs. The greatest proportion of the work is consultative, rather than instructive. The teacher-consultant travels from school to school and often from county to county to work with personnel. Since traveling time is significant, little time remains for direct instruction with the student.

The teacher-consultant model works best for students who work independently and require minimal skills training. The program is least effective for students who require intensive skills training or lack coping behaviors for study in a regular classroom.

Barraga, Natalie C. *Visual Handicaps and Learning.* Belmont, Calif.: Wadsworth Publishing Company Inc., 1976.
Scholl, Geraldine, ed. *Foundations of Education for Blind and Visually Handicapped Children and Youth.* New York: American Foundation for the Blind, 1986.

tear system The tear or nasolacrimal system is the system that the eye uses to produce, maintain and eliminate tears from the eye. Tears protect, nourish, and moisturize the eye. Without proper tear function, as in dry eye, the CORNEA and CONJUNCTIVA may become dry and develop disorders.

In the normal eye, the tear film is made up of three layers, which are produced by the lacrimal gland and accessory lacrimal glands and cells. The lacrimal glands are located in the ORBIT and inner eyelid. The accessory glands and cells are located in the conjunctiva.

The top layer of tears is formed by the secretion of the meibomian glands and is oily in nature. The second layer is composed of watery tears from the lacrimal glands, and the third layer, which lies next to the cornea, is of mucouslike consistency and is produced by accessory glands. The layers are maintained by constant blinking and are all necessary for proper health of the eye.

Tears are constantly being produced and drained from the eye. They drain through lacrimal puncta, holes in each inner corner of the upper and lower lids. The tears are gathered in the lacrimal sac, an organ at the junction of the nose and lower lid. The tears then pass under the tissue to drainage ducts in the nasal cavity.

The nasolacrimal system is subject to functional disorders, obstructions and infections that may result in WET EYE, DRY EYE, or DACRYOCYSTITIS. Inadequate drainage of tears leads to wet eye. Wet eye may be a congenital or acquired condition. Congenital wet eye occurs as a result of obstructions to the nasolacrimal ducts. Symptoms include tearing, crusting of the lids or eyelashes, mucous discharge, and inflammation of the lacrimal sac.

Obstructions often clear spontaneously within the first 12 months of life. After this time, obstructions are cleared surgically by simple probe and irrigation or silicone intubation procedures or the more serious surgical procedure, dacryocystorhinostomy, which connects the lacrimal sac to the nasal cavity.

Acquired obstructions usually occur in middle age, and most commonly among women. Tearing becomes severe and annoying. The simple procedures of probe and irrigation or silicone intubation are often ineffective, and a dacryocystorhinostomy is indicated.

The condition of dry eye may occur as a result of poor tear production (called keratoconjunctivitis sicca), poor tear quality, or inadequate blinking, which leaves the eye open to the drying elements or which does not properly wet the entire surface of the eye.

Symptoms of dry eye include burning, irritation, redness, and loss of corneal luster. Conditions that can cause dry eye include SARCOIDOSIS, rheumatoid arthritis, vitamin-A deficiency, pemphigoid, TRACHOMA, Stevens-Johnson syndrome, chemical burns, neuroparalytic and exposure KERATITIS, and AGING.

Dry eye may lead to corneal damage, permanent corneal scarring, and opacification. Once the cornea has opacified, vision is lost.

Treatment of dry eye includes treating the underlying cause or disease and the administration of artificial tears. In some cases, ANTIBIOTICS may be prescribed, and the use of home vaporizers or humidifiers may be advised. Surgery may be performed to close the tear drainage ducts to ensure better utilization of reduced tear production. If the cornea is severely scarred and vision is lost, a CORNEAL TRANSPLANT, or keratoplasty, may be indicated. However, those with dry eye conditions are generally poor candidates for a successful corneal transplantation.

Dacryocystitis is an inflammation of the tear drainage sac caused by an infection. It usually affects one eye only and may become a chronic disorder. It is most commonly found in adult females, and may be caused congenitally, from a blockage or obstruction of the tear duct or from a trauma or injury. The resulting infection is caused most often by bacteria such as *Staphylococcus aureus* and beta-hemolytic streptococcus, and by fungi such as *Candida albicans*. Symptoms may include constant tearing, swelling, discharge, and tenderness of the eye. A culture of the discharge may identify the infecting agent.

Dacryocystitis is usually treated with warm compresses and topical or systemic antibiotics. Blocked nasolacrimal ducts of infants may be massaged to encourage dilation. If the duct fails to open, it may require probe and irrigation therapy. If the condition produces an abscess, it may be drained.

technology   See COMPUTERS.

telebraille   A braille telephone device for deaf-blind persons. Manufactured by TELESENSORY SYSTEMS, INC., the device is a modified TDD (telecommunications device for the deaf) system, which provides braille input and output. The system contains a standard TDD, including a standard alphabet keyboard and visual character display, plus a braille keyboard and refreshable braille display.

The telebraille can be used to communicate with other standard TDDs over telephone lines or as an aid in communication for deaf-blind persons. In a conversation, the sighted person types words onto the standard TDD unit. The text is translated into braille and is read by the deaf-blind person on the refreshable display. To reply, the deaf-blind person types words on the braille keyboard, they are translated to text and read by the sighted person on the visual display. There have been several versions of the telebraille. The latest is TeleBraille III.

Telephone Pioneers of America   A service-oriented fraternal group made up of current and retired employees with 15 or more years of service within the telephone industry. Established in 1911, the membership has grown to 800,000 members and maintains a budget of $4 million.

The organization sustains three goals: fellowship, loyalty, and service. Fellowship and loyalty goals are met by providing opportunities for telephone employees to develop friendships, accurately preserve the history of telephone technology, and acknowledge the contributions of members.

Service programs provide services to the disabled, including braille transcription, talking book recording, support of eye banks, and development and repair of communication, mobility, and recreational aids. Additional programs encompass volunteer hospital services, work with the elderly, education, safety and health programs, and collection drives.

Telephone Pioneers of America maintains 84 chapters in the United States, Canada, and Mexico. They hold a yearly convention and print a quarterly publication, *The Telephone Pioneer*.

Contact:

Telephone Pioneers of America
930 15th Street, Suite 1200
Denver, CO 80202
303-571-1200 (ph)
303-572-0520 (fax)
www.telephone-pioneers.org

Telesensory Systems, Inc.   (TSI)   A company that designs, manufactures, and markets equipment for blind and visually impaired persons. The company was founded in 1970 when four members of the electrical engineering department at Stanford University developed the technology that was the basis for the Optacon, a portable electronic print-reading device that was the company's first product. The Optacon was developed specifically to help the visually impaired daughter of one of the inventors.

Today, the company provides personal computers, scanners, speech-output systems, video magnifiers, braille-based computer systems, braille printers, and closed-circuit television systems. TSI has more than 300 dealers, distributors, and resellers across the United States, and its products are available in 50 countries around the world. It maintains sales offices in London, Paris, New York, Detroit, Tampa, and Phoenix.

Contact:

Telesensory Systems Inc.
520 Almanor Ave.
Sunnyvale, CA 94086
408-616-8700 (ph)
408-616-8720 (fax)
www.telesensory.com

terminology   There is no complete consensus on terms concerning the topic of blindness and vision impairment. Rehabilitation experts, doctors, educators, legislators, and other leaders in the field determine and define terminology according to their own preferences and viewpoints.

Over the past 150 years, visual impairments have been described by numerous terms, including medically blind, economically blind, braille blind, educationally blind, functionally blind, partially seeing, partially blind, vocationally blind, legally blind, low vision, visually defective, visually handicapped, visually impaired, visually disabled, and visually limited. In recent years, those involved in the field of blindness and vision impairment have made strides to standardize terms to eliminate confusion or misinterpretation. The following definitions combine common aspects of terms drawn from a variety of sources.

An *impairment* refers to a recognizable defect or malfunctioning of an organ or any part of the body, such as an eye. The defect or malfunction can be diagnosed and defined by a medical doctor. A visually impaired person may range from an individual with no sight to someone with low vision.

A *disability* is the effect the impairment has on the individual to function. It is the limitation, restriction, or disadvantage due to the malfunction.

The word *handicap* stems from "cap in hand," a reference to beggars. Because of this negative connotation, the word *disability* is often the preferred term. A handicap may be defined as a disadvantage in the performance of tasks as a result of expectations or attitudes about the impairment. Disabilities are not necessarily handicaps. When the term visually handicapped is applied to a child it usually refers to the requirement for special educational provisions due to the sight loss.

Visually limited refers to an individual's difficulty in using vision under average circumstances. A visually limited person may be able to see with corrective lenses or optical aids.

Blind is a term many reserve for those with no vision or light perception only. Legally blind is a term defined by the federal government to determine eligibility for benefits. Legal blindness involves central visual acuity of 20/200 or less in the better eye with correction or a field of vision of 20 degrees or less in the better eye with correction.

Partially sighted or *partially seeing* is defined as a central visual acuity between 20/70 and 20/200 in the better eye with correction. *Low vision* is defined as a central visual acuity of between 20/50 and 20/200 in the better eye with correction or a visual field of 20 to 40 degrees or less in the better eye with correction. Low vision, partially sighted, and visually impaired are often used interchangeably to describe individuals with some usable vision, regardless of how little.

Fully sighted individuals are those who have correctable vision to 20/20. The terminology does not include a term for those individuals with correctable vision between 20/20 and 20/50. These people fall between the definitions for the terms fully sighted or low vision.

American Foundation for the Blind. *Low Vision Questions and Answers.* New York: AFB, 1987.

Barraga, Natalie C. *Visual Handicaps and Learning.* Belmont, California: Wadsworth Publishing Company Inc., 1976.

ERIC Clearinghouse on Handicapped and Gifted Children. *ERIC Digest: Visual Impairments.* Reston, Virginia: ERIC, 1982.

Foundation for the Junior Blind. *California Services for Persons with Visual Impairments.* Los Angeles: FJB, 1987.

Kelley, Jerry D., ed. *Recreational Programming for Visually Impaired Children and Youth.* New York: American Foundation for the Blind, 1981.

National Association for Visually Handicapped. *Problems of the Partially Sighted.* New York: NAVH, 1980.

National Information Center for Handicapped Children and Youth. *General Information about Handicaps and People with Handicaps.* Washington, D.C.: NICHC, 1982.

Scholl, Geraldine T. *Foundations of Education for Blind and Visually Handicapped Children and Youth.* New York: American Foundation for the Blind, 1986.

thermoform   A thermoform machine or duplicator is a device that heats a sheet of plastic paper, called BRAILON, so that it may be molded to whatever shape is placed beneath it. Thermoform machines produce copies of braille and can be used to create raised-line maps or graphs. The user places a sheet of thermoform plastic over a page of braille or topographical material and inserts it into the machine. The duplicator reproduces the material onto the Brailon sheet.

Timolol   A drug, in the form of timoptic eye drops or Blocadren tablets, prescribed for open-angle GLAUCOMA and high blood pressure. The drug is a beta-adrenergic blocking agent that also decreases the amount of fluid produced within the eye and increases the fluid elimination rate. The drug has been found to lower intraocular pressure by 26 to 38 percent.

Timolol should not be used by pregnant or nursing women or those who cannot tolerate oral beta-blocking drugs. Care should be exercised by those with upper respiratory disorders such as asthma, hay fever, or allergies. Some patients may suffer side effects that include decreased heart rate, increased possibility of congestive heart failure, lowered blood pressure, insomnia, tingling in the arms or legs, dizziness, depression, and fatigue. Patients may also experience visual problems, including hallucinations, disorientation, personality change, memory loss, and abdominal disorders including diarrhea, constipation, cramps, nausea or vomiting. Reactions such as sore throat, fever, blood system disorders, or upper respiratory difficulties indicate an allergy to the drug.

Psychotropic or psychiatric drugs may interact with Timolol to cause serious problems. Timolol raises the effectiveness of antidiabetic medications. Physicians of diabetics taking Timolol may need to reduce present dosages of insulin or oral medication while the patient is taking Timolol. Timolol also lowers the effectiveness of digitalis, so physicians of heart-disease patients may need to increase the dosage of digitalis while the patient takes Timolol. Timolol may also interact with certain prescription blood pressure medications and over-the-counter cold remedies. These should not be taken with Timolol without a physician's advice.

Symptoms of Timolol overdose include heart failure, decreased heart rate and blood pressure, and upper respiratory problems. Overdose patients require proper treatment at a hospital emergency room. Timolol should be decreased slowly, over a period of time. Abrupt discontinuance can cause serious problems.

tobacco amblyopia   A condition in which the vision is lost due to the use of tobacco. The toxic effects of tobacco constrict the vessels of the body and interfere with circulation. As a result, the OPTIC NERVE swells, a condition known as optic neuritis.

Early symptoms of tobacco amblyopia include painless blurring or loss of central vision that may be accompanied by numbness or tingling in the fingers. If allowed to progress, the blurring may spread to the peripheral visual fields, and optic nerve damage may result. Reduction or elimination of tobacco usage in conjunction with proper nutrition usually restores vision. Patients may be instructed to supplement the diet with additional vitamins, such as B_{12}.

tomography   Also known as computerized axial tomography, tomography is a test that records the way tissues react when exposed to X rays. The computerized process measures the resistance of the soft tissues to the passage of the rays and translates the measurements to pictures on film or video screen. The process intensifies and contrasts sections of the eye, eye orbit and brain, which are indistinguishable with X rays alone.

The process is a computer scan that can isolate segments of the eye as slight as three millimeters thick. It can outline the CRYSTALLINE LENS apart from the surrounding AQUEOUS FLUID and point out tumors to the back of the eye, such as in the CHOROID, which would be invisible to standard X rays. Computerized axial tomography can often be used as a safer alternative to more expensive and risky procedures that require hospitalization, such as injection of air or radiopaque dyes.

tonography A test to determine the fluid pressure within the eye, called intraocular pressure. The test is conducted as part of the routine annual eye examination.

A *tonometer* is used to conduct the test. This is a small instrument probe that is attached to a biomicroscope or slit lamp. The biomicroscope is an instrument that illuminates and magnifies the front part of the eye. The examiner looks through the biomicroscope as the test is conducted.

The test is painless. The eyes are prepared by first inserting anesthetic drops. Next, the examiner gently touches a strip of paper laced with fluorescein dye to the inside of each lower lid. The released orange dye mixes with the eye's tears and covers the CORNEA.

The examiner shines a blue light on each eye and then gently touches the cornea with the tonometer. When the probe touches the cornea, a pattern is created in the dye. The intraocular pressure is measured by the amount of force needed to create the pattern. A normal reading varies from 14 to 21. A higher reading may indicate the presence of GLAUCOMA. The procedure is regularly performed as a glaucoma screening test and often is a step in presurgical evaluations to determine whether surgery is immediately prudent.

tonometer See TONOGRAPHY.

toxic amblyopia A condition in which vision is lost as a result of the absorption of toxic agents or the deficiency of nutrients. The condition, also known as nutritional amblyopia, is usually bilateral, and although in the case of wood alcohol and arsenic poisoning the vision loss is irreparable, it generally tends not to be permanent.

Some poisons induce a central vision blurring or scotoma, a blind spot. These include tobacco, ethyl alcohol, methyl alcohol, carbon disulphide, halogenated hydrocarbons, aromatic amino and nitrocompounds, sedatives such as barbiturates, opium, and morphine, anti-infective compounds and other drugs, and the metals lead and thallium.

Other compounds produce a reduction of the peripheral field, or tunnel vision. These include organic arsenic, quinine, carbon tetrachloride, methyl iodide, and the drugs salicylic acid, hydrocupreine derivatives, ergot, and aspidium.

Alcohol and tobacco amblyopia are common conditions. Overuse of either compound affects the OPTIC NERVE and OPTIC DISK, causing optic atrophy. A slow, progressive loss of central vision and, often, color vision follows. Both conditions are associated with poor nutrition or diet, which also affects ocular function. Treatment with VITAMINS and minerals as well as reduction of alcohol and tobacco use often restores vision.

Vitamin and mineral deficiencies are linked to nutritional amblyopia. Lack of vitamin A in the diet causes blindness. A lack of zinc prevents the body from using adequate vitamin A stored in the body. Thiamine and B_{12} deficiencies may cause optic neuropathy and vision loss. Generally, intensive vitamin therapy and proper nutrition can restore lost vision.

toxocariasis An infection caused by dog tapeworm eggs called *Toxocara canis*. Human infection occurs with ingestion of infected fecal material. An estimated 10,000 cases of toxocariasis occur annually in humans in the United States.

The larvae causes acute CHORIORETINITIS, an inflammation of the CHOROID and RETINA. The infection spreads rapidly, involving the VITREOUS and clouding it with inflammatory cells. As the center portion of the globe becomes involved, the condition is termed ENDOPHTHALMITIS. Complete loss of sight in the affected eye may result. The condition may be treated with steroids, and VITREC-TOMY (removal and replacement of the vitreous) may be performed in advanced cases.

toxoplasmosis   An infection caused by the parasite *Toxoplasma gondii,* a protozoan carried by wild or domesticated animals such as cats. Toxoplasmosis causes CHOROIDITIS (or posterior uveitis), an inflammation of the CHOROID. More than 60 million people in the United States are probably infected with the toxoplasma parasite, according to the Division of Parasitic Diseases of the Centers for Disease Control and Prevention. Very few people develop symptoms, however, because the immune system keeps the parasite from causing illness.

Toxoplasmosis occurs when the parasite infects the body and enters the blood stream through ingestion of infected material. Adult infection is usually moderate, but the parasite may be transmitted through the placenta and can cause serious infections in children. Congenital toxoplasmosis affects the brain and eyes and may cause epilepsy or mental developmental problems. Both eyes may develop choroiditis or CHORIORETINITIS of the macular region, a vision-threatening disorder.

The *Toxoplasma* parasite lives in fundus lesions of the eye, which can be dye tested to confirm a diagnosis. However, the diagnosis must be carefully made since a large portion of the population has been infected with the parasite at some time even though they may be unaware of any symptoms of the infection.

Symptoms of toxoplasmosis chorioretinitis or choroiditis include blurred vision and the appearance of floaters, possibly preceded by a fever. Treatment of the condition is unsatisfactory but may include systemic steroids or a combination of steroids and antibiotics if the infection threatens the macular region of the retina.

Most cases resolve themselves over time, leaving chorioretinal scarring near the macula. Recurrences are common and tend to originate on the borders of scarred areas.

See UVEITIS.

toys and games   Although many familiar toys and games played by sighted individuals are appro-priate for use by those with little or no vision, others, which have been specially adapted, are available through adaptive-aids catalogs and organizations that serve the visually impaired.

Many games differ little from the original versions and merely require tactile markings for numbers, letters, or space delineation to be adaptable. Others are original games specially designed for the needs and goals of the visually impaired.

Board and card games are adapted with raised dots, braille, large print, a change in playing pieces or some other type of tactile marking. Playing cards are printed in large print, braille, or a combination of the two for use by both sighted and visually impaired players.

Checkers is played on an adapted board with raised and recessed squares using square and round playing pieces. Chess is played on a similar board which may be drilled to hold pegs projecting from under the chess pieces. Since each piece is distinguishable by shape, the only adaptation may be a point on top to distinguish the white from the black.

Many popular games such as Monopoly, Scrabble, bingo, backgammon, cribbage, dice, dominoes, Chinese checkers and tic tac toe have been modified with large print, braille, or shape changes for use by the blind and visually impaired. Board games can be adapted at home by adding glue dots or lines that harden when dry or large-print or braille labels.

Puzzles are available in a variety of forms ranging from children's puzzles, which chime or play a tune when the pieces are in place, to large-print crossword puzzles, to the tactually marked Rubik's Cube.

Balls of all types, including basketballs and outdoor game balls, are available with bells or electronic beepers placed inside to alert the visually impaired user as to the location of the ball. Other adaptations for sports exist, including a bowling rail, which is placed next to the aisle as a bannister guide for visually impaired bowlers.

Educational toys and games for children are available in a myriad of designs. They range from simple tactual clocks to more sophisticated toys, such as the Flexi-Formboard (developed at SMITH-KETTLEWELL EYE RESEARCH INSTITUTE, available from

Adaptive Communication Systems), which contains plastic shapes that fit into a corresponding puzzle board. Placing a shape in its correct location on the board activates a battery-operated toy.

Other such games include modules to teach fine motor skills, braille and large-print spelling machines, math and reading games, bright or fluorescent materials to stimulate visual interest in children with low vision, sensory-stimulation games, biology and science models, and TACTILE MAPS and globes. (See SPORTS AND RECREATION.)

trabeculectomy A surgical procedure performed to treat open-angle GLAUCOMA, a condition in which the intraocular pressure builds within the eye to cause damage and vision loss.

Intraocular pressure is controlled by the flow of AQUEOUS FLUID, a watery liquid that flows through the ANTERIOR CHAMBER, nourishing the avascular LENS and CORNEA and carrying away waste. The intraocular pressure rises when the aqueous fluid of the anterior chamber is unable to properly drain from the eye through the trabecular meshwork.

A trabeculectomy bypasses the damaged meshwork drainage systems and creates a new drainage duct from the eye. During the procedure, the SCLERA, or white part of the eye, is dissected to make a "trapdoor" opening or flap. A block of tissue as thick as the sclera and corneal tissue and containing trabeculum is removed.

Often, an IRIDECTOMY is then performed. A peripheral iridectomy is the removal of a peripheral section of IRIS blocking the anterior angle and deterring aqueous fluid drainage.

After the iridectomy, the opening is sutured shut in a loose stitch that will serve as a trapdoor drainage canal for the aqueous and relieve the intraocular buildup. The conjunctival covering of the sclera is then stitched closed.

A trabeculectomy is performed with local or general anesthesia in a hospital operating room. The procedure usually takes less than an hour. The patient remains hospitalized for up to three days, and eye drops are prescribed for up to one month. Heavy lifting, bending or strenuous activity is not permitted for one month. The results of trabeculectomy surgery vary greatly, depending on factors

such as inflammation, scarring, and healing of the drain.

Complications associated with trabeculectomy include flattened anterior chambers, scarring of the drainage site (which results in continued glaucoma), infection, inflammation, and hemorrhage. Approximately one-third of all trabeculectomy patients develop CATARACTS. (See SURGICAL PROCEDURES.)

trachoma A contagious disease of the eyelids, CONJUNCTIVA and CORNEA. It is a leading cause of blindness in the world and may affect over 500 million people. It has caused blindness in about 6 million people according to the World Health Organization. While practically unknown in the United States, the infection is widespread in underdeveloped countries with poor sanitation and medical care.

Trachoma is caused by the bacteria *Chlamydia trachomatis* and may be linked to bacterial infections caused by agents Koch-Weeks bacillus, Morax Axenfeld diplobacillus, and the gonococcus bacillus. It thrives in overcrowded conditions in which a lack of clean water and poor sewage disposal, sanitation, and hygiene exist. In such conditions, the highly communicable disease may infect an entire community.

The infection attacks both eyes, scarring the conjunctiva inside the eyelid and eventually spreading to the cornea. Initial symptoms include pain, oversensitivity to light, and impaired vision. The eye produces a surplus of tears and a discharge. Muscle spasms develop in the eyelids, and the eyelashes turn inward, which further inflames the cornea. As the cornea becomes more scarred, it becomes more opaque, and blindness may result.

Trachoma can be successfully treated in the early stages with sulpha drugs, ANTIBIOTICS, or surgery. Advanced stages of the disease resist treatment and often result in blindness. A drug called azithromycin is being used in some countries, with good results. Trachoma can be prevented by improving sanitary conditions, such as the water supply, personal hygiene, and medical care. (See WORLD BLINDNESS.)

Transceptor Technologies, Inc.   A company that produces the Personal Companion, a voice-driven communication system designed to aid the blind, visually impaired, and physically disabled user. The companion reads newspapers, personal correspondence and records, enters checkbook data, takes notes, files information, and dials and answers the telephone.

The Personal Companion is activated by the user's voice when spoken through the microphone. Through voice commands, the user accesses the Library for electronic national information networks, the Phone Management System (which automatically dials, receives calls, and takes messages), a calculator for arithmetic functions, the Notepad to take notes and make lists, the Date Book to record appointments and set reminders, the Appliance Controller (which turns any appliance on or off), and the Bank Book for recording information on both savings and checking accounts.

Model 100 is designed for the blind and contains no monitor. Model 100/M is designed with a monitor that displays regular or large print for visually impaired or physically impaired users. Model 100/MPC allows running of IBM-PC compatible software.

Contact:

Transceptor Technologies, Inc.
2001 Commonwealth, Suite 205
Ann Arbor, MI 48105
313-996-1899

transportation laws   Congress has enacted legislation that protects the rights of disabled persons, including those with visual impairments, to use public transportation.

As amended in 1970, the Urban Mass Transportation Act of 1964 (UMTA) requires that mass transportation facilities and services be designed to accommodate use by elderly and disabled persons. A program of grants and loans was authorized in the act to fund such facilities and services.

The act established three programs:

1. The Mass Transportation Technology Research and Demonstration Program funds projects of national priority, including accessibility to mass transportation by elderly and disabled persons.
2. The Urban Mass Transportation Technical Studies Program funds grants for planning, engineering, and designing mass-transportation projects, including those specially designed with accommodation for elderly and disabled passengers in mind.
3. The Urban Mass Transportation Demonstration Grants Program funds demonstration projects that improve accessibility using innovative methods.

The National Mass Transportation Assistance Act of 1974 amended the Urban Mass Transportation formula-grant program by requiring project applicants to set fares for elderly and disabled passengers traveling at nonpeak hours at one-half the normal, peak-hour fare price. The amendment allowed local transportation systems which transport elderly and disabled persons for free to remain eligible for federal formula-grant aid.

The Surface Transportation and Uniform Relocation Assistance Act of 1987 required the Secretary of Transportation to conduct a feasibility study for standards development for UMTA-funded programs concerning tactile aids to improve accessibility to blind and visually impaired passengers.

The Omnibus Budget Reconciliation Act of 1987 founded a three-year demonstration project operated by the Easter Seal Society to improve accessibility to transportation for disabled persons. The program uses UMTA funds to develop methods for identifying disabled persons within the community, outreach strategies, and training programs for transit operators and disabled persons.

The Surface Transportation and Uniform Relocation Assistance Act of 1987 authorized a 95 percent federal share of the cost for specific capital improvement projects (excluding those required by federal law) that improve accessibility to elderly and disabled persons using mass transportation. The act authorized grant assistance for programs that concern human-resource needs relating to mass transportation.

The Federal-Aid Highway Act of 1973 authorized use of highway improvement funds to improve accessibility to disabled and elderly passengers using transportation facilities.

The Rail Passenger Service Act as amended by the Amtrak Improvement Act of 1973 founded the National Railroad Passenger Corporation. The corporation is responsible for taking all necessary steps to ensure accessibility to disabled and elderly persons on all intercity transportation and on passenger trains operated by the corporation.

The Federal Aviation Act of 1958 as amended in 1986 by the Air Carrier Access Act prohibits discrimination against disabled persons in the use of air transportation. The act directed the Department of Transportation to promulgate regulations ensuring nondiscrimination "consistent with the safe carriage of all passengers on air carriers."

The Americans with Disabilities Act of 1989, a bill passed by the senate and the House of Representatives in fall 1990, addresses the issue of public services including public transportation. It mandates that all new transportation facilities and services (not including air travel) must be accessible to disabled persons and that all new buses and trains solicited 30 days after enactment of the bill must be accessible.

U.S. Department of Education. *Summary of Existing Legislation Affecting Persons with Disabilities.* Washington, D.C.: USDE, 1988.

transpupillary thermotherapy (TTT) A new experimental laser treatment for patients who have the wet form of age-related macular degeneration, especially those who have a condition known as occult choroidal neovascularization.

Occult choroidal neovascularization is a condition in which the abnormal blood vessels that grow beneath the macula in the wet form of age-related macular degeneration are hidden beneath layers of tissue. Because a doctor must be able to see the abnormal vessels in order to treat them with traditional laser therapy or PHOTODYNAMIC THERAPY, patients with occult choroidal neovascularization were considered unsuitable for those treatments.

TTT involves using a low-intensity laser to apply heat to the area in which the abnormal blood vessels are growing. The heat raises the temperature of the retina, causing the blood in the ab-

normal vessels to clot. This stops the blood vessels from leaking, and reduces the size of lesions in the area of the blood vessels. This is beneficial because the fluid and blood that leak from the vessels damage the light-sensitive photoreceptor cells in the macula.

Trials showed that about 20 percent of the 15 patients who participated in a pilot study experienced a slight improvement in vision. All but a few patients showed a notable decline in the thickness of the retina, which doctors say indicates that the growth and leakage of new blood vessels had been stopped—at least temporarily. Researchers are continuing to move forward with TTT and say that the procedure appears to be promising in the area of treatments for macular degeneration.

trauma Ocular trauma is any injury to the eye. Ocular trauma, even seemingly minor injuries, should be examined promptly and thoroughly by a physician. A trauma may be blunt (concussive) or perforating (invading the inner eye). An estimated half million serious eye injuries occur each year, with 25,000 of them resulting in blindness.

The eyelids are often the first line of defense in an injury, and if closed in time can minimize the severity of the injury. However, in protecting the eye, the eyelids are often damaged. A contusion, or blunt blow from a ball or fist, will result in hemorrhaging and swelling under the skin. This will appear as a "black eye" and will heal itself.

Minor cuts to the eyelids that are located away from the lid margin often do not require stitching. However, cuts that involve the eyelid margin are considered serious and may require surgical repair performed in an hospital operating room.

Care must be taken during examination and treatment to ensure that the eyelid properly closes. If left uncovered, the cornea could become damaged, and loss of vision may result.

Nasolacrimal (tear duct) injuries may result in constant tearing and must be surgically repaired. Often the area must be allowed to partially heal before final surgery can be performed. In this case, and in minor injuries of the nasolacrimal area, a tiny silicone tube is inserted into the tear duct to ensure correct healing.

The CONJUNCTIVA and the CORNEA are subject to injury by foreign bodies, lacerations and burns. The conjunctiva is the membrane that covers the white part of the eye (SCLERA) and the inside of the eyelids. The cornea is the clear protective covering of the eye.

Foreign bodies may become lodged in the conjunctiva or cornea. Conjunctival foreign bodies usually wash out of the eye by the flushing action of the tears. However, foreign bodies that imbed in the cornea are painful and require removal by a physician.

Minor lacerations to the conjunctiva are usually not treated. Lacerations that produce significant bleeding in the sclera should be examined for a more serious injury. Nonperforating lacerations such as scratches and abrasions, including those caused by overwear of contact lenses, cause pain to the cornea but are usually self-healing. In the case of corneal abrasion, the cornea can be comfortably examined with anesthetic drops, but the continued use of the drops is discouraged since they delay healing. Treatment may include antibiotic drops and temporary eye patching.

Chemical burns to the cornea are serious and vision threatening. The burns cause permanent, severe corneal scarring, which precludes vision. Burns caused by acid or lye should be flushed immediately and profusely with water. The eyes must receive emergency care by an ophthalmologist.

Thermal burns such as those caused by sunlight are generally not serious to the cornea and are self-healing or treated with antibiotic drops. There may be substantial pain, however, and the lids may be burned and require treatment.

Blunt injuries can also cause damage to portions of the inner eye. Hyphema, hemorrhaging into the anterior chamber of the eye can be caused by injury. The patient is usually instructed to rest prone for up to three days to prevent secondary bleeding, which may cause GLAUCOMA. Blood staining of the cornea may be permanent and cause an opacity that interferes with vision.

Contusion may cause radial tears or splits in the IRIS and CILIARY BODY from the sclera. This may reduce the angle of the ANTERIOR CHAMBER and contribute to or cause glaucoma.

Severe contusion involving the LENS may cause CATARACT, although the process of opacification set in motion by the injury may take years to mature and be noticeable. A blow may also cause the lens to become completely dislocated or subluxated (partially displaced). A displaced lens is associated with secondary glaucoma.

The VITREOUS may hemorrhage or become detached after a blunt injury. Vitreal hemorrhages generally are self-limiting, but a detached vitreous can result in a retinal tear or detached retina.

The retina may hemorrhage and develop macular edema as a result of a contusion. Blows to the eye may result in retinal tears which could lead to a retinal detachment.

Blunt injuries may cause tears in the choroid, optic atrophy, and hemorrhaging into the optic nerve sheath, conditions that can result in permanent vision loss.

Severe contusion injuries such as automobile accidents may involve the side of the cheek and one eye. This often results in a blow-out fracture of the orbit. The orbit is forced backwards, the orbital floor is fractured, and the bone is displaced downward. A plastic implant is placed in the floor of the orbit to correct the situation.

Perforating wounds pass the cornea and enter the inner eye. Perforating injuries are caused by pointed instruments such as scissors, darts, sharp tools, or glass. Any perforating wound is considered an emergency and may be subject to infection. The prognosis for the health of the eye and the preservation of the vision depends on the depth of the wound and the care taken to clean and repair the wound. If the wound penetrates the cornea alone, it may be cleaned and sutured with excellent prognosis.

If the lens has been breached, cataract or aphakia (an eye without a lens) may eventually become the result. If the eye is further invaded, retinal damage and detachment are possible.

Perforating injuries are treated immediately with a preventative tetanus injection and systemic and local antibiotics. X rays are often ordered to locate the presence of foreign bodies in the wound. Foreign bodies that breach the inner eye can cause infection and blindness.

Metal particles associated with some occupations can cause iron salt deposits to gather in the eye and result in blindness. The particles can be removed with a surgical procedure that employs a magnet.

Pellets from pellet guns cause massive damage to the eye upon entry. The entire eye is usually enucleated, or removed. Some glass or plastic particles that enter the eye may be of materials that are well tolerated by the eye and do not require removal.

Sympathetic ophthalmia must be considered after any perforation injury. This condition involves the spread of inflammation from a steadily inflamed eye to the uninjured eye over a period of two weeks.

The infected eye may be removed during the two-week period, to prevent sympathetic ophthalmia. If the condition develops after the two week period it may be treated with steroids but may continue to recur. (See INJURIES, PREVENTION OF BLINDNESS.)

Galloway, N. R. *Common Eye Diseases and Their Management.* Berlin: Springer-Verlag, 1985.

Reynolds, James D. *Ocular Trauma.* HealthNet Library. Columbus: CompuServe, 1989.

Rhode, Stephen J., and Stephen P. Ginsberg. *Ophthalmic Technology.* New York: Raven Press, 1987.

travel aids   See ELECTRONIC TRAVEL AIDS.

TravelVision   An organization that provides orientation and mobility training for visually impaired people and their families. It was founded by Kathy Zelaya, who is certified by the state of California in clinical rehabilitative services. TravelVision also offers information about long canes, guide dogs, and other mobility devices, plus a detailed history of the orientation and mobility program. Its staff trains health care workers how to best assist blind and visually impaired patients.

TravelVision staff are available to conduct orientation and mobility training in the visually impaired person's own environment.

Contact:

TravelVision
P.O. Box 10763
Glendale, CA 91209-0763
818 551-0890
http://kathyz.home.mindspring.com

trephine   A surgical instrument used in ophthalmologic procedures. The metal instrument looks much like a small, round cookie cutter attached to a handle. The round section comes in various diameter sizes, ranging from three to five millimeters. The size of the trephine is etched onto the handle for identification.

The trephine is generally used as a marker. When pressed gently onto the CORNEA, it makes a distinct, temporary indentation for the surgeon to follow. The trephine is used in corneal transplant surgery to mark duplicate sections of cornea from host and donor, and in RADIAL KERATOTOMY (RK) surgery, to mark the optical zone for radial cuts.

trichiasis   A condition in which the eyelashes grow inward into the eye. The lashes rub against the CORNEA, causing pain and infection. This may occur spontaneously or be caused by an injury, infection, or disease such as trachoma. The lashes can be removed with epilating forceps to immediately remedy the disorder. If regrowth is a problem, the lash roots can be destroyed by electrolysis.

trifluridine   An antimetabolite drug used in the treatment of ocular herpes. It is also known by the names TFT, F3T, and Viroptic. Trifluridine, along with idoxuridine, was one of the first drugs developed to treat herpes keratitis, an inflammation of the CORNEA caused by the herpes virus.

Trifluridine is a toxic drug since it is activated by the enzymes contained in healthy human cells. Since it cannot differentiate between healthy and viral cells, it may attack and destroy normal cells along with the unwanted viral cells. Because of its toxicity, trifluridine is not to be taken intravenously. It is available in ointment or drop form only.

Trifluridine drops are used nine times per day for a period of two to three weeks.

Trifluridine is not a cure for herpes keratitis. It is effective only when the virus is active in the body. It is ineffective during periods when the virus is latent or inactive.

trifocal lenses   Three lens prescriptions put into one pair of contact lenses or eyeglasses. Trifocal lenses are prescribed when bifocals are not sufficient for clear vision at all distances. Those who need trifocals are usually over 40 and suffering from PRESBYOPIA, aging of the eyes. As the eye ages, it loses the ability to bring close objects into focus.

The three sections of the trifocal include a reading section for close work, a distance section for seeing objects five feet away or farther, and a section for the midrange between the two.

The placement and size of the segments within the lens frame is determined by the wearer's needs. The largest section is generally the one most often used.

Trifocal wearers must develop head and eye movements in conjunction with their new lenses. It may be necessary to move the head up or down in order to match the section of lens to the object viewed.

tumors   Tissue growths that can form in any part of the body and eye. Tumors may be malignant (cancerous) or benign (noncancerous).

Malignant tumors carry specific characteristics. The cells of these tumors differ from the cells of the encompassing tissue, tend to grow quickly and uncontrollably, do not stop growing once they have reached a particular size, and tend to spread or metastasize to other parts of the body. Malignant tumors may be life threatening.

Three common malignant tumors found in the eye are MALIGNANT MELANOMA, RETINOBLASTOMA, and metastatic tumors. All are serious disorders that benefit from early diagnosis and treatment.

Malignant melanoma is a tumor that develops from the melanin-laden cells in the CHOROID, IRIS or CILIARY BODY. The tumor may develop spontaneously or from a mole. This type of tumor usually grows and metastasizes at a slow rate and generally affects one eye only.

Symptoms of melanoma include redness, inflammation, vision loss, GLAUCOMA, and distortion of the PUPIL. Melanoma is usually treated by enucleation, or removal of the eye, but may be subjected to chemotherapy or radiation treatments during a period of observation. The cause of melanoma is unknown.

Retinoblastoma is a malignant tumor of the retina found in young children. The tumor spreads rapidly and may metastasize up the OPTIC NERVE to the brain.

The tumor is hereditary or may develop sporadically. The more common sporadic type usually is limited to one eye and appears at approximately two years of age. The hereditary type often affects both eyes, appears near one year of age, and can be passed to future generations.

Symptoms of retinoblastoma include redness, pain, inflammation, crossed eyes, and change in pupil color. Immediate treatment includes enucleation. In cases in which both eyes are involved, the more affected eye may be removed and the less affected treated with radiation, chemotherapy, or cryotherapy (freezing treatments).

Retinoblastoma has one of the highest rates of spontaneous regression, but little is known about the causes for regression. The development of the tumor is caused by the absence of paired retinoblastoma genes on the 13th chromosome, a condition that may occur through heredity or environmental conditions.

Metastatic tumors are malignant tumors that originate in another organ of the body and metastasize to the eye. Metastatic tumors affect both eyes approximately 25 percent of the time.

Symptoms of the secondary ocular tumor may be apparent before those of the primary tumor. Symptoms may involve pain, redness, glaucoma, and vision loss or interference. Once a diagnosis has been made, the primary tumor is appropriately treated. Treatment of the ocular tumor may involve surgery, chemotherapy or radiation treatment.

Basal-cell carcinoma and squamous-cell carcinoma are two similar-looking malignant tumors found on the eyelids. They each first appear as a small bump and then develop into a saucer-shape with a raised rim.

The tumor is removed and sent for biopsy to determine the identity of type. If left untreated, the basal-cell carcinoma may spread to the underlying bone but rarely metastasizes further. Advanced basal-cell carcinoma is treated with radiation therapy.

Squamous cell carcinoma is a more serious tumor. It may metastasize to the lymph nodes of the upper or lower lids. This type of carcinoma may be treated with chemotherapy or radiation treatment.

Rhabdomyosarcoma is a rare malignant tumor of the ORBIT. It affects children and is characterized by rapid growth. Early treatment with radiation gives the best hope for a cure.

Benign tumors differ little from encompassing tissue, grow more slowly than malignant tumors and often stop growing at a certain point. Benign tumors do not spread to other parts of the body. In the case of benign ocular tumor, the growth may be left intact if it does not interfere with sight.

Benign tumors may develop in any part of the eye. The strawberry nevus and the cavernous hemangioma are two commonly found in the eyelids. The nevus, or strawberry nevus, is a tumor that appears as a pinkish or red raised mark on the skin. It is present at birth but is often undetectable until later in life when it starts to grow. It rarely becomes malignant and may spontaneously regress. The nevus may be left untreated.

The cavernous hemangioma is a deeper tumor that may appear as a blue raised area on the lid. The tumor tends to expand during periods of crying. This tumor may spontaneously regress or may be treated by freezing methods.

Benign tumors of the orbit include the pseudotumor, or a mass of inflamed tissue found in the orbit. Symptoms of pseudotumor are EXOPHTHALMOS, or bulging forward of the eyes, and double vision. If a biopsy reveals nonmalignant tissue, the tumor may be treated with steroids.

See CANCER.

tunnel vision   The common term for the reduced field of vision seen when a severe loss of peripheral or side vision occurs. Commonly, a loss of night vision accompanies tunnel vision since the rods, which are responsible for night vision, are less numerous in the area of central vision.

A peripheral field defect affecting all but 10 degrees of central vision results in mobility difficulties but may not limit reading capabilities. A loss affecting all but 5 degrees of central vision exposes only the foveal (center portion of the MACULA or sharpest sight of vision) area. This affects mobility and reading capabilities. Since the FOVEA contains no rods, this loss renders the individual night blind.

Peripheral-field loss involving tunnel vision may be caused by RETINITIS PIGMENTOSA, GLAUCOMA, OPTIC ATROPHY, TRAUMA, TUMORS, Leber's disease, toxic conditions due to drugs, proliferative retinopathy, and vascular diseases.

Optical aids to benefit those with tunnel vision include prescriptive lenses, contact lenses, intraocular lenses, field-expansion devices, or illumination aids. Prescriptive or contact lenses ensure that the remaining central vision is as clear as possible. Intraocular lenses provide the best possible central vision correction for aphakic (without a natural lens) patients.

Field expansion or widening devices employ reverse telescopic systems, separate lens loupes, and prism systems. Reverse telescopic systems minify the image seen so that more visual information is included in the residual field. These devices produce a distortion that some users find distracting.

Separate loupes, or swing-down, small lenses, are attached to the prescription lenses frame of some individuals. By rotating the eye, the individual can use the lens to expand the visual field.

PRISMS such as the Fresnel prism are incorporated into prescription lenses or pressed onto uncorrective spectacles in sections above and below, or to the sides of the usable central visual field. By moving the eyes or the head slightly, the user can see through the prisms into the restricted field.

Illumination aids are used to by those with night blindness to improve or amplify the available light in the visual field. One such aid, the Night Vision Aid (NVA), is an optical device that amplifies available low light up to 800 times within the remaining field, thus improving mobility.

ultrasonography   The use of sonic waves in ophthalmologic tests. High-frequency sound waves are used to probe and view the inner eye when other instruments prove ineffective. The sonic waves are directed to the eye, and the echoing sounds are translated into a picture of it.

Ultrasonography is used to examine the tissues of the eye for the presence of tumors, retinal detachments or fractures. Ultrasonography may be performed after GLAUCOMA surgery to review results. It is used to take measurements of the eye or to determine the health of the underlying RETINA in presurgical tests for CATARACT surgery.

The A-SCAN applies ultrasonography to measure the length of the eye to determine the correct strength of intraocular lens needed for cataract surgery. The B-SCAN uses the sound waves to view a retina obscured by a dense cataract.

unemployment   See EMPLOYMENT, EMPLOYMENT DISINCENTIVES.

Uniform Anatomical Gift Act   (UAGA)   Legislation that allows for the donation of the body or body parts, including eyes and CORNEAS, for transplantation or research. It was approved by the National Conference of Commissioners on Uniform State Laws in 1968. Since that time, all 50 states and the District of Columbia have adopted some form of this act.

The act permits any individual over 18 years of age and of sound mind to donate his entire body or parts of his body to any organ bank, hospital, medical school, surgeon, or physician. It further allows a donor to specify an individual as the recipient of the organs for therapy or transplantation.

The gift or donation can be specified in a written will or document. The document may be as simple as a card carried by the donor or, as is offered in 43 states, a signed section of the driver's license. However, family members must confirm the donation at the time of death, so it is important that they be notified in advance of intent to donate.

The document or card need not be filed with or delivered to a government agency. The only requirement needed to validate the document is the written intention of the donor, his signature, and the signatures of two witnesses. The document becomes invalidated when it is destroyed or mutilated. The act also allows the next of kin of the deceased to donate all or part of the cadaver, unless the donor left documentation to the contrary.

The UAGA also contains a section that permits a medical examiner or coroner to remove body parts from a cadaver for use in transplantation or therapy. The act lists specific actions to be taken by the official before removal. Within the limits of time needed to maintain the usefulness of the part, the official must make a reasonable effort to locate and examine the donor's medical records and provide the next of kin with the opportunity to approve or deny the donation.

Twenty-two states have medical examiner sections included in their laws. Of these, 12 require the medical examiner to take the specified steps before removal. The remaining 10 do not require the official to examine the medical records or notify the next of kin.

Two court cases, *Georgia Lions Eye Bank Inc. v. Lavant* and *Florida v. Powell*, established the constitutionality of the removal of body parts (in these cases, corneas) without the notification and approval of the next of kin. The court noted the significant increase in available tissue to the donor pool resulting from enactment of thc law as stated.

Statistics were presented that showed that the number of corneal donations increased. In Florida, 3,000 corneas were available for transplants in 1985 as compared with 500 that were available in 1976. The statistics also showed that the percentage and numbers of usable corneas for transplantation increased with the medical examiner law. Normal corneal tissue donations are often unsuitable for transplantation due to the advanced age of the average donor. In comparison, up to 85 percent of tissue obtained under medical examiner laws is acceptable for transplantation. In this decade, of the 185,000 corneal transplants performed, 100,000 used tissue obtained under the medical examiner laws.

The Uniform Anatomical Gift Act has been criticized for unresolved issues such as the lack of procedure for determining who may receive unspecified donations and the lack of criteria for dctcrmining the moment of death. As the law stands, one doctor is required to determine the moment of death. This doctor is not allowed to participate in the process of removing or transplanting donor parts.

Other countries, such as France, Czechoslovakia, and Portugal, require two doctors to determine the time of death as a protection for the donor. Some states, including California, Virginia, and Kansas, have included statutes that specify the moment of death as the time of brain death.

United States Association for Blind Athletes (USABA)

A national volunteer, nonprofit organization that provides opportunities for athletic participation and competition to blind and visually impaired athletes regardless of age or degree of impairment. It was established in 1976 following the 1976 Olympiad for the Physically Disabled, the first games to include the blind.

USABA is the only organization to sponsor local, state, regional, national, and international competitions for the blind and visually impaired. Through its state chapters, the 3,000 members compete in nine sports, which include wrestling, track and field, tandem cycling, swimming, power lifting, judo, gymnastics, goal ball, and Nordic and alpine skiing.

USABA trains, coaches, and prepares blind athletes for national and international competition. It sponsors clinics and workshops for coaches, athletes, and volunteers in leadership and skills development. The association works to promote independence and ability through athletic contest and plays a critical role in mainstreaming blind persons into regular education and physical education courses.

USABA offers memberships to both sighted and visually impaired persons interested in supporting sports competition and participation. It publishes the newsletter *Insight*.

In 2000, four USABA athletes achieved national ranking in three sports. One of them was runner Marla Runyan, who became the first legally blind person ever to qualify for a U.S. Olympic team.

Contact:

United States Association for Blind Athletes
33 N. Institute Street
Brown Hall, Suite O15
Colorado Springs, CO 80903
719-630-0422 (ph)
719-630-0616 (fax)
www.usaba.org

United States Housing Act of 1937

As amended, the Housing Act of 1937 established programs that help disabled and elderly individuals acquire acceptable housing. Section 8, or the Lower Income Housing Assistance program, is a rent-subsidy program designed to assist low-income families and develop an economic mix within neighborhoods. Title IV of the act establishes congregate housing, a mixture of residential care and personal services, for disabled or elderly persons.

Single, disabled individuals are included in the act's definition of a low-income family. A disabled person, as defined by the act, is one who has a permanent or long-term impairment that hinders independent living and who would benefit from improved housing.

Section 8 was designed to encourage the building and renovation of low-income housing such as privately or publicly developed new or considerably renovated housing, or new state-supported housing. Although this was its original intent, the program is most often used to supplement rent on existing housing.

Rent subsidies, or housing-assistance payments, are direct payments made to private home owners or public housing agencies that provide safe, clean, suitable housing for eligible needy families. Eligible families must pay up to 30 percent of their net income for rent. The rent subsidy compensates the owner for the difference between the fair market rent amount and the resident's payment.

Housing vouchers are also offered under Section 8. The voucher program authorizes housing payments to owners who provide safe, clean, suitable housing for very-low-income families. Eligible families pay up to 30 percent of their net income toward rent. The voucher makes up the difference between this payment and the local payment standard, or amount paid for rents in comparable housing in that region.

The main difference between the voucher system and rent subsidy is that the rent for the housing is not kept to a fair market price, but rather, is negotiated between the landlord and the tenant. Also, the voucher program is restricted to 5 years, whereas the rent-subsidy program lasts 15 years. In 1998, about 1.4 million households participated in the Section 8 program.

Congregate housing services were designed to allow disabled individuals who cannot live independently to live within their own residence and avoid institutionalization. The program contracts with public-housing agencies or disabled/elderly housing sponsors that qualify under Section 202 of the act.

The three- to five-year contracts direct the contractor to provide a minimum of two meals per day, seven days per week. Other necessary social and personal services that the contractor may provide include grooming, transportation, or housekeeping. Contractors who serve the disabled must confer with disability organizations such as rehabilitation and vocational agencies, developmental-disabilities councils, and state mental-health or mental-rehabilitation organizations.

U.S. Department of Education. *Summary of Existing Legislation Affecting Persons with Disabilities.* Washington, D.C.: USDE, 1988.

universities   There are no universities or colleges exclusively for blind or visually impaired students. It is generally considered desirable for them to attend the same institutions of higher learning as nondisabled students. Section 504 of the Rehabilitation Act of 1973 mandates that no qualified disabled individual can be excluded solely on the basis of disability from participation in any program, including educational programs, that receive federal financial support.

Although programs vary on campuses across the country, most offer a number of "core" services: interpreters, readers, notetakers, counselors, and tutors. These services are usually available from a university or college Office of Disabled Student Services. Many university programs rely on federal, state, and private grants to expand services for disabled students. There is a trend for higher education institutions to offer specialized technology to meet the educational and employment needs of the disabled students they serve.

The Center on Disabilities at California State University, Northridge (CSUN), near Los Angeles, is widely regarded as a model for other university programs. CSUN serves a disabled student body of approximately 3 percent of the entire student population, a figure twice that of the national average.

In addition to offering core services, CSUN's Office of Disabled Student Services has taken a leadership role in delivering technological services to the disabled student body and the professionals who serve them. This office has established a Technology Group, a critical mass of programs and professional personnel, that:

- Conducts one of the largest conferences in the world on the subject of Technology and Persons with Disabilities. Some scholarships are available for parents and persons with disabilities, making it one of the most accessible conferences in the country for these groups.

- Established a Computer Access Lab offering the latest in peripherals (braille printers, speech synthesizers) and software such as the VISTA large-print program for blind and visually impaired users.

- Conducts training in technology for rehabilitation counselors and employers throughout California, Arizona, Nevada, Guam, Saipan, and American Samoa.

- Conducts engineering research through projects such as the Universal Access System, which provides access to any computer through a laptop computer.
- Hosts a monthly radio show on KIEV (Los Angeles) on the subject of Technology and Persons with Disabilities.

Other CSUN-sponsored conferences include those concerning learning disabilities, art for disabled persons, and employment-related topics.

Students entering universities or colleges may receive funding for personal readers or educational materials from the state agency for the blind. Federal transition services offered through state commissions for the blind or vocational-rehabilitation agencies are a federal priority but are not mandated.

Contact:

CSUN Center on Disabilities
1811 Nordhoff Street
Northridge, CA 91330-8340
818-677-2578 (voice and TTY)
818-677-4929 (fax)
www.csun.edu/cod

Urban Mass Transportation Act (UMTA) As amended in 1970, the Urban Mass Transportation Act of 1964 (UMTA) requires that mass transportation facilities and services be designed to accommodate use by elderly and disabled persons. A program of grants and loans was authorized in the act to fund such facilities and services.

The act established three programs:

1. The Mass Transportation Technology Research and Demonstration Program funds projects of national priority, including accessibility to mass transportation by elderly and disabled persons.
2. The Urban Mass Transportation Technical Studies Program funds grants for planning, engineering, and designing mass-transportation projects, including those specially designed with accommodation for elderly and disabled passengers in mind.

3. The Urban Mass Transportation Demonstration Grants Program funds demonstration projects that improve accessibility using innovative methods.

The National Mass Transportation Assistance Act of 1974 amended the Urban Mass Transportation formula-grant program by requiring project applicants to set fares for elderly and disabled passengers traveling at nonpeak hours at one-half the normal peak-hour fare price. The amendment allowed local transportation systems that transport elderly and disabled persons for free to remain eligible for federal formula-grant aid.

The Surface Transportation and Uniform Relocation Assistance Act of 1987 required the Secretary of Transportation to conduct a feasibility study for standards development for UMTA-funded programs concerning tactile aids to improve accessibility to blind and visually impaired passengers.

The Omnibus Budget Reconciliation Act of 1987 founded a three-year demonstration project operated by the Easter Seal Society to improve accessibility to transportation for disabled persons. The program uses UMTA funds to develop methods for identifying disabled persons within the community and training programs for transit operators and disabled persons.

The Intermodal Surface Transportation Efficiency Act of 1991, signed into law by President George H. W. Bush, allocated funds for public ground transportation, provided it complied with the Americans with Disabilities Act.

U.S. Department of Education. *Summary of Existing Legislation Affecting Persons with Disabilities.* Washington, D.C.: USDE, 1988.

Usher's syndrome An inherited condition combining a serious hearing loss and a progressive loss of vision caused by RETINITIS PIGMENTOSA (RP). According to the RP FOUNDATION FIGHTING BLINDNESS, there are between 10,000 and 15,000 people with Usher's syndrome in the United States. It is the major cause of deaf-blindness.

There are three known types of Usher's syndrome. Type I individuals are born with a profound hearing loss and retinitis pigmentosa. Individuals with Type II are born with a mild to moderate hearing loss and generally have a less severe form of RP. Type III Usher's syndrome is characterized by hearing loss and vision loss due to RP that are both progressive.

Retinitis pigmentosa is characterized by a degeneration of the RODS AND CONES (light-sensitive cells) of the RETINA. The retina of the eye receives the reflected light from an object, and the rods and cones translate the light into electrical impulses that the retina sends to the brain through the OPTIC NERVE. The brain changes the impulses into an image.

The rods function in low light or darkness and are responsible for detecting movement and shape. They are scattered throughout the retina and are accountable for peripheral or side vision. The cones discern detail and color and require light to work effectively. They are concentrated into the central section of the retina, the MACULA, and are responsible for central vision.

Retinitis pigmentosa attacks the rods first, then the cones. As the disease progresses, night vision diminishes and peripheral or side vision is lost. Over long periods of time, central vision is affected. The vision loss may not be apparent for several years. Tunnel vision and night blindness may become noticeable during adolescence, and progressively worsen.

Roughly 30 percent of those with retinitis pigmentosa report a hearing loss, some of whom may be considered to have Usher's syndrome. Usher's syndrome accounts for up to 3 percent of all cases of profound deafness. The hearing loss is caused by a malfunction in the sensory cells of the inner ear by an unknown cause. The loss is generally present at birth or follows shortly after birth.

Usher's syndrome can be diagnosed. The hearing loss is easily detected with audiometric testing. RP can be diagnosed by the characteristic changes that take place in the retina. Tests such as an electroretinogram and a visual-field test may be performed to confirm the diagnosis.

Usher's syndrome affects individuals of all races, ethnic and cultural backgrounds and is equally prevalent among males and females. It is a recessively inherited disorder that requires the necessary gene from both the mother and father. A

pairing of two carriers of the gene results in a one in four chance of producing Usher's syndrome. A pairing of a carrier and a noncarrier of the gene seldom results in Usher's syndrome, but the gene is passed on to future generations. At present, there is no method for determining a gene carrier other than tracing family history of the disease. Genetic counseling may be beneficial in prevention of the disease.

Scientists have made significant progress in the late 1990s to learn more about the defects that cause Usher's syndrome. Researchers think there are nine different genes that contain mutations that cause various types of Usher's syndrome. They are currently working to develop rodent models of Usher's syndrome that will help them understand how the genes function and how mutations in the gene lead to the hearing and vision loss that is typical of the disease.

There is no cure for Usher's syndrome or retinitis pigmentosa although a specified amount of vitamin A has been found to slow the progression of RP in some people. The hearing loss tends to remain stable, but since it is an inner ear loss, surgery is not possible to restore hearing. Some individuals without any residual hearing have been candidates for cochlear implants. Many of those with residual hearing have benefited from hearing aids.

The progressive sight loss is untreatable. Each case is unique and unpredictable. The retina may degenerate rapidly or over a period of decades. Usually, some central vision is maintained through middle age. Most Usher's syndrome patients who become legally blind retain some central vision.

Cataracts, a clouding of the eye's lens, may develop in patients with RP and Usher's syndrome. If the CATARACT is removable, the surgery does not improve retinal degeneration but can restore the visual acuity lost to the opacity of the cataract.

In the research for a cure or treatment for Usher's syndrome and retinitis pigmentosa, experiments and studies involving DMSO applications and light deprivation have had less than satisfactory results. Usher's syndrome patients may maximize their residual vision with low-vision aids. Optical aids such as Corning or NOIR glasses, telescopes, microscopes, and night-vision aids may be useful. Nonoptical and electronic aids such as the Wide Angle Mobility Light, large print, talking computers, and closed-circuit television may further independence. However, these low-vision aids cannot restore vision that has been lost to RP or Usher's syndrome.

Annala, L. "Facing the Future with Usher's Syndrome." Workshop on Usher's syndrome (December 2–3, 1976). Helen Keller National Center, Sands Point, NY.

Boardman, L. "My Son has Usher's Syndrome." *The Deaf-Blind American.* (June 1985): pp. 50–60.

The Foundation Fighting Blindness. *Usher Syndrome Gene Identified.* Hunt Valley, Md.: The Foundation for Fighting Blindness, 2001.

Pimentel, A. "Handling the Upper, Secondary and College Usher's Syndrome Student." Workshop on Usher's syndrome (December 2–3, 1976). Helen Keller National Center, Sands Point, NY.

Roehrig, A. "Living with Usher's Syndrome." Workshop on Usher's syndrome (December 2–3, 1976). Helen Keller National Center, Sands Point, NY.

RP Foundation Fighting Blindness. *Answers to Your Questions about Usher's Syndrome.* Baltimore, Maryland: RPFFB, 1988.

Vernon, McCay, Joann A. Boughman and Linda Annala. "Considerations in Diagnosing Usher's Syndrome: RP and Hearing Loss." *Journal of Visual Impairment and Blindness,* 76 (1982): 258–261.

uvea　The uvea, or uveal tract, is a heavily vascularized layer that supplies blood to the eye. It includes the melanin-pigmented portions of the eye: the IRIS and CILIARY BODY in the front of the eye and the CHOROID to the back of the eye.

The iris is the colored portion of the eye. It controls the size of the PUPIL, which regulates the amount of light that enters the eye. The ciliary body lies just behind the iris and is attached to the LENS of the eye. The ciliary body produces AQUEOUS FLUID and moves the lens to focus properly. The choroid is a layer of blood vessels between the RETINA and the SCLERA, or white part of the eye. It nourishes and supports the eye.

Disorders of the uvea may include inflammations, injuries or infections. A common disorder, UVEITIS, is an inflammation of the uveal tract. It can be caused by an injury or other illness present in the body or can appear spontaneously from an unknown cause. In addition, each section of the uvea is subject to inflammation, including IRITIS CYCLITIS and CHOROIDITIS.

uveitis　An inflammation of the uveal tract of the eye. The uveal tract includes the IRIS, the CILIARY BODY, and the CHOROID. The entire tract is highly vascularized and contains the pigment melanin, which is also found in the skin. Uveitis may occur because of an injury, in connection with another disease of the eye or body, or spontaneously. The disorder is usually categorized as either anterior or posterior uveitis.

Anterior uveitis (or IRIDOCYCLITIS) occurs when the inflammation involves the iris and the ciliary body. The iris is the colored part of the eye. It controls the PUPIL, which opens and shuts to regulate the light that enters the eye. The ciliary body lies behind the iris and is connected to the LENS of the eye. The ciliary body produces AQUEOUS FLUID and moves the lens to focus the eye properly. Symptoms of anterior uveitis include redness, light sensitivity, blurred vision, and extreme pain, especially when focusing on near objects. A thorough ophthalmologic examination may be needed to determine the cause of uveitis. Additional tests such as X rays of the chest, skull or sinuses, blood tests, and examinations for arthritis or other diseases may be necessary.

Usually, a specific cause for anterior uveitis is not found, and the condition is determined to have occurred spontaneously. Other diseases and disorders may cause uveitis and include arthritis, tuberculosis, SARCOIDOSIS, sinus disorders, venereal disease, ulcerative colitis, and injuries.

The prognosis for anterior uveitis is generally good, unless the eye develops complications due to recurrences. Recurrent uveitis may result in CATARACTS or secondary GLAUCOMA due to increased intraocular pressure. Mild anterior uveitis is treated with the application of steroid eye drops to reduce the inflammation. Acute uveitis may be treated with steroid pills or injections. In both cases, cycloplegics, drops that widen the pupil, such as atropine sulfate, may be prescribed to restrict the focusing power of the inflamed eye and allow for a rest period.

Posterior uveitis involves the choroid and is also called CHOROIDITIS. The choroid is a layer of blood vessels between the RETINA and the SCLERA, or white part of the eye. The choroid nourishes and supports the eye.

Posterior uveitis is not usually as painful as anterior uveitis. There may be redness of the eye, blurred or lost vision, light sensitivity, and the appearance of floaters (small dark spots that seem to float through the field of vision). If the uveitis remains in the area of peripheral vision, the symptoms may not be noticed.

Posterior uveitis, like anterior uveitis, may occur spontaneously. It has been associated with toxoplasmosis, tuberculosis, sarcoidosis, venereal disease, viruses, and injuries. If untreated, posterior uveitis can spread from the choroid to the retina and the VITREOUS. If the inflammation involves the MACULA, permanent central vision loss may occur. When the inflammation spreads into the vitreous and entails the center of the globe, the condition is called endophthalmitis, which may be treated with ANTIBIOTICS and possibly reversed. Treatment for posterior uveitis includes steroid eye drops or pills. In more serious cases, immunosuppressive medications may be used. (See IRITIS.)

In 1990 researchers at the University of Iowa identified a gene defect that they believe is the cause of a new clinical syndrome they call hereditary uveitis. The proper name of the syndrome is autosomal dominant neovascular inflammatory vitreoretinopathy (ADNIV). Many of the features of the syndrome are common to those found in uveitis.

In 1992, researchers established that the gene that causes ADNIV is located on the long arm of chromosome 11. They are still working, however, to isolate the particular gene that they believe causes ADNIV.

venereal disease Any disease of the genitals, usually contracted by sexual contact. Some venereal diseases, or sexually transmitted diseases (STDs), such as gonorrhea, syphilis, herpes, and nongonococcal urethritis can cause eye disease and vision loss.

In the United States, gonorrhea is the second most reported communicable disease to the Centers for Disease Control and Prevention; chlamydial infections are first. In 1997, there were 324,901 cases reported. This is a drop from the mid- to late 1980s, when nearly a million cases were reported each year. Researchers say the disease may have been more prevalent during the latter part of the 1980s because doctors were treating it with antibiotics to which the disease had become resistant. The Centers for Disease Control recommended in its 1998 Sexually Transmitted Disease Treatment Guideline that only highly effective antimicrobial agents be used to treat gonorrhea.

Gonorrhea is caused by the gonococcus bacteria and may result in blindness when contracted congenitally. The disease is passed from mother to child during birth. As the infant moves through the birth canal, the infant's eyes come into contact with the gonococcus bacteria growing in or near the cervix and become infected.

The infection, called gonococcal ophthalmia, or OPHTHALMIA NEONATORUM in the case of the newborns, causes severe CONJUNCTIVITIS. First symptoms include swelling and redness of the CORNEA, CONJUNCTIVA and eyelids. Without treatment, the condition may progress to damage the cornea and result in blindness.

Adults may contract gonococcal ophthalmia by introducing the eyes to anything carrying the bacteria. Adults exhibit more serious signs of the infection than do infants, and may develop a severe puslike discharge. The organism may invade the cornea and cause blindness. Gonorrhea in adults may be diagnosed from a Gram's stain or a cervical culture.

Treatment for gonococcal ophthalmia involves use of local antibiotic drops or ointments such as penicillin or tetracycline. Systemic or injected ANTIBIOTICS may also be prescribed.

At one time, congenital gonorrhea was the leading cause of blindness in children. The legislation all states requiring the administration of silver nitrate drops, or comparable antibiotics, to the eyes of all new born infants has drastically reduced its incidence.

SYPHILIS is a venereal disease caused by the spirochete *Treponema pallidum*. The disease may cause ocular disorders, both congenitally and after birth. Syphilis is contracted congenitally from the infected mother to the child through the womb after the fourth month of pregnancy when the spirochete can pass through the placenta. Congenital syphilis may result in vision loss and ocular impairment, deafness, dental defects, mental retardation, organ damage, and death.

Ocular damage may involve severe KERATITIS, or corneal inflammation and chorioretinal scarring. Although the infection is present at birth, the keratitis may develop later in life between ages five and 25. Severe keratitis may be treated with medication but may result in corneal opacification and PHOTOPHOBIA.

Syphilis contracted after birth can cause chorioretinal scarring, IRITIS (or inflammation of the iris) and OPTIC NERVE atrophy or degeneration.

Syphilis can be diagnosed with a Wasserman test, a blood test to determine the presence of the spirochete in the blood. An eye examination may also determine the presence of the disease and is often used to confirm the diagnosis.

Syphilis is treated with antibiotics, and ocular disorders are treated with medication. If treated in the early stages, the damage due to syphilis may be mild.

Congenital syphilis can be prevented if the disease of the mother is treated and controlled before the fifth month of pregnancy. Toward this purpose, most states have developed laws that require testing for syphilis at the beginning of each pregnancy.

HERPES SIMPLEX is a virus that is accountable for most corneal blindness due to infection in the United States. Herpes simplex is one of four types of herpes virus and may infect the genitals, skin, brain, and eyes. The other types of herpes virus are herpes zoster, cytomegalovirus, and Epstein-Barr virus.

Herpes simplex virus cells usually enter the body through the mouth, genitals, or eyes. In the past, those infections that occurred above the waist were commonly referred to as Type I, and those below the waist were referred to as Type II. However, the above- and below-the-waist categorizations are used less commonly, because Type I herpes is now frequently seen below the waist and Type II is increasingly diagnosed above the waist.

Herpes simplex may infect the eyes in one of three ways: congenitally, primarily, or recurrently. Congenital herpes is contracted by infants during birth. If the mother has active genital herpes, the infant may become exposed to the virus when the water breaks or when traveling through the birth canal.

Congenital herpes may result in permanent damage to the eyes, brain, liver, or kidneys, or in death. Ocular damage may involve the RETINA, conjunctiva, optic nerve, LENS, and cornea. Congenital herpes may be prevented by a Caesarean section birth if the mother is aware of an active herpes infection.

Primary herpes infection of the eyes is rare in adults and generally occurs only in children or adolescents. The symptoms include fever, fatigue, swollen eyelids, conjunctivitis, and a blistering rash around the eyes. The infection is usually mild and short-lived. It can be treated with antiviral eye drops or ointments.

Recurrent ocular herpes are eye infections, usually involving only one eye, that happen as a result of a reawakening of the dormant herpes virus. The virus, which may have first infected the mouth, travels to the fifth nerve ganglion, the trigeminal, where it remains dormant. The fifth ganglion has connecting fibers to the upper part of the face, including the eyes. On reactivation, the virus travels back up these fibers and infects the eye.

A recurrent infection is typified by redness, pain, and a watery discharge of the eye. Herpes keratitis, or corneal infection, iritis, GLAUCOMA, and CATARACTS may result from this infection. As the eye attempts to heal itself, corneal scarring may develop, followed by loss of vision. Each recurrence increases the possibility of scarring and vision loss.

Herpes keratitis is treated with the drugs vidarabine, TRIFLURIDINE, IDOXURIDINE, and ACYCLOVIR, antiviral eye drops or ointments. These drugs are not a cure for herpes. They stop the reproduction of viral cells but cannot rid the body of the virus. During periods of dormancy, the drugs are ineffective in fighting the virus.

Severe scarring is treated with CORTISONE eye drops. Cortisone is a steroid that may actually worsen the herpes infection and is therefore used only for short periods of time. Severe vision loss due to scarring may in some cases be corrected with a corneal transplant, or keratoplasty.

Nongonococcal urethritis, NGU, is a venereal disease caused most often by two organisms, *Chlamydia trachomatis* and plasma urealyticum. NGU causes inflammation of the urethra in men and cystitis and pelvic inflammatory disease (PID) in women.

NGU may infect the eyes of adults when the eyes are exposed to the live infection, or congenitally as the infant travels through the birth canal. When the eyes become infected, conjunctivitis results. If left untreated, the infection could lead to corneal scarring and blindness. Symptoms of NGU conjunctivitis are similar to those of gonococcal conjunctivitis and include redness, swelling, and a pus discharge. Those with symptoms of NGU are given a Gram's stain test to rule out gonorrhea. If the culture from the stain is negative for gonorrhea, treatment for NGU is prescribed. Treatment involves local administration of antibiotics such as chlortetracycline ointment and oral antibiotics.

venous occlusion   A condition that results from a blockage to a retinal vein. The disease usually involves the central retinal vein, or CRV. The damage to the RETINA occurs when blood flows into the eye from the undamaged arteries but cannot flow from the eye due to the blockage. Hemorrhaging and swelling occur, and vision is damaged.

The condition may occur suddenly or over a period of days. The vision may regress to 20/400 or worse, but there is rarely accompanying pain. The cause of the disease is unknown, but it is suspected that it occurs as a result of an intraluminal thrombosis, or a blood clot in the lamina cribrosa of the OPTIC NERVE.

Because of the high occurrence of CRV obstruction and ARTERIOSCLEROSIS of the central retinal artery, it is believed that arteriosclerosis may lead to the obstruction. Open-angle GLAUCOMA, orbital or global trauma, and optic-nerve or orbital tumors may also lead to occlusion.

Treatment for venous occlusion includes therapy for the underlying cause, if apparent, and may include anticoagulation medications and photocoagulation therapy. Laser surgery may be advised to help reduce macular swelling, prevent abnormal growth of new vessels, or prevent bleeding. It is not, however, always successful. Once a venous occlusion has occurred, vision loss can be permanent. Complications of venous occlusion include neovascular glaucoma (20 percent chance), neovascularization, and RETINAL DETACHMENT.

Branch-vein occlusion occurs because the vein crosses over a hard arteriosclerotic arteriole (small part of an artery that ends in capillaries). It can cause central vision loss, neovascularization and glaucoma.

VersaBraille   See PAPERLESS BRAILLE.

veterans   According to the Blinded Veterans Association, there are approximately 120,000 visually impaired veterans in the United States. Many more veterans become blind or visually impaired each year due to common eye diseases such as AGE-RELATED MACULOPATHY, GLAUCOMA, and RETINITIS PIGMENTOSA.

The U.S. Department of Veterans Affairs (VA) provides a wide range of benefits to American veterans, including those with vision impairments, and their families. The vision loss does not need to occur during military service in order for a veteran to qualify for benefits.

Veterans who receive an honorable discharge are eligible for all benefits, including educational benefits. Those receiving general discharges qualify for all benefits except educational. Those who receive dishonorable and bad-conduct discharges are not eligible for veterans benefits. Those who receive other than honorable discharges may or may not qualify for some benefits. These cases are reviewed individually by the VA. Veterans rated nonservice-connected are required to complete an income questionnaire (means test) when applying for medical care and may be denied medical care depending on the results.

Those who originally enlisted after September 7, 1980, and those who entered military service after October 16, 1981, must complete the shorter of two possible terms in order to qualify for benefits: either 24 months of continuous active duty or the full period for which the individual was called to active duty. This does not apply to veterans with a service-connected disability or who were discharged near the end of an enlistment term because of a disability incurred or aggravated in the line of duty or due to hardship.

The U.S. Department of Veterans Affairs provides the benefits through three major offices:

1. The Veterans Benefits Administration administers compensation, pensions, GI loans, insurance, education, and job-training programs, including vocational-rehabilitation and disability benefits. The Veterans Administration operates the Blind Rehabilitation Service, which administers programs for blinded veterans at VA Blind Rehabilitation Centers and Clinics.
2. The National Cemetery System administers death benefits. These include burial expenses and compensation to surviving spouses and children.

3. The Veterans Health Services and Research Administration administers health-care benefits, such as hospitalization, nursing-home care, domiciliary care, outpatient medical and dental treatment, beneficiary travel, alcohol- and drug-dependency treatment, Agent Orange or nuclear radiation exposure treatment, prosthetic appliances, readjustment counseling centers, medical care for dependents, overseas benefits, appeals, and blind aids and services.

Aids and services are available to blind veterans who are eligible for medical services. Veterans are considered blind if they meet the specifications of legal blindness. Most blind veterans qualify for an annual review by the Visual Impairment Services Team (VIST), adjustment to blindness training, home improvements and structural alterations to homes, low-vision aids and training, approved electronic and mechanical aids for the blind (as well as their repair and replacement), and dog guides and the cost of the dog's medical care.

In order to inform blind veterans of the benefits available to them, Congress chartered the Blinded Veterans Association (BVA) to serve veterans with severe vision loss. The organization works through a field service program and an outreach employment program to help veterans obtain services, benefits, rehabilitation training, and employment. (See BLINDED VETERANS ASSOCIATION and REHABILITATION.)

Another group, the Blinded American Veterans Foundation (BAVF), was formed in 1985 by three American veterans who had lost their sight while serving in Korea and Vietnam. The BAVF has three primary goals: research, rehabilitation, and reemployment. It does not maintain a membership, but serves as a clearinghouse for research and educational efforts and advancements.

The BAVF supports medical research concerning blindness and other sensory disabilities, participates in outreach programs to learn the needs and concerns of veterans with sensory disabilities, and conducts informational programs directed at government, business, and the general public. It also has developed a national volunteer corps to help veterans with sensory disabilities.

The BAVF funded the research and development of the Americane, a sensory aid that has been certified by the Department of Veterans Affairs and distributed to more than 2,500 blind veterans.

Contact:

The Blinded American Veterans Foundation
P.O. Box 65900
Washington, DC 20035-5900
www.bavf.org

The Blinded Veterans Association
477 H Street
Northwest Washington, DC 20001-2694
202-371-8880
www.bva.org

vidarabine   See ARA-A.

Viroptic   See TRIFLURIDINE.

visual acuity   The measurement of the amount of detail an individual sees in relation to the amount of detail someone with normal vision sees. Visual acuity is stated as an equation with 20 as the first number, a slash mark and a second number of either 15, 20, 25, 30, 40, 50, 70, 100 or 200, such as 20/20. The first number of the equation, 20, indicates the distance at which the measurement is taken. The second number indicates the distance at which a normally sighted person can see specific detail or print.

Normal or "perfect" vision is written as 20/20. Someone with 20/20 vision sees detail at 20 feet that a normally sighted person sees at 20 feet. Someone with 20/100 vision sees detail at 20 feet that someone with normal vision could see at 100 feet.

The eye chart usually used for the visual acuity test is called the SNELLEN CHART. Using this chart as a measurement, the individual can be given a visual acuity range from 20/15 to 20/200. A measurement of 20/200 means that the individual was only able to see the largest letter on the chart, the big E.

The term *count fingers* refers to an individual who cannot see the big E, but who can count the number of fingers the examiner holds up. *Hand motion* is the term used to describe someone who cannot see the separate fingers, but who can discern some movement when the hand is waved.

Light perception, or LP, describes the person who can perceive only light or its absence. NLP, or no light perception, refers to one who is unable to discern any light.

Visual-acuity measurements help describe legal definitions for blindness. These classifications determine eligibility for federal benefits. Someone with corrected vision of 20/50 in the better eye is classified as having LOW VISION. An individual with corrected vision of 20/200 in the better eye is classified as LEGALLY BLIND.

visual aids See ADAPTIVE AIDS.

visual field The area in which a person can see. This area or field is measured in degrees. A person with normal vision can see objects within a field of about 150 degrees with one eye and 180 degrees with both eyes when looking straight ahead. The central 60 degrees seen by both eyes is called CENTRAL VISION. It is also known as "seeing" vision, because it is the vision you use to look directly at something.

The vision on either side of these 60 degrees is called PERIPHERAL VISION. This is the vision surrounding what you are looking at. It describes side vision, or the things you see out of the "corner of your eye." Peripheral vision is also called "traveling" vision.

A loss of visual field can occur in the central vision, the peripheral vision or both. An individual with a visual field of 40 to 20 degrees of a possible 180 in the better eye is classified as having LOW VISION. Someone with a field of 20 degrees or less of the possible 180 in the better eye is classified LEGALLY BLIND.

visual impairment A term that describes a recognizable defect or malfunctioning of the eye. Impairments are diagnosed and defined by a medical doctor. Visual impairments range from total blindness to low vision.

The term *visually impaired* is also used frequently to describe those persons who have sight loss in one or both eyes but are not legally blind. Legally blind persons have a visual acuity of 20/200 or less in the better eye after correction or a visual field of less than 20 in the better eye after correction.

According to National Eye Institute, there are approximately 14 million persons who are visually impaired in the United States. That is about one in every 20 people. Worldwide, it is estimated that 135 million people are visually impaired.

The majority of visually impaired persons are male between the ages of 25 and 64. Most of those with severe impairments are female and 65 or older.

CATARACT is a leading cause of all degrees of visual impairment. Age-related macular degeneration is the leading cause of vision impairment among people who are 75 and older. It is the most common cause of new visual impairment in those 65 and older. Injury, GLAUCOMA, and congenital causes are commonly responsible for lesser impairments, whereas diabetes and cardiovascular diseases are commonly responsible for severe impairments. (See BLINDNESS.)

Prevent Blindness America. "Age-Related Macular Degeneration FAQ." www.preventblindness.org: 2001.
National Eye Institute of the National Institutes of Health. "Low Vision." www.nei.nih.gov/nehep/faqs.htm#2: 2000.

vitamins Vitamins are essential to the health of the eyes and maintenance of vision. Vitamin A, or retinol, is an element most closely tied to vision. The retina contains light sensitive RODS AND CONES, which receive light and provide information about the seen object. This information is converted by the RETINA to electrical impulses sent to the brain. The brain translates the impulses into an image.

The cones are responsible for central vision, detail, and color, and require light to function. The rods are responsible for peripheral vision and function in low light.

The rods contain the pigment rhodopsin, or visual purple, which is chemically very similar to vitamin A. When light strikes a rod, the rhodopsin is broken down and used up. In order to make new rhodopsin and continue to function, the rod must draw on vitamin A within the body. Without replenishment of vitamin A, the rod will eventually be destroyed.

The first sign of vitamin-A deficiency is night blindness. In dim light the eye depends on the rods to maintain vision. When the rods are not functioning, night blindness occurs.

Vitamin-A deficiency causes XEROPHTHALMIA, a leading cause of blindness in developing countries of the world. According to Helen Keller International, xerophthalmia impairs the vision of 5 million to 10 million children annually, and causes irreparable blindness to 500,000 of these.

Vitamin A is found in yellow vegetables such as carrots and is stored in the body for long periods of time in the liver. A normal diet that includes vegetables and vitamin A-rich foods will prevent vitamin-A deficiency.

Vitamin-B deficiency may cause vision loss. A deficiency of thiamine, vitamin B_1, affects the OPTIC NERVE, which carries the electrical impulses to the brain, thus interrupting or interfering with the message. This condition, referred to as nutritional AMBLYOPIA, produces scotomas, or blind spots, in the field of vision. Thiamine supplements can often correct and restore vision lost to B_1 deficiency.

Vitamin-B_2 (riboflavin) deficiency may cause cornea disease or KERATITIS, and vitamin-B_6 (pyridoxine) deficiency may cause vascular congestion and corneal neovascularization. Vitamin-B_{12} deficiency, or pernicious anemia, is associated with RETROBULBAR NEURITIS (swelling of the optic nerve). Treatment with adequate dosages of these vitamins usually reverses or improves the conditions caused by their lack.

Vitamin C, in large doses, has been shown to be effective in drawing fluid away from the eye and reducing elevated intraocular pressure associated with GLAUCOMA. It is not used as a treatment for glaucoma but rather as a diet supplement.

Vitamin C may be effective in the prevention of CATARACTS and retinal disorders such as DIABETIC RETINOPATHY and AGE-RELATED MACULOPATHY. Cataracts and retinal damage may be caused by an excess of free radicals, chemicals that are generated by a normal body process called oxidation. Since vitamin C is an antioxidant, a diet containing vitamin C may decelerate the process of developing cataracts or retinal disorders. Because subsequent research and studies in this area differ in their conclusions, this theory remains controversial.

Vitamin-C deficiency, or scurvy, may lead to ocular hemorrhage. For any hemorrhage of the eye not related to DIABETES, hypertension or another cause may be investigated as a symptom of scurvy. Vitamin-C treatment may produce results in a week.

An excess of vitamin D may cause opacities in the CORNEA or CONJUNCTIVA and scleral calcification. Overdosage in infancy may produce optic atrophy, optic neuritis, or convergent STRABISMUS.

Researchers at the Department of Newborn Medicine at the Royal Alexandra Hospital in Edmonton, Alberta, have found that a dose of vitamin E given within 12 hours of birth may reduce the incidence of severe forms of RETINOPATHY OF PREMATURITY. This has not been confirmed in other studies and remains an unproven controversial form of treatment.

Supplements of vitamins A, C, and E may be prescribed in combination to retard the progression of diabetic retinopathy, age-related maculopathy, and cataracts, help maintain the health of blood cells and vessels of the retina, and assist in the healing process after surgery.

Zinc is necessary to healthy vision and is contained in the highest concentration in the body in the retina. Zinc allows vitamin A to be released from the liver and is used in the process of metabolism in the retina. Since a zinc deficiency prevents the body from using the available vitamin A, it may cause the same effects as a vitamin-A deficiency.

Vitamin products that claim to help guard against age-related macular degeneration and other diseases are available. Most doctors, however, warn that vitamins, while important in maintaining eye health, are not miracle cures for eye diseases.

Carden, Robert G. "Vitamins for Healthier Eyes." *Let's Live,* September 1984, pp. 10–11.

Editors of Prevention Magazine. *Prevention's New Encyclopedia of Common Diseases.* Emmaus, Pennsylvania: Rodale Press, 1984.

Havener, William H. *Ocular Pharmacology.* St. Louis: C.V. Mosby Company, 1970.

Helen Keller International. *Facts About Helen Keller International.* New York: HKI, 1987.

Vaughn, Lewis, ed. *The Complete Book of Vitamins and Minerals for Health.* Emmaus, Pennsylvania: Rodale Press, 1988.

Yukin, John. *The Penguin Encyclopedia of Nutrition.* New York: Viking Press, 1985.

vitrectomy   A surgical procedure in which the VITREOUS of the eye is removed and replaced. The vitreous is the clear, gel-like substance that fills the back section of the eye and supplies support to the entire eyeball. The vitreous must remain clear to function properly. It may become clouded due to infection, injury, or RETINAL DETACHMENT, or as a complication of other diseases, such as SICKLE CELL DISEASE and DIABETIC RETINOPATHY. These conditions often result in hemorrhaging into the vitreous, formation of new blood vessels and scar tissue and clouding of the vitreous.

Once the vitreous is obscured, a loss of vision results. Vitreous hemorrhaging can spontaneously resolve itself, but if the underlying condition is not arrested, it may continue to cloud the vitreous and destroy vision. In some cases, vitrectomy can restore or improve vision. This microsurgery involves the use of a VISC, a vitreous infusion suction cutter. This specialized instrument is inserted into the eye through the CILIARY BODY. The motor-driven VISC illuminates the inside of the eye, separates and removes the vitreous and replaces it with a sterile saline solution.

According to the National Institute of Health, vitrectomy improves vision in over 60 percent of all cases. The procedure is being studied for use in treatment of corneal and macular edema, acute inflammation, and severe penetrating eye injuries.

vitreous   A clear gel-like substance within the back of the eye between the LENS and the RETINA. If fills approximately 80 percent of the volume of the eye and gives support to the other organs within.

Light passes through the CORNEA and the ANTERIOR CHAMBER filled with AQUEOUS FLUID and enters the back of the eye through the PUPIL. It then passes through the lens and the vitreous and is focused onto the retina. The retina is a light-sensitive layer that receives and encodes light information and sends it via the OPTIC NERVE to the brain, where the information is translated into an image. In order for light to be focused on the retina, the vitreous must remain clear. When the vitreous becomes obscured or cloudy, vision may be lost.

The vitreous can become clouded due to many conditions and diseases. This clouding is frequently associated with hemorrhaging due to injuries, DIABETES, SICKLE-CELL DISEASE, or RETINAL DETACHMENT.

DIABETIC RETINOPATHY is a complication of diabetes in which the retinal blood vessels deteriorate and hemorrhage into the vitreous. As new blood vessels form, the vitreous may become inflamed and develop vitreous membranes. As the membranes contract, a process called traction, they may cause the retina to detach from the underlying epithelial layer.

In other types of retinal detachments, the vitreous may accumulate under the retina causing it to bulge forward and detach, or it may flow into a retinal hole or tear and float the retina away from the epithelial layer.

Sickle-cell anemia is a disease in which the blood vessels of the retina develop small aneurysms and hemorrhages. New vessels may develop that also leak into the vitreous to further obscure it.

RETINITIS PIGMENTOSA produces changes in the vitreous. In the early stages, the vitreous may appear clouded by evenly distributed dustlike particles. Later, opaque sections may develop, or the vitreous may collapse within the orbit.

Occasionally, an obscured vitreous may spontaneously clear. However, if the underlying cause is not arrested, it may continue to cloud the vitreous and destroy vision. Some instances of obscured vitreous can be treated with a vitrectomy. This is a surgical procedure in which the cloudy vitreous and its scar tissue are drained from the eye and replaced with a clear solution. Vitrectomy improves vision in over 60 percent of the cases.

The vitreous is also subject to inflammation. When the inflammation involves the vitreous, posterior uveal tract, and much of the center of the globe, the condition is called ENDOPHTHALMITIS. This may occur after an injury or ophthalmologic surgery.

ANTIBIOTICS are often injected into the vitreous to combat the infection. Unfortunately, the antibiotics may diffuse from the vitreous into the retina and poison this organ. As endophthalmitis spreads to the entire eye, it becomes a condition called PANOPHTHALMITIS. As panophthalmitis destroys the eye, it shrinks and may require removal.

As the eye ages, the vitreous gel liquefies and shrinks. This may lead to posterior vitreous detachment in which the vitreous collapses from above and separates from the retina. Although there are often no symptoms of posterior vitreous detachment, it can cause retinal tears or traction, reduced vision or the appearance of light flashes or floaters.

Floaters are bits of debris that float in the vitreous and appear in the field of vision. Floaters occur in normal vision and are not considered a serious symptom unless they appear suddenly in great numbers.

vocational aids   Any devices that allow an individual to perform any facet of a job. Vocational aids are often called sensory aids, because frequently they are devices that compensate for a loss of one of the senses.

Vocational aids for visually impaired individuals compensate for a lack of vision or a reduced field of vision. The aid may be an adapted form of an old device that has been marked with raised dots, braille, or large print. It may have an auditory signal or voice output component, or may be designed in a new form to compensate for the user's lack of sight.

Vocational aids may be categorized by type, including:

- BRAILLE devices, such as a brailler or braille typewriter, a braille shorthand machine, braillex (which records braille information in digitized form), digicassette (which records and stores braille on magnetic tape from a braille keyboard), or paperless braille (which records and stores braille information to discs).

- Calculators, such as those that provide a braille paper tape or printout of the display, electronic tone calculators that sound out a series of beeps to indicate a number, and talking calculators.

- Computers and computer-related items, such as punched-card readers (which enable users to determine characters on punched computer cards), voice-prompting automatic data-entry terminals, braille printers and embossers (which interface with computers), talking computer terminals or software with speech output or synthesis, or talking telephone directories (which respond vocally to typed requests).

- Magnifying aids, such as simple hand-held MAGNIFIERS or mounted magnifiers, loupes, bioptics, telescopic devices, and CLOSED-CIRCUIT TELEVISION (CCTV) systems.

- Illumination aids, which may be as simple as replacing low-wattage bulbs with higher-wattage light bulbs, may also include devices to reduce glare and flicker, special lamps, or hand-held flashlight magnifiers.

- Measuring aids, such as circuit testers (which emit a tone when a circuit or test cable attachment is complete), talking frequency measurers, auditory meter readers, brailled calipers, auditory or tactile dial indicators, electronic levels, tactually marked protractors, saw guides and tape measure, and auditory thermometers or pressure gages.

- Reading aids, such as the Kurzweil Personal Reader, the Optacon, and speech output for the Optacon.

- Recorders, such as cassette recorders and playback machines with variable-speed playback or time-compression systems.

- Tactile aids, such as the Sensory Quill, raised-line drawing kits, tactile maps, phone adaptors for determining tactually which lines on a multiline phone are activated, or Lamp Activated Signal Terminal for telephone system workers.

- Organizational aids, such as large-print or braille label makers, talking label makers, and file folders differentiated by color.

- Time-keeping aids, such as raised-dot marked watches, talking clocks, metronomes, and raised-dot or talking stop watches.

- Tools, including adaptive chiseling guides, dovetailing guides, drill positioners, tactually marked framing squares, light probes for determining indicator lights, and copy holders.

Vocational Education Act The Vocational Education Act of 1963 established the first permanent system to fund state vocational education through public schools. Amendments to the act in 1968 required each state to apply 10 percent of the funds received to programs specially designed for handicapped students.

In 1976, the act was amended to require states to match 50 percent of the funds received with state funds that must be applied to disability services. These funds were further earmarked to be used to assist disabled students to participate in nondisabled vocational programs and reduce segregation of programs. Funded states were also directed to create vocational education procedures and plans in compliance with the policies described in the act.

As rewritten in 1984, the act, known as the Carl D. Perkins Vocational Education Act of 1984 includes two major parts, Titles II and III. Title II, parts A and B, award state grants, and Title III funds special services and programs.

Part A of Title II establishes the Vocational Education Opportunities program, which receives the majority of state grantfunding allocated by Congress. Part B establishes the Innovation and Expansion grant program, which receives the remainder of the appropriated funds.

States receiving Part A monies must earmark 10 percent or more for vocational-education services for disabled students. Disabled students must be afforded equal opportunities in recruitment, registration and placement. They must be allowed equal opportunity in course choices and apprenticeship programs. Courses must be held in the least restrictive facility in compliance with the Education of the Handicapped Act.

Vocational programs supported by federal funds must provide each disabled student with a written evaluation concerning his interests, skills, and needs as they apply to a vocational-education program. The state must supply any needed adaptive equipment, curriculum materials or facilities. The programs must provide special guidance or career development counseling, as well as transitional employment counseling by professionally trained instructors. The state is required to pay one-half of the cost for supplemental disability services.

Under Title IV of the act, grants are awarded for research into improving and expanding vocational education to targeted groups of students, including those with disabilities. The act also assists the National Center for Research in Vocational Education and the National Institute of Education in programs these institutions coordinate for disabled persons.

The act was further amended in 1998 to include technical education. The current act is known as the Carl D. Perkins Vocational Education Act of 1998, or Perkins III.

EducationDaily.com. Carl D. Perkins Vocational and Applied Technology Education Amendments of 1998. www.educationdaily.com/FTP/Laws: 1998.

U.S. Department of Education. *Summary of Existing Legislation Affecting Persons with Disabilities.* Washington, D.C.: USDE, 1988.

vocational rehabilitation Vocational rehabilitation services are programs that provide vocational training or support to disabled individuals from federal, state, or private agencies. Vocational rehabilitation enables visually impaired individuals to continue employment or train for new work. Vocational rehabilitation may be offered through a public or private residential school, within a program of special education in a public school, through an organization for the blind, by a private rehabilitation facility, by a sheltered workshop, through correspondence courses or by state rehabilitation agencies.

All 50 states administer programs of vocational rehabilitation and DAILY LIVING SKILLS for the purpose of enabling disabled individuals to become independent, employed, integrated members of society. These agencies are listed under various names, such as Department of Rehabilitation; Commission for the Visually Handicapped: State Services for the Blind and Visually Impaired; and the Bureau of the Blind.

Each state program varies according to the range of services and training available and the amount of financial assistance provided. Services may include medical and vocational diagnostic services, rehabilitation training, physical restoration, braille instruction, communication-skills training, books and training supplies, transportation allowance, reader services for the blind, vocational rehabilitation, job-placement services, postemployment services, procurement of job-related equipment and occupational licenses, ADAPTIVE AIDS evaluation, and selection, counseling, and family-member services.

Legally blind individuals may qualify for state rehabilitation services if they can provide certification of disability, if the disability results in a substantial handicap to employment, and if the state has a reasonable expectation that the recipient will get or hold a job as a result of vocational training.

Rehabilitation services are available at little or no cost to the individual. Some aspects of the rehabilitation program may require financial contribution by the individual. In some states, services such as psychological counseling, equipment purchase, transportation to school, or school tuition may be financed by the state or a combination of the state, the individual, and grants or loans.

In all state programs, each individual's case is carefully evaluated by a vocational-rehabilitation counselor for the blind with input from the disabled individual. College-trained vocational-rehabilitation specialists evaluate existing skills and aptitudes, evaluate and recommend occupations, outline needed skills, provide vocational-skills training and education, and recommend and provide training in the use of vocational aids or devices.

Every eligible individual is given an Individualized Written Plan that outlines the rehabilitation goals, the individual's skills and needs, and the process that will be taken to meet those needs.

The plan may provide for a medical examination to ascertain the extent and limitations of the disability, in order to assess suitable employment possibilities. Medical treatment or equipment, including surgery, psychiatric counseling, hospital services, prostheses, and eyeglasses, may be provided to reduce or alleviate the disability and improve productivity on the job.

Guidance counseling may be suggested to assess the individual's potential for rehabilitation, independent living, and appropriate employment. Job training may be provided at home, rehabilitation centers, trade schools, or on-the-job settings.

Educational tuition and expenses may be supplied if college is necessary to the vocational rehabilitation. The plan may furnish financial assistance during the rehabilitation process, as well as transportation costs, job referral and placement services, and job modification or reevaluation services.

Vocational-rehabilitation training may result in disabled individuals being employed in the mainstream of industry. These individuals earn and work at the same level of productivity as their sighted peers. Others may be employed in a Business Enterprise Program (BEP). These are usually vending, short order or cafeteria-style stands, or small businesses that are given priority for operation within federal facilities such as post offices, federal offices, or military institutions. The BEP is administered through the state vocational-rehabilitation agency and is supported by federal funds.

An individual may work in a sheltered workshop. A sheltered workshop is any place of employment that protects employment of the disabled. The individual may also be employed at home as a homemaker and family care provider.

The success of vocational-rehabilitation training varies by individual. The extent of the visual loss, the time in life when the loss occurred, and the abilities and aptitude of the individual all affect the outcome. The length of time for rehabilitation services also differs and may continue six months or longer.

American Foundation for the Blind. *An Introduction to Blindness Services in the United States.* www.afb.org/into_document_view.asp?documentid=930, 2001.

American Foundation for the Blind. *Rehabilitation Services.* New York: AFB, 1988.

California Department of Rehabilitation. *Client Information Booklet.* Sacramento: CDR, 1987.

California Department of Rehabilitation. *Rehabilitation is Here to Help.* Sacramento: CDR, 1986.

Lions Club International. *Rehabilitation of the Blind.* Oak Brook, Illinois: LCIRB, 1984.

National Association for Visually Handicapped. *The Adult Partially Seeing.* New York: NAVH, 1984.

VTEK   See TELESENSORY SYSTEMS INC.

Wagner-Peyser Act The Wagner-Peyser Act of 1933, as currently amended, established a state and federal employment security program to find jobs for the unemployed and qualified workers for employers. Amendments to the act in 1954 required a designated staff person within each employment-services office to help disabled individuals find employment or training.

Further amendments to the act were made in 1982, by the Job Training Partnership Act (JTPA), and again in 1998 by the Workforce Investment Act of 1998. The 1982 amendments established a coordinated effort between local JTPA programs and state employment services and offered Wagner-Peyser funding incentives to states assisting targeted populations, including disabled persons. The 1998 amendments specified that job training programs must be managed at the local level where employers' needs are best understood, and gives more control to individuals to choose the services they require.

Disabled persons are described in the act as those who have a physical, mental, or emotional disability, including drug or alcohol dependence, which hinders employment. Employment services to the disabled strive to provide equal opportunity for employment and equal wages, the highest level of employment possible given the individual's skills, suitable accommodation to the job or work station, and an occupation that will not endanger the individual or others.

U.S. Department of Education. *Summary of Existing Legislation Affecting Persons with Disabilities.* Washington, D.C.: USDE, 1988.

U.S. Department of Labor. Workforce Investment Act of 1998. www.workforce.org, 1999.

Weihenmayer, Eric Eric Weihenmayer is a blind speaker, writer, and adventurer who in 2001 became the first blind person to climb Mount Everest, the highest peak on Earth. Weihenmayer, who was born in 1969, began the climb in March and reached the summit shortly after midnight on May 25. He relied on his sense of touch and followed other climbers who wore bells during the ascent.

Born with retinoscheses, a degenerative eye disorder, Weihenmayer knew as a child that he would become blind by the time he was 13. He credits his family with helping him to develop and keep a positive outlook and to overcome the disadvantages that resulted from his blindness.

In addition to mountain climbing, Weihenmayer enjoys acrobatic skydiving, scuba-diving, long-distance biking, running marathons, skiing, ice climbing, and rock climbing. He is determined that his blindness will not stop him from attaining his goals and has become an inspiration for blind people all around the world. The National Federal of the Blind sponsored Weihenmayer's Everest climb.

Weihenmayer has become well known to corporations and schools as an inspirational speaker. He has been featured in *Life, People, Sports Illustrated, Inside Edition, The Today Show, Good Morning America,* the Learning Channel, and many other newspapers, magazines, radio, and television shows. He recently completed his first book, *Touch the Top of the World: A Blind Man's Journey to Climb Further than the Eye Can See.* He lives in Englewood, Colorado, with his wife, Ellie, and daughter, Emma.

Western Blind Rehabilitation Center (WBRC) A blind rehabilitation center founded in 1967 by the United States Department of Veterans Affairs. The

32-bed inpatient facility serves 14 western states, the largest geographic area designated by the VA.

The WBRC program is available to any legally blind, honorably discharged veteran. The average age of veterans entering the program is near 60, but individuals of any age may be eligible.

Current figures from WBRC indicate that over 20,000 legally blind veterans in the 14 states are served by the WBRC. The number of those served is expected to triple in the future due to the aging of veterans and age-related vision-limiting conditions.

The program offered by the WBRC has four parts: living skills, manual skills, orientation and mobility, and visual skills. Living skills consists of training to perform daily tasks independently. It covers personal care, home management, communications, kitchen skills, and a computer-reading-aids program.

The manual skills section concerns sensory development, organizational skills, and self-confidence. Activities such as woodworking, leather projects, copper tooling, and home mechanics improve tactual perception, bimanual coordination, finger dexterity, and hand-foot coordination.

Orientation and mobility teaches independent traveling and safety skills. Long-cane travel skills, techniques for using electronic travel aids, and low-vision travel evaluations are included.

Visual skills consists of instruction for veterans with low vision. It introduces low-vision aids and devices and nonoptical aids. Optometry services develop and provide an individualized vision rehabilitation plan.

The facility also offers psychological counseling, social services, family training, nutrition and dietetics counseling, nursing and medical services, and recreation therapy.

Contact:

Western Blind Rehabilitation Center 124
Veterans Affairs Medical Center
3801 Miranda Avenue
Palo Alto, CA 94304
650-493-5000
www.palo-alto.med.va.gov

wet eye   a condition in which the eye contains an overabundance of tears due to inadequate tear drainage. It may be an annoying condition but rarely affects visual acuity.

Tears are constantly being produced and drained from the eye. They drain through lacrimal puncta, holes in each inner corner of the upper and lower lids. The tears are gathered in the lacrimal sac, an organ at the junction of the nose and lower lid. The tears then pass under the tissue to drainage ducts in the nasal cavity.

When the tears fail to drain adequately, wet eye occurs. This may be a congenital or acquired condition. Congenital wet eye occurs as a result of obstructions to the nasolacrimal ducts. Symptoms include tearing, crusting of the lids or eyelashes, mucous discharge, and inflammation of the lacrimal sac.

Obstructions often clear spontaneously within the first 12 months of life. After this time, obstructions are cleared surgically by simple probe and irrigation, silicone intubation procedures, or the more serious surgical procedure of dacryocystorhinostomy.

The probe and irrigation procedure is a five-minute operation that involves syringing the obstructed area under general anesthetic. The silicone intubation consists of inserting and looping a tiny silicone tube through the tear-duct system to link the upper and lower puncta. The tube is tied and left in the tear-duct system for several months. A dacryocystorhinostomy is a surgical operation that connects the lacrimal sac to the nasal cavity.

Acquired obstructions usually occur in middle age, and most commonly among women. Tearing becomes severe and annoying. The simple procedures of probe and irrigation or silicone intubation are often ineffective, and a dacryocystorhinostomy is indicated.

work opportunity tax credit (WOTC)   A federal tax incentive aimed at getting employers to hire individuals from seven groups that are seen as disadvantaged for employment purposes according to government guidelines. The WOTC replaces the targeted jobs tax credit, which had expired at the end of 1994. The new program went into effect September 30, 1996.

The groups targeted as disadvantaged for employment purposes are qualified veterans, qualified food-stamp recipients, qualified ex-felons, and qualified youth during the summer months. Also, it includes vocational rehabilitation referrals, which include workers with a physical or mental handicap; high-risk youth; and some workers who recently received some types of federal assistance.

Employers who choose to employ the WOTC may claim a credit of 35 percent of qualified first-year wages paid to an employee from one of the designated targeted groups. Tax credits generally range from a maximum of $2,100 for a full-time worker and $1,050 for a qualified summer employee.

world blindness Blindness is an international problem that exists in both developed and developing countries. Because of differences in methods used to gather statistics and differences in definitions of blindness, statistics measuring the number of blind persons in the world vary. According to 2001 statistics from the World Health Organization (WHO), there are an estimated 40 million to 45 million blind people in the world. WHO projects the number will double by the year 2025, unless decisive public health action is taken.

Blindness is more prevalent in developing countries, where up to 85 percent of the population may have little or no access to hospitals in urban areas. Throughout Africa, South America, and Asia, blindness rates are increasing with the growth of the population. Four major causes of blindness in developing countries are CATARACT, TRACHOMA, XEROPHTHALMIA, and ONCHOCERCIASIS. Cataract is the leading cause of blindness in all parts of the world. In developed countries, sight is restored with cataract surgery and extraction. In developing countries, an estimated 16 million adults have cataract-induced vision loss due to lack of trained personnel and facilities to perform cataract surgery. In most countries of Africa and Asia, cataracts account for half of all blindness.

Cataract is any opacity in the eye's normally CRYSTALLINE LENS. The vision may be completely obstructed in specific areas of the visual field.

Cataracts commonly worsen progressively over time.

The most common form, senile cataract, is a natural result of aging, although heredity, nutrition, general health and environment may influence the onset. There is no preventative treatment for senile cataracts, but they can be removed surgically. In developing countries, cataract extraction is often performed in mobile clinics or surgery units operated by mission or governmental agencies.

Trachoma, a contagious ocular disease caused by a chlamydial eye infection, may have a prevalence of as much as 500 million people worldwide and has caused blindness in about 6 million people. The infection causing the disease is due to the TRIC agent *Chlamydia trachomatis*. The infection is linked to bacterial infections caused by agents Koch-Weeks bacillus, Morax Axenfeld diplobacillus, and the gonococcus bacillus. Trachoma thrives in overcrowded conditions in which poor sewage disposal, sanitation, and personal hygiene, along with a lack of clean water supply, exist. In such conditions, this highly communicable disease may infect an entire community.

The disease first appears as a form of CONJUNCTIVITIS on the inside of the upper eyelids, later followed by symptoms of irritation, light sensitivity, and tearing. As the infection progresses to the CORNEA, it may cause ulceration leading to scarring, opacification, and vision loss.

Trachoma is treated with topical antibiotic eye ointment for several weeks. However, vision loss due to corneal scarring may be irreversible. Trachoma is prevented by improving environmental factors such as providing a clean water supply and employing simple methods of good personal hygiene.

XEROPHTHALMIA is the leading cause of blindness in children of developing countries. According to Helen Keller International, xerophthalmia annually affects 5 million to 10 million children in the world and completely destroys the vision in 350,000 of these per year. The disease occurs worldwide but is found most commonly in Asia and Africa. Children under six years of age are at greatest risk.

Xerophthalmia results from a lack of vitamin A in the diet. It occurs as a result of malnutrition and is closely associated with measles, diarrhea, and acute respiratory infection in vitamin-A-deficient children. Early symptoms include night blindness and Bitot's spots, a result of the drying of the CONJUNCTIVA leading to a sloughing of conjunctival epithelial cells.

The disease causes fundamental changes in the conjunctiva and cornea, which can lead to blindness. In severe cases, the cornea ulcerates and can perforate, causing AQUEOUS FLUID loss and collapse of the ANTERIOR CHAMBER. The cornea becomes opaque, and the eyeball is destroyed.

Xerophthalmia can be detected during an eye examination or by electroretinogram, a method impractical in field work. Treatment of the disease consists of three megadoses of 200,000 IU vitamin A by mouth, coupled with a protein- and calorie-rich diet, and treatment of any accompanying systemic infection.

One 200,000 IU vitamin-A dosage may be administered twice a year as a preventative measure. Other preventatives include enrichment with vitamin A of a commonly ingested staple such as tea or sugar, nutrition education and improvement in diet.

ONCHOCERCIASIS is a disease caused by the filarial worm, *Onchocerca volvulus*, transmitted by the Simulium blackfly. The disease occurs mainly in West Equatorial Africa, Central America, and South America. It is estimated to have infected over 18 million people and blinded an estimated 270,000 people. Visual impairment is projected for 20 percent of all those infected.

Onchocerciasis occurs when the worm infests the human body. The human becomes host to the worm, which may live up to 15 years within the body's skin, organs, and blood.

The disease causes corneal inflammation, or KERATITIS, corneal scarring, and vision loss. The inflammation can also cause chronic IRIDOCYCLITIS and GLAUCOMA.

Prior to 1986, there was no effective medical treatment for onchocerciasis. Prevention of the disease consisted of vector control, using insecticides to rid the community of the worms, avoidance of breeding sites such as rivers and open waterways, wearing protective clothing, and excising of skin nodules that contain the worms.

Since 1986, human trials have shown that a drug, ivermectin, discovered by Merck, Sharp and Dohme Inc., is highly effective in killing the microfilariae in humans and does so with few adverse reactions. The drug is available for worldwide distribution from Merck, Sharp and Dohme Inc., free of charge to onchocerciasis-control programs under the trade name Mectizan.

World blindness can be addressed by strengthening infrastructures and training health workers in the community being served. Indigenous people can be trained to become community health workers. The workers can maintain health-screening projects to diagnose and treat eye diseases in the earliest stages. Health education and awareness programs can improve personal hygiene, environmental conditions, sanitation, and nutrition. Mobile teams and surgical units can provide specialized treatment, surgery, and follow-up care.

Bath, Patricia E. "Blindness Prevention Through Programs of Community Ophthalmology in Developing Countries." In *Ophthalmology*. Vol. 2. Edited by K. Shimizu and J. Oosterhuis. Amsterdam: Excerpta Medica, 1979.

Cupak, K. "The Importance of Eye Camps in Underdeveloped Countries." In *Ophthalmology*. Vol. 2. Edited by K. Shimizu and J. Oosterhuis. Amsterdam: Excerpta Medica, 1979.

Helen Keller International. *Facts About Helen Keller International.* New York: HKI, 1987.

Helen Keller International. Diseases/causes.www.hki.org/diseases/index.html, 2000.

Phillips, Calbert I. *Basic Clinical Ophthalmology.* London: Pitman Publishers Limited, 1984.

World Health Organization. *Available Data On Blindness (Update 2000).* New York: WHO, 1987.

World Blind Sailing Championship   A competition started in 1992, when it was hosted by a blind group in New Zealand. The championship was held again in 1994 in Australia and in 1997 in England. Sailing is an activity in which blind people can participate and excel. In 1999, 29 four-person teams participated in the championships held that year in Miami.

A team includes two visually impaired crew and two sighted guides. One of the visually impaired persons is the helmsman, responsible for steering the boat around the course. The other controls the foredeck. The sighted guides, who are experienced sailboat racers, give verbal instructions to the visually impaired crew.

World Health Organization (WHO) A specialized agency, founded in 1948 by the United Nations, for improving world health levels that will permit all citizens of the world to lead a socially productive life.

Through cooperation with its member states, WHO maintains advisory and technical activities around the world, including research, technical assistance, establishment of international health-level standards, health-information dissemination and statistics collection, and aid to victims of natural disasters.

WHO provides aid and assistance at the country's request. It establishes health programs and services, provides and trains health and medical technicians and supports national health programs of disease control. WHO priorities include maternal and child health care, elimination of malnutrition, promotion of mass immunization of preventable diseases, provision of safe water supplies, and control of malaria, tuberculosis, smallpox, and leprosy.

The World Health Assembly serves as the legislative body and is formed of representatives from the member states. The assembly meets annually to determine budget and policy decisions that are enacted by an executive board. A director-general manages a secretariat in Geneva, Switzerland.

Contact:

World Health Organization
1211 Geneva 27
Switzerland
(+00-41-22) 791-21-11
www.who.int

Xalatan   See EYE DROPS.

xanthelasma   Yellow plaques that form on the eyelid. The plaques consist of fat deposits and suggest that the body may be unable to process fats or cholesterol. Xanthelasma occasionally accompanies DIABETES, hypercholesterolemia, and histiocytosis. The blood should be tested for cholesterol and treated by diet or medication as indicated.

The condition is harmless and does not affect vision. Xanthelasma may be removed but may recur.

X-Chrom lens   See CONTACT LENSES.

xerophthalmia   A disease caused by a vitamin-A deficiency in the diet. It may occur as a result of malnutrition, protein malnutrition, or diarrhea. Early symptoms of the disorder include night blindness, conjunctivitis, and tearing.

Xerophthalmia is the second leading cause of blindness in the world and a leading cause of blindness in children in third world countries. Helen Keller International cites that xerophthalmia visually impairs 5 million to 10 million children worldwide each year and blinds 350,000 of these. Although the disease occurs worldwide, it is most concentrated in Southern Asia and Northern Saharan Africa. Children under six years of age are at greatest risk.

The disease causes fundamental changes in the CORNEA, CONJUNCTIVA, and anterior segments of the eye, which can lead to blindness. In severe cases, the cornea is perforated and AQUEOUS FLUID is lost. As a result, the ANTERIOR CHAMBER flattens, the IRIS adheres to the cornea, and the eyeball is destroyed. Xerophthalmia can be detected during a corneal examination or by electroretinogram, a method impractical in field work. Treatment of the disease consists of megadoses of 200,000 IU of vitamin A by mouth, coupled with a protein- and calorie-rich diet, and treatment of any accompanying systemic infection.

The vitamin-A dosage may be administered twice a year as a preventive measure. Other preventatives include enrichment of a commonly ingested staple such as tea or sugar with tasteless form of vitamin A, nutritional education, and improvement in diet.

Bath, Patricia E. "Blindness Prevention Through Programs of Community Ophthalmology in Developing Countries." In *Ophthalmology*. Vol. 2. Edited by K. Shimizu and J. Oosterhuis. Amsterdam: Excerpta Medica, 1979.

Cupak, K. "The Importance of Eye Camps in Underdeveloped Countries." In *Ophthalmology*. Vol. 2. Edited by K. Shimizu and J. Oosterhuis. Amsterdam: Excerpta Medica, 1979.

Helen Keller International. *Facts About Helen Keller International*. New York: HKI, 1988.

Phillips, Calbert I. *Basic Clinical Ophthalmology*. London: Pitman Publishers Limited, 1984.

World Health Organization. *Available Data On Blindness (Update 2000)*. New York: WHO, 2000.

YAG laser The YAG, or Neodymium: Yttrium-Aluminum-Garnet, laser is used in the postsurgical treatment of CATARACT-removal patients. After extracapsular cataract surgery, many patients experience opacification of the cataract capsule left behind in the eye. The YAG laser is used to create an opening in the capsule to restore vision.

The physician focuses the laser to a fine point on the capsule and releases a series of 500,000 watt explosions of energy that destroy the capsular matter. Because the laser can be so minutely focused, the physician can aim the beam accurately and avoid surrounding tissue or an intraocular lens resting on the opaque capsule.

The procedure is quick and painless and is most often performed without local anesthesia. The patient is able to walk or drive home after treatment.

The YAG laser is unique in its ability to perform this procedure because, unlike other lasers, it is not dependent on pigmented tissue to be effective. The argon and other lasers depend on pigment such as that found in the IRIS of the eye or in blood flowing through blood vessels in tissue. The pigmented tissue absorbs the energy from the argon laser and is destroyed. However, cataracts or their remaining capsules contain no pigmentation and are immune to the power of the argon laser.

In the past, when the postoperative vision declined due to this clouding of the capsule, a second surgery, a posterior capsulectomy, was necessary to restore good vision. The YAG approach is viewed as a safer, quicker procedure with fewer possible complications.

Z

zonule The zonules, or zonule of Zinn, is the group of thin, tightly drawn fibers that hold the lens in place in the EYE. The thousands of thread-like fibers are attached to the ciliary muscle and work with the muscle to change the shape of the LENS.

In order to focus on objects at different distances, the lens must adjust or accommodate. To focus on a near object, the lens must thicken and bulge forward. The ciliary muscle contracts, allowing the zonule to slacken and the lens to thicken and protrude forward. To focus on a distant object, the lens must flatten. The ciliary muscle expands, the zonule is pulled taut, and the lens flattens.

Zovirax See ACYCLOVIR.

APPENDIXES

APPENDIX I
COMPANIES

American Thermoform
  Corporation
1758 Brackett Street
La Verne, CA 91750
800-331-3676; fax 909-593-8001
http://www.atcbrleqp.com

Arkenstone, Inc.
555 Oakmead Parkway
Sunnyvale, CA 94086
800-444-4443; fax 408-328-8467
http://www.arkenstone.org

Artic Technologies
55 Park Street
Troy, MI 48083-2753
248-588-7370; fax 248-588-2650
http://www.artictech.com

Bavisoft
P.O. Box 8
Dewitt, NY 13214
http://www.bavisoft.com

Berkeley Systems, Inc.
1700 Shattuck Avenue
Berkeley, CA 94709
415-540-5535; fax 415-540-5115

BIT Corporation
52 Roland Street
Boston, MA 02129
617-666-2488; fax 617-666-4646

Blazie Engineering
105 East Jarrettsville Road
Forest Hill, MD 21050
410-893-9333; fax 410-836-5040
http://www.blazie.com

Duxbury Systems, Inc.
270 Littleton Road
Unit 6
Westford, MA 01886-3523

978-692-3000; fax 978-692-7912
http://www.duxburysystems.com

Enabling Technologies Company
1601 Northeast Braille Place
Jensen Beach, FL 34957
561-225-3687; fax 561-225-3299
http://www.brailer.com

Henter-Joyce, Inc.
11800 31st Court North Street
St. Petersburg, FL 33716
800-336-5658;
    fax 813-803-8001
http://www.hj.com

HumanWare, Inc.
6245 King Road
Loomis, CA 95650
800-722-3393
http://www.humanware.com

IBM Accessibility Center
11400 Burnett Road
Building 901, Room 5D-014
Austin, TX 78758
www.ibm.com/able

Independent Living Aids
200 Robbins Lane
Jericho, NY 11753
800-537-2118; fax 516-937-3906
http://www.independentliving.
  com

Lernout & Hauspie
52 Third Avenue
Burlington, MA 01803
781-203-5000; fax 781-238-0986
http://www.lhsl.com

LS&S Group, Inc.
P.O. Box 673
Northbrook, IL 60065

1-800-468-4789; fax 847-498-
  1482
http://www.lsgroup.com

NanoPac, Inc.
4823 South Sheridan Road
Suite 302
Tulsa, OK 74145-5717
918-665-0329; fax 918-665-0361
http://www.nanopac.com

Noir Medical Technologies
P.O. Box 159
South Lyon, MI 48178
1-800-521-9746; fax 734-769-
  1708

Talking Computers, Inc.
140 Little Falls Church Road
Suite 205
Falls Church, VA 22046
703-241-8224 or 1-800-458-6338

Telesensory Corporation
520 Almanor Avenue
Sunnyvale, CA 94086
408-616-8700; fax 408-616-8720
http://www.telesensory.com

Tojek & Associates
17355 Mierow Lane
Brookfield, WI 53005
414-784-4979

Transceptor Technologies, Inc.
2001 Commonwealth Boulevard
Suite 205
Ann Arbor, MI 48105
313-996-1899

Vision Technology, Inc.
8501 Delport Drive
St. Louis, MO 63114-5905
1-800-560-7226; fax 314-890-8383
http://www.visiontechinc.com

APPENDIX II
DISABILITY DATABASES

ABLEDATA
8401 Colesville Road
Suite 200
Silver Spring, MD 20910
800-227-0216
http://www.abledata.com/index.
  htm

Accent on Information
P.O. Box 700
Bloomington, IL 61701
309-378-2961; fax 309-378-4420

Ageline
American Association of Retired
  Persons
601 E Street NW
Washington, DC 20049
800-424-3410
http://www.aarp.org

Assistive Device Database System
Assistive Device Resource Center
California State University
6000 J Street
Sacramento, CA 95819
916-278-6916

BRS Information Technologies
1200 Route 7
Latham, NY 12110
518-783-7251

Combined Health Information
  Database (CHID)
National Institutes of Health
Box CHID
9000 Rockville Pike
Bethesda, MD 20892

301-468-6555
http://chid.nih.gov

CompuServe
232 N. Main Street
Marysville, Ohio
937-642-0002
http://www.compuserve.com

CTG (Closing the Gap) Solutions
P.O. Box 68
Henderson, MN 56044
507-248-3294; fax 507-248-3810
http://www.closingthegap.com

Dialog Information Services
3460 Hillview Avenue
Palo Alto, CA 94304
1-800-324-2564

Easter Seals Project ACTION
700 Thirteenth Street, NW
Suite 200
Washington, DC 20005
202-347-3066; fax 202-347-4157
http://www.projectaction.org

ERIC
Educational Resources Information Center
U.S. Department of Education
Office of Educational Research
  and Improvement
National Library of Education
555 New Jersey Avenue, NW
Washington, DC 20208-5721
202-219-2289
http://www.ed.gov

Job Accommodation Network
  (JAN)
West Virginia University
P.O. Box 6080
Morgantown, WV 26506
800-526-7234
http://janweb.idci.wvu.edu

MEDLINEplus
National Library of Medicine
8600 Rockville Pike
Bethesda, MD 20894
301-594-5983 or 1-888-346-3656
http://www.medlineplus.gov

The National Rehabilitation Information Center (NARIC)
1010 Wayne Avenue
Suite 800
Silver Spring, MD 20910
301-562-2400; fax 301-562-2401
http://www.naric/com

SPECIALNET
GTE Educational Network
  Services
5525 MacAuthur Boulevard
Suite 320
Irving, TX 75038
800-927-3000 or 214-751-0964
www.gte.net

APPENDIX III
DOG-GUIDE SCHOOLS

Canine Companions for
  Independence
P.O. Box 446
Santa Rosa, CA 95402-0446
866-224-3647 or 1-800-572-2275
http://www.caninecompanions.org

Eye Dog Foundation for the
  Blind, Inc.
512 N. Larchmont Boulevard
Los Angeles, CA 90004
602-276-0051

Fidelco Guide Dog Foundation,
  Inc.
P.O. Box 142
Bloomfield, CT 06002
203-243-5200; fax 203-243-7215

Guide Dog Foundation for the
  Blind, Inc.
371 East Jericho Turnpike
Smithtown, NY 11787

516-265-2121; fax 516-361-5192
http://www.guidedogs.com

Guiding Eyes for the Blind, Inc.
611 Granite Springs Road
Yorktown Heights, NY 10598
914-245-4024; fax 914-245-1609
http://www.guiding-eyes.org

Guide Dogs of America
13445 Glenoaks Boulevard
Sylmar, CA 91342
818-362-5834; fax 818-362-6870

Leader Dogs for the Blind
1039 Rochester Road
Rochester, MI 48063
810-651-9011; fax 810-651-5812
http://www.leaderdog.org

Pilot Dogs, Inc.
625 West Town Street
Columbus, OH 43215
614-221-6367; fax 614-221-1577

Seeing Eye, Inc.
P.O. Box 375
Morristown, NJ 07960
1-800-539-4425
http://www.seeingeye.org

Southeast Guide Dogs, Inc.
4210 77th Street East
Palmetto, FL 33561
813-729-5665; fax 813-729-6646
http://www.guidedogs.org

Upstate Guide Dog Association
P.O. Box 165
Hamlin, NY 14464
716-964-8815

APPENDIX IV
FEDERAL AGENCIES

U.S. DEPARTMENT OF EDUCATION

Center for Libraries and
  Educational Improvement
400 Maryland Avenue, SW
Room 613
Washington, DC 20202
202-254-6572

Clearinghouse on Handicapped
  and Gifted Children
1920 Association Drive
Reston, VA 22091
703-620-3660

Division of Blind and Visually
  Impaired
330 C Street, SW
Washington, DC 20202
202-732-1316

National Council on the
  Handicapped
330 C Street, SW
Room 3118
Washington, DC 20202
202-453-3846

National Institute on Disability
  and Rehabilitation Research
400 Maryland Avenue, SW
Washington, DC 20202
202-205-5666; TDD
  202-205-4756

Office of Special Education and
  Rehabilitative Services
330 C Street, SW
Room 3132
Washington, DC 20202
202-732-1241

Office of Special Education
  Programs
330 C Street, SW
Room 3086
Washington, DC 20202
202-732-1007

Office of the Secretary
400 Maryland Avenue, SW
Washington, DC 20202
202-732-3000

Rehabilitative Services Administration
330 C Street, SW
Washington, DC 20202
202-732-1282

U.S. DEPARTMENT OF HEALTH AND HUMAN SERVICES

Administration for Children,
  Youth, and Families
Donahoe Building
400 Sixth Street, SW
Washington, DC 20024
202-755-7762

Administration on Aging
North Building, Room 4760
200 Independence Avenue, SW
Washington, DC 20201
202-245-0724

Health Care Financing
  Administration
200 Independence Avenue, SW
Washington, DC 20201
202-245-6726

Health Resources and Services
  Administration

Bureau of Health Professions
5600 Fishers Lane
Rockville, MD 20857
301-443-5794

Health Services Administration/
  Division for Maternal and
  Child Health
Bureau of Health Care Delivery
  and Assistance
5600 Fishers Lane
Room 605
Rockville, MD 20857
301-443-2170

National Center for Health
  Statistics
3700 East-West Highway
Hyattsville, MD 20782
301-436-8500

National Institutes of Health/
  National Eye Institute
Building 31, Room Ao3
Bethesda, MD 20892
301-496-2234

Office of Human Development
  Services
200 Independence Avenue, SW
Room 309F
Washington, DC 20201
202-245-7246

Office of Policy Planning and
  Legislation
200 Independence Avenue, SW
Room 306E
Washington, DC 20201
202-245-7027

Office of the Secretary
200 Independence Avenue, SW
Room 615F
Washington, DC 20201
202-245-7000

Social Security Administration
6401 Security Boulevard
Baltimore, MD 21235
301-965-1234

U.S. DEPARTMENT OF LABOR

Employment Standards Administration
Branch of Special Employment
200 Constitution Avenue, NW
Washington, DC 20210
202-523-8727

Office of Federal Contract
Compliance Programs
200 Constitution Avenue, NW
Washington, DC 20210
202-523-9475

Office of the Secretary
200 Constitution Avenue, NW
Washington, DC 20210
202-523-8165

U.S. Employment Service
Patrick Henry Building
601 D Street, NW
Washington, DC 20213
202-376-6750

VETERANS ADMINISTRATION

Blind Rehabilitation Service
810 Vermont Avenue, NW
Washington, DC 20420
202-233-3232

Department of Medicine and
Surgery
810 Vermont Avenue, NW
Washington, DC 20420
202-223-2596

Department of Veterans Benefits
810 Vermont Avenue, NW
Washington, DC 20420
202-233-2044

Office of the Administrator
810 Vermont Avenue, NW
Washington, DC 20420
202-223-3775

OTHER AGENCIES

Architectural and Transportation
Barriers Compliance Board
1111 18th Street, NW
Suite 501
Washington, DC 20036
202-653-7834

Committee for Purchase from the
Blind and Other Severely
Handicapped
Crystal Square 5
Suite 1107
1755 Jefferson Davis Highway
Arlington, VA 22202-3509
703-557-1145

Equal Employment Opportunity
Commission
Office of Legal Counsel
2401 E Street, NW
Room 222
Washington, DC 20507
202-634-6460

Library of Congress National
Library Service for the Blind
and Physically Handicapped

1291 Taylor Street, NW
Washington, DC 20542
202-287-5100 or 1-800-424-9100

President's Committee on
Employment of People with
Disabilities
1111 20th Street, NW
Washington, DC 20036
202-653-5044

Small Business Administration
1441 L Street, NW
Washington, DC 20416
202-653-6605

U.S. Department of Justice
Civil Rights Division/Coordination
and Review Section
10th Street and Constitution
Avenue, NW
Washington, DC 20530
202-633-2151 or 202-724-7678
(TDD)

U.S. Office of Personnel
Management
Governmentwide Selective Placement Programs Division
1900 E Street, NW
Room 5A09
Washington, DC 20415
202-632-5491

APPENDIX V
NATIONAL ORGANIZATIONS

Affiliated Leadership League
1030 15th Street, NW
Suite 468
Washington, DC 20005
202-775-8261

American Academy of Ophthalmology
P.O. Box 7424
San Francisco, CA 94120
415-561-8500
http://www.eyenet.org

American Association for Pedi-
atric Ophthalmology and
Strabismus
P.O. Box 193832
San Francisco, CA 94119
415-561-8505

American Association of Certified
Orthoptists
St. Louis Children's Hospital Eye
Center
One Children's Plaza
Room 2, South 89
St. Louis, MO 63110
314-454-2122
http://www.orthoptics.org

American Association of the
Deaf-Blind
814 Thayer Avenue
Silver Spring, MD 20910

American Council of the Blind
1155 15th Street, NW
Washington, DC 20005
202-467-5081
http://www.acb.org

American Council on Rural
Special Education
Kansas State University

2323 Anderson Avenue
Suite 226
Manhattan, KS 66502
785-532-2737
http://www.ksu.edu/acres

American Diabetes Association
National Service Center
P.O. Box 25757
1600 Duke Street
Alexandria, VA 22313
703-549-1500 or 1-800-232-3472

American Foundation for the
Blind
11 Penn Plaza
Suite 300
New York, NY 10001
212-502-7660 or 800-232-5463;
TDD 212-502-7662
http://www.afb.org

American Optometric Association
243 North Lindbergh Boulevard
St. Louis, MO 63141
314-991-4100 or 1-800-365-2219
http://www.aoanet.org

American Society of Cataract and
Refractive Surgery
4000 Legato Road
Suite 850
Fairfax, VA 22030
703-591-2220; fax 703-591-0614
http://www.ascrs.org

American Society of Contempo-
rary Medicine, Surgery and
Ophthalmology
820 North Orleans Street
Suite 208
Chicago, IL 60610
312-440-0699

Associated Services for the Blind
911 Walnut Street
Philadelphia, PA 19107
215-627-0600

Association for Education and
Rehabilitation of the Blind and
Visually Impaired
206 North Washington Street,
Suite 320
Alexandria, VA 22314
703-548-1884

Association for Macular Diseases
210 East 64th Street
New York, NY 10021
212-605-3719

The Association for Persons with
Severe Handicaps
29 W. Susquehanna Avenue
Suite 210
Baltimore, MD 21204
410-828-8274 or 800-482-8274;
TDD 410-828-1306
http://www.tash.org

Association of Radio Reading
Services
University of South Florida,
WRB 209
Tampa, FL 33620
813-974-4193

Association on Handicapped
Student Service Programs in
Postsecondary Education
P.O. Box 21192
Columbus, OH 43221
614-488-4872

Blind Children's Center
4120 Marathon Street
P.O. Box 29159

Los Angeles, CA 90029
213-664-2153

Blind Children's Fund
230 Central Street
Auburndale, MA 02166
617-332-4014

Blind Outdoor Leisure Development
533 East Main Street
Aspen, CO 81611
303-925-8922

Blinded Veterans Association
477 H Street, NW
Washington, DC 20001
202-371-8880 or 800-669-7079

Braille Institute of America
741 North Vermont Avenue
Los Angeles, CA 90029
323-663-1111 or 800-272-4533
http://www.brailleinstitute.org

Corneal Dystrophy Foundation
1926 Hidden Creek Drive
Kingwood, TX 77339
713-358-4227

Council for Exceptional Children
1110 North Glebe Road
Suite 300
Arlington, VA 22201
703-620-3660 or 888-221-6830;
    TDD 703-264-9446
http://www.cec.sped.org

Council of Citizens with
    Low Vision
1400 North Drake Road
Kalamazoo, MI 49007
616-381-9566

Delta Gamma Foundation
3250 Riverside Drive
Columbus, OH 43221
614-481-8169
http://www.deltagamma.org

Eye Bank Association of America
    Inc.
1725 Eye Street, NW
Suite 308
Washington, DC 20005
202-775-4999

Eye Bank for Sight Restoration
210 East 64th Street
New York, NY 10021
212-980-6700

Eye Research Institute of the
    Retina Foundation
20 Stanford Road
Boston, MA 02114
617-742-3140

Fight for Sight
381 Park Avenue South
Suite 809
New York, NY 10016
212-679-6060

Foundation Fighting Blindness
11435 Cronhill Drive
Owings Mills, MD 21117-2220
410-568-0150 or 1-888-394-
    3937; TDD 1-800-683-5551
http://www.blindness.org

Friends of Eye Research
99 West Cedar Street
Boston, MA 02114
617-523-0303

Glaucoma Research Foundation
200 Pine Street
Suite 200
San Francisco, CA 94104
415-986-3162 or 800-826-6693
http://www.glaucoma.org

Guide Dog Users
14311 Astrodome Drive
Silver Springs, MD 20906
310-598-5771 or 888-858-1008
http://gdui.org

Helen Keller International
90 Washington Street
15th Floor
New York, NY 10006
212-943-0890
http://www.hki.org

Helen Keller National Center for
    Deaf-Blind Youth and Adults
111 Middle Neck Road
Sands Point, NY 11050
516-944-8900;
    TDD 516-944-8637
http://www.helenkeller.org

International Eye Foundation
7801 Norfolk Avenue
Bethesda, MD 20814
301-986-1830
http://www.iefusa.org

International Institute for Visually
    Impaired, 0-7
311 W. Broadway
Suite 1
Mount Pleasant, MI 48854
989-779-9966; fax 989-779-0015
http://www.blindchildrenfund.org

International Society on
    Metabolic Eye Disease
1125 Park Avenue
New York, NY 10128
212-427-1246

In Touch Networks
15 West 65th Street
New York, NY 10023
212-769-6270 or 800-456-3166

Joint Commission on Allied
    Health Personnel in
    Ophthalmology
2025 Woodlane Drive
St. Paul, MN 55125
651-731-2944 or 800-284-3937
http://www.jcahop.org

Joslin Diabetes Center
One Joslin Place
Boston, MA 02215
617-732-2400
http://www.joslin.org

Knights Templar Eye Foundation
5097 North Elston Avenue
Chicago, IL 60630
773-205-3838

Lions Club International
300 22nd Street
Oak Brook, IL 60570
630-571-5466
http://www.lionsclubs.org

March of Dimes Birth Defects
    Foundation
1275 Mamaroneck Avenue
White Plains, NY 10605
914-428-7100
http://www.modimes.org

Maynard Listener Library
171 Washington Street
Taunton, MA 02780
617-823-3783

Myasthenia Gravis Foundation
123 West Madison Street
Suite 800
Chicago, IL 60602
312-853-0522 or 800-541-5454
http://www.myasthenia.org

Myopia International Research
    Foundation
1265 Broadway
Room 608
New York, NY 10001
212-684-2777

National Accreditation Council for
    Agencies Serving the Blind and
    Legally Visually Handicapped
260 Northland Boulevard
Cincinnati, OH 45246
513-772-8449

National Association for Parents
    of Children with Visual
    Impairments
P.O. Box 317
Watertown, MA 02272
617-972-7444 or 800-562-6265

National Association for Visually
    Handicapped
22 W. 21st Street
New York, NY 10010
212-889-3141
http://www.navh.org

National Association of Blind
    Teachers
c/o American Council of the
    Blind
1155 15th Street, NW
Washington, DC 20005
202-467-5081

National Association of State
    Directors of Special Education
Suite 320
1800 Diagonal Road
Alexandria, VA 22314
703-519-3800; TDD 703-519-
    7008
http://www.nasdse.org

National Association of Vision
    Professionals Prevention of
    Blindness Society
1774 Church Street, NW
Washington, DC 20036
202-234-1010
http://www.members.tripod.com/
    charlie216

National Braille Association
3 Town Line Circle
Rochester, NY 14623
716-427-8260
http://www.nationalbraille.org

National Council of Private
    Agencies for the Blind
8770 Manchester Road
St. Louis, MO 63069
314-968-9000

National Council of State
    Agencies for the Blind
1213 29th Street, NW
Washington, DC 20007
202-333-5841

National Easter Seals Society
230 West Monroe
Suite 1800
Chicago, IL 60606
312-726-6200 or 800-221-6827;
    TDD 312-726-4258
http://www.easter-seals.org

National Eye Institute
2020 Vision Place
Bethesda, MD 20892
301-496-5248
http://www.nei.nih.gov

National Eye Research Foundation
910 Skokie Boulevard
Northbrook, IL 60062
847-564-6522
http://www.nerf.org

National Federation of the Blind
1800 Johnson Street
Baltimore, MD 21230
410-659-9314
http://www.nfb.org

National Glaucoma Research
    Program of the American
    Health Assistance Foundation

15825 Shady Grove Road
Suite 140
Rockville, MD 20850
301-948-3244
http://www.ahaf.org

National Industries for the Blind
1901 North Beauregard Street
Suite 200
Alexandria, VA 22311
703-998-0770
http://www.nib.org

National Multiple Sclerosis
    Society
733 Third Avenue
Sixth Floor
New York, NY 10017
212-986-3240
http://www.nmss.org

National Rehabilitation
    Information Center
1010 Wayne Avenue
Suite 800
Silver Spring, MD 20910
1-800-346-2742 or 301-562-
    2403
http://www.naric.com

National Society to Prevent
    Blindness
4200 California Street
#101
San Francisco, CA 94118-1314
415-387-0934; fax 415-387-1689
http://www.eyeinfo.org

New Eyes for the Needy
P.O. Box 332
549 Millburn Avenue
Short Hills, NJ 07078
201-376-4903

ODPHP (Office of Disease
    Prevention and Health
    Promotion)
Office of Public Health and Sci-
    ence
200 Independence Avenue, SW,
    Room 738G
Washington, DC 20201
202-401-6295; fax 202-205-9478
http://www.odphp.osophs.dhhs.
    gov

Opticians Association of America
7023 Little River Turnpike
Suite 207
Annadale, VA 22003
703-916-8856
http://www.opticians.org

Randolph-Sheppard Vendors of
   America
1808 Faith Place
#B
Terrytown, LA 70056
504-368-7785 or 800-467-5299
http://www.acb.org/rsva

Recording for the Blind
20 Roszel Road
Princeton, NJ 08540
609-452-0606 or 1-800-883-7201
http://www.rfbd.org

Research to Prevent Blindness
645 Madison Avenue
New York, NY 10022

212-752-4333 or 800-621-0026
http://www.rpbusa.org

Smith-Kettlewell Eye Research
   Institute
2318 Fillmore Street
San Francisco, CA 94115
415-345-2000
http://www.ski.org

Taping for the Blind
3935 Essex Lane
Houston, TX 77027
713-622-2767

Telephone Pioneers of America
930 15th Street
Suite 1200
Denver, CO 80202
303-571-1200;
   fax 303-572-0520
http://www.telephone-
   pioneers.org

United States Association for
   Blind Athletes
33 North Institute Street
Colorado Springs, CO 80903
719-630-0422
http://www.usaba.org

United States Braille Chess
   Association
428 West Lima Street
Findlay, OH 45840
419-422-2833
http://www.crisscrosstech.com/
   usbca

Vision Council of America: Better
   Vision Institute
1700 Diagonal Road
Suite 500
Alexandria, VA 22314
703-548-4560 or 877-642-3253
http://www.visionsite.org

APPENDIX VI
SCHOOLS FOR BLIND AND
VISUALLY IMPAIRED STUDENTS (BY STATE)

ALABAMA

Alabama Institute for Deaf and
  Blind
205 East South Street
Talladega, AL 35160
256-761-3259
http://www.aidb.state.al.us

Southwest Alabama Regional
  School for the Deaf and Blind
8901 Airport Boulevard
Mobile, AL 36608-9503
334-633-0241

ARIZONA

Arizona State Schools for the
  Deaf and the Blind
1200 West Speedway Boulevard
Tucson, AZ 85745
520-770-3700; TTD/TTY 520-770-
  3213
http://www.asdb.org

ARKANSAS

Arkansas School for the Blind
2600 West Markham
Little Rock, AR 72203
1-800-362-1810; TTD/TTY 501-
  296-1833

CALIFORNIA

Blind Children's Learning Center
18542-B Vanderlip Avenue
Santa Ana, CA 92705
714-573-8888
http://www.blindkids.org

Blind Children's Center
4120 Marathon Street
Los Angeles, CA 90029
323-664-2153
http://www.blindcntr.org

California School for the Blind
500 Walnut Avenue
Fremont, CA 94536
510-794-3800
http://goldmine.cde.ca.gov/csmt/
  apendd.html

Palomar College Adapted Computer Training Center
1140 Mission Road
Sand Marcos, CA 92069
760-744-1150; TDD/TTY 760-
  471-8506
http://www.palomar.edu

COLORADO

Colorado School for the Deaf and
  the Blind
33 North Institute Street
Colorado Springs, CO 80903-3599
719-578-2100; TDD/TTY 719-
  577-2101
http://www.csdb.org

CONNECTICUT

Connecticut Institute for the
  Blind/Oak Hill School
120 Holcomb Street
Hartford, CT 06112
860-242-2274
http://www.ciboakhill.org/
  index.htm

FLORIDA

Florida School for the Deaf and
  Blind
207 North San Marco Avenue
St. Augustine, FL 32084
904-827-2200 or 1-800-344-3732
http://www.fsdb.k12.fl.us

GEORGIA

Georgia Academy for the Blind
2895 Vineville Avenue
Macon, GA 31204
478-751-6083
http://www.gabmacon.org

IDAHO

Idaho School for the Deaf and
  Blind
1450 Main Street
Gooding, ID 83330
208-934-4457
http://www.isdb.state.id.us

ILLINOIS

Hadley School for the Blind
700 Elm Street
Winnetka, IL 60093
847-446-8111 or 1-800-323-
  4238; TDD/TYY 847-441-8111
http://www.hadley-school.org

Hope School
50 Hazel Lane
Springfield, IL 62705-5810
217-585-5437; TTD/
  TTY 217-529-5766
http://www.thehopeschool.org

Illinois School for the Visually
 Impaired
658 East State Street
Jacksonville, IL 62650
217-479-4400
http://www.il.us/agency/dhs/isvi.
 htm

Philip J. Rock Center and School
818 DuPage Boulevard
Glen Ellyn, IL 60137
630-790-2474 or 1-800-771-
 1158; TDD/TTY 630-790-4723
http://www.project-reach-illi-
 nois.org

INDIANA

Gary Community School
 Corporation
Lew Wallace Building
Suite B122
415 West 45th Avenue
Gary, IN 46408
219-980-6305

Indiana School for the Blind
7725 North College Avenue
Indianapolis, IN 46240
317-253-1481

IOWA

Iowa Braille and Sight-Saving
 School
1002 G Avenue
Vinton, IA 52349
319-472-5221 or 1-800-645-4579
http://www.iowa-braille.k12.ia.us

KANSAS

Kansas State School for the Blind
1100 State Avenue
Kansas City, KS 66102
913-281-3308 or 1-800-572-5463
http://www.kssb.net

KENTUCKY

Kentucky School for the Blind
1867 Frankfort Avenue
Louisville, KY 40206
502-897-1583
http://www.ksb.k12.ky.us

LOUISIANA

Louisiana School for the Visually
 Impaired
1120 Government Street
Baton Rouge, LA 70802-4897
225-342-8694

MARYLAND

Maryland School for the Blind
3501 Taylor Avenue
Baltimore, MD 21236-4499
410-444-5000 or 800-400-4915;
 TDD/TTY 410-319-5703
http://www.mdschblind.org

Ruth Parker Eason School
648 Old Mill Road
Millersville, MD 21108-1373
410-222-3815

MASSACHUSETTS

Perkins School for the Blind
175 North Beacon Street
Watertown, MA 02472
617-924-3434
http://www.perkins.pvt.k12.
 ma.us

MICHIGAN

Michigan School for the Blind
1667 Miller Road
Flint, MI 48503-5096
810-257-1420 or 1-800-622-6730
 ext. 420
http://www.msdb.k12.mi.us

MINNESOTA

Minnesota State Academy for
 the Blind
P.O. Box 68
Fairbault, MN 55021
507-333-4800 or 1-800-657-3634
http://www.msab.state.mn.us

MISSISSIPPI

Mississippi School for the Blind
1252 Eastover Drive
Jackson, MS 39211

601-984-8200; TTD/TTY 601-984-
 8097
http://www2.mde.k12.ms.us/msb

MISSOURI

Blue Springs Special Services
 Center
2103 West Vesper
Blue Springs, MO 64015
816-224-1360

Children's Center for the Visually
 Impaired
3101 Main Street
Kansas City, MO 64111-1921
816-333-3166

Missouri School for the Blind
3815 Magnolia Avenue
St. Louis, MO 63110
314-776-4320 or 1-800-622-5672
http://www.msb.k12.mo.us

MONTANA

Montana School for the Deaf
 and Blind
3911 Central Avenue
Great Falls, MT 59405
406-771-6000
http://www.sdb.mt.us

NEBRASKA

Nebraska Center for the Education of Children who are Blind
 or Visually Impaired
824 Tenth Avenue
Nebraska City, NE 68410
402-873-5513 or 1-800-826-
 4355
http://www.ncecbvi.org

NEW JERSEY

LIFT
P.O. Box 4264
Warren, NJ 07059
908-707-9840 or 1-800-552-5438
http://www.lift-inc.org

Matheny School and Hospital
Main Street
Peapack, NJ 07977

908-234-0011
http://www.matheny.org

St. Joseph's School for the Blind
253 Baldwin Avenue
Jersey City, NJ 07306
201-653-0578 or 1-800-457-8563
http://school.nj.com/school/sjsb

NEW MEXICO

New Mexico School for the
  Visually Handicapped
1900 North White Sands
  Boulevard
Alamogordo, NM 88310
505-437-3505 or 1-800-437-
  3505
http://www.nmsvh.k12.nm.us

NEW YORK

Lavelle School for the Blind
3830 Paulding Avenue
Bronx, NY 10469
718-882-1212

New York Institute for Special
  Education
999 Pelham Parkway
Bronx, NY 10469
718-519-7000; TDD/
  TTY 718-519-6196
http://www.nyise.org

New York State School for
  the Blind
2A Richmond Avenue
Batavia, NY 14020
716-343-5384 or (toll-free)
  1-877-697-7382
http://web.nysed.gov/vesid/nyssb.
  htm

NORTH CAROLINA

Governor Morehead School
2303 Mail Service Center
301 Ashe Avenue
Administration Building
Raleigh, NC 27699-2303
919-733-6381
http://www.governormorehead.
  net

NORTH DAKOTA

North Dakota Vision Services:
  School for the Blind
500 Stanford Road
Grand Forks, ND 58203-2799
701-795-2708 or 1-800-421-
  1181
http://www.ndsb.k12.nd.us

OHIO

Ohio State School for the Blind
5220 North High Street
Columbus, OH 43214
614-752-1152

OKLAHOMA

Oklahoma School for the Blind
3300 Gibson Street
Muskogee, OK 74403
918-781-8200 or (toll-free)
  1-877-229-7136
http://www.osb.k12.ok.us/index/
  html

OREGON

Oregon School for the Blind
700 Church Street, SE
Salem, OR 97301
503-378-3820

PENNSYLVANIA

Overbrook School for the Blind
6333 Malvern Avenue
Philadelphia, PA 19151-2597
215-877-0313

Royer-Greaves School for
  the Blind
118 South Valley Road
Paoli, PA 19301-1444
610-644-1810
http://royer-greavesschoolforblind.
  com

Western Pennsylvania School for
  Blind Children
201 North Bellefield Avenue
Pittsburgh, PA 15213-1499
412-621-0100

SOUTH CAROLINA

South Carolina School for the
  Deaf and the Blind
355 Cedar Springs Road
Spartanburg, SC 29302
864-585-7711 or (toll-free)
  1-888-447-2732; TDD/
  TTY 803-798-4936
http://www.scsdb.k12.sc.us

SOUTH DAKOTA

South Dakota School for the
  Blind and Visually Impaired
423 17th Avenue SE
Aberdeen, SD 57401
605-626-2580 or (toll-free)
  1-888-275-3814; TDD/
  TTY 605-626-7829
http://www.sdsbvi.sdbor.edu/

TENNESSEE

Tennessee School for the Blind
115 Stewarts Ferry Pike
Nashville, TN 37214
615-231-7340
http://volweb.utk.edu/Schools/
  tsb/

TEXAS

Texas School for the Blind and
  Visually Impaired
1100 West 45th Street
Austin, TX 78756-3494
512-454-8631 or 1-800-872-5273;
  TDD/TTY 512-206-9188
http://www.tsbvi.edu

UTAH

Utah School for the Blind
742 Harrison Boulevard
Ogden, UT 84404
801-629-4700 or 1-800-990-9328;
  TDD/TTY 801-629-4701
http://www.usdb.k12.ut.us

VIRGINIA

Virginia School for the Deaf and
  Blind at Staunton

P.O. Box 2069
Staunton, VA 24402
540-332-9000 or 1-800-522-8732

Virginia School for the Deaf,
  Blind and Multi-Disabled
  at Hampton
700 Shell Road
Hampton, VA 23661-2299
757-247-2050
http://www.vsdbh.org

WASHINGTON

Washington State School for
  the Blind
2214 East 13th Street
Vancouver, WA 98661-4120
360-696-6321
http://www.wssb.wa.gov

WEST VIRGINIA

West Virginia Schools for the Deaf
  and Blind

301 East Main Street
Romney, WV 26757
304-822-4800

WISCONSIN

Wisconsin Center for the Blind
  and Visually Impaired
1700 West State Street
Janesville, WI 53546
608-758-6146 or 1-800-832-
  9784; TDD/TTY 608-758-6127

APPENDIX VII
PERIODICALS

ABLA Newsletter
American Blind Lawyers
  Association
P.O. Box 1590
Indianola, MS 38751
662-887-5398

ACB Parents Newsletter
Council of Citizens with Low
  Vision
5707 Brockton Drive
Suite 302
Indianapolis, IN 46220
317-254-1332 or 800-733-2258

AER Report
Association for Education and
  Rehabilitation of the Blind and
  Visually Impaired
4600 Duke Street
Suite 430
Alexandria, VA 22304
703-823-9690 or 877-492-2708
http://www.aerbvi.com

AFB News
American Foundation for
  the Blind
11 Penn Plaza
Suite 300
New York, NY 10001
212-502-7660 or 800-232-5463;
  TDD 212-502-7662
http://www.afb.org

*American Council of the Blind
  Federal Employees News Council
  of Citizens with Low Vision*
5707 Brockton Drive
Suite 302
Indianapolis, IN 46220
317-254-1332 or 800-733-2258

*The American Lupus Society
  Quarterly*
The American Lupus Society
23751 Madison Street
Torrance, CA 90505
213-373-1335

American Rehabilitation
U.S. Department of Education
Mary Switzer Building
Room 3212
330 C Street, SW
Washington, DC 20202
202-205-5482

*Blindness, Visual Impairment,
  Deaf-Blindness, Semiannual
  Listing of Current Literature*
Association for Education of the
  Visually Handicapped
Room 700
919 Walnut Street
Philadelphia, PA 19107

The Blind Teacher
American Council of the Blind
1155 15th Street NW
Suite 1004
Washington, DC 20005
202-467-5081 or 800-424-8666;
  fax 202-467-5085
http://www.acb.org

Braille Book Review
National Library Service for the
  Blind and Physically Handicapped
1291 Taylor Street, NW
Washington, DC 20542
202-707-5100
http://www.loc.gov./uls

Braille Forum
American Council of the Blind
1155 15th Street, NW
Suite 1004
Washington, DC 20005
202-467-5081 or 800-424-8666;
  fax 202-467-5085
http://www.acb.org

The Braille Mirror
Braille Institute of America
741 N. Vermont Avenue
Los Angeles, CA 90029
323-663-1111
http://www.brailleinstitute.com

Braille Memorandum
Braille Revival League
1010 Vermont Avenue, NW
Washington, DC 20005

Braille Monitor
National Federation of the Blind
1800 Johnson Street
Baltimore, MD 21230
410-659-9314
http://www.afb.org

CCB Outlook
Canadian Council of the Blind
396 Cooper Street
Suite 401
Ottawa, Ontario K2P 2H7 Canada
613-567-0311 or 877-304-0968

CCLV Newsletter
Council of Citizens with Low
  Vision
5707 Brockton Drive
Suite 302
Indianapolis, IN 46220
317-254-1332 or 800-733-2258

Deaf Blind New Summary
Xavier Society for the Blind
154 East 23rd Street
New York, NY 10010
212-473-7800

Deafblind Weekly
Xavier Society for the Blind
154 East 23rd Street
New York, NY 10010
212-473-7800

Diabetes '90
American Diabetes Association
1701 Beauregard Street
Alexandria, VA 22314
703-549-1500 or 800-342-2383
http://www.diabetes.org

Diabetes Self-Management
R.A. Rapaport Publishing Inc.
150 West 22nd Street
New York, NY 10011

Dialogue
Dialogue Publications Inc.
3100 South Oak Park Avenue
Berwyn, IL 60402

*Education of the Visually
   Handicapped*
Heldref Publications
4000 Albemarle Street, NW
Washington, DC 20016

Encore
Division for the Blind and
   Visually Handicapped
Library of Congress
1291 Taylor, NW
Washington, DC 20542
202-707-5100
http://www.loc.gov/nls

Exceptional Children
Council for Exceptional Children
1110 North Glebe Road
Suite 300
Arlington, VA 22201
703-620-3660 or 888-221-6830;
   TDD 703-264-9446
http://www.cec.sped.org

Free Press
Wisconsin School for the Visually
   Handicapped

American Printing House for
   the Blind
1700 W. State Street
Jamesville, WI 53545
608-755-2977 or 1-800-832-9784

Guide Dog News
Guide Dogs for the Blind
350 Los Ranchitos Road
San Rafael, CA 94903
415-499-4000 or 800-295-4050
http://www.guidedogs.com

Heresay
Association of Radio Reading
   Services
National Office
4200 Wisconsin Avenue, NW
Suite 106-346
Washington, DC 20016
202-347-0955

HKI Report
Helen Keller International
90 Washington Street
15th Floor
New York, NY 10006
212-943-0890
http://www.hki.org

Inside MS
National Multiple Sclerosis
   Society
205 East 42nd Street
New York, NY 10017-5706
212-986-3240

Insight
Prevent Blindness News
National Society for the Prevention of Blindness
500 E. Remington Road
Schaumburg, IL 60173
312-843-2020

Insight
John Milton Society for the Blind
   in Canada
40 St. Clair Avenue, E.
#202
Toronto, ON M4T 1M9 Canada
416-960-3953

*International Eye Foundation
   Newsletter*

International Eye Foundation
7801 Norfolk Avenue
Bethesda, MD 20814

Jottings
Gospel Association for the Blind
7850 South U.S. Highway 1
Bunnell, FL 32110
904-586-5885

*Journal of Visual Impairment and
   Blindness*
American Foundation for
   the Blind
11 Penn Plaza
Suite 300
New York, NY 10001
212-502-7660 or 800-232-5463;
   TDD 212-502-7662
http://www.afb.org

Journal of Visual Rehabilitation
Media Productions and
   Marketing Inc.
2440 O Street
Suite 202
Lincoln, NE 68510
402-474-2676

Log of the Bridgetender
Friends in Art of ACB
Council of Citizens with Low
   Vision
5707 Brockton Drive
Suite 302
Indianapolis, IN 46220
317-254-1332 or 800-733-2258

Long Cane News Letter
Boston College
140 Commonwealth Avenue
Chestnut Hill, MA 02167

Lutheran Braille Evangelism Bulletin
Lutheran Braille Evangelism
   Association
1740 Eugene Street
White Bear Lake, MN 55110
651-426-0469

Mainstream
Pennsylvania Association for
   the Blind
2843 North Front Street

Harrisburg, PA 17110
http://www.pablind.org

MS Quarterly Report
Demos Publications
156 Fifth Avenue
Suite 1018
New York, NY 10010
212-255-8768

NARIC Quarterly
National Rehabilitation
    Information Center
8455 Colesville Road
Suite 935
Silver Spring, MD 20910-3319

NBA Bulletin
National Braille Association
3 Townline Circle
Rochester, NY 14623
716-427-8260
http://www.members.aol.com/
    nbaoffice/index.htm

*News About Library Services for the
    Blind and Physically Handicapped*
SC State Library—DBPH
301 Gervais Street
P.O. Box 821
Columbia, SC 29202
803-737-9970 or 1-800-922-
    7818

NEWSBITS
Talking Computers Inc.
140 Little Falls Road
Suite 205
Falls Church, VA 22046
1-800-458-6338

Opportunity
National Industries for the Blind
1901 North Beauregard Street
Alexandria, VA 22311
703-998-0770
http://www.nib.org

Paw Tracks
Council of Citizens with
    Low Vision
5707 Brockton Drive
Suite 302
Indianapolis, IN 46220
317-254-1332 or 800-733-2258

*Pilot Guide Dog Foundation
    Newsletter*
Pilot Guide Dog Alumni
    Foundation
1123 Wolfram Street
Chicago, IL 60657
312-671-1336

Recording for the Blind News
20 Roszel Road
Princeton, NJ 08540
609-452-0606 or 1-800-221-4792

Reflections
Council of Citizens with
    Low Vision
5707 Brockton Drive
Suite 302
Indianapolis, IN 46220
317-254-1332 or 800-733-2258

Scene
Braille Institute of America
741 N. Vermont Avenue
Los Angeles, CA 90029
323-663-1111
http://brailleinstitute.org

Seeing Eye Guide, The
Seeing Eye Inc.
Washington Valley Road
Morristown, NJ 07960
973-539-4425 or 800-539-4425
http://www.seeingeye.org

Sightsaving
National Society for the
    Prevention of Blindness
79 Madison Avenue
New York, NY 10016

*Smith-Kettlewell Technical File: A
    Quarterly Journal for the Blind
    and Visually Impaired*
Smith-Kettlewell Eye Research
    Foundation
2318 Fillmore Street
San Francisco, CA 94115
415-345-2000
http://www.ski.org

Standard-Bearer
National Accreditation Council for
    Agencies Serving the Blind
260 Northland Boulevard

Suite 223
Cincinnati, OH 45246
513-772-8449

Student Advocate
National Alliance of Blind
    Students
1010 Vermont Avenue, NW
Suite 1100
Washington, DC 20005
202-393-3666 or 1-800-425-8666

Talking Book Topics
National Library Service for the
    Blind and Physically
    Handicapped
Library of Congress
1291 Taylor Street, NW
Washington, DC 20542
202-707-5100
http://www.gov.nls

Towers
Overbrook School for the Blind
6333 Malvern Avenue
Philadelphia, PA 19151

Update
National Library Service for the
    Blind and Physically
    Handicapped
Library of Congress
1291 Taylor Street, NW
Washington, DC 20542
202-707-5100
http://www.loc.gov/nls

USABA Newsletter
U.S. Association for Blind
    Athletes
33 North Institute Street
Colorado Springs, CO 80903
719-630-0422
http://www.usaba.org

Utah Eagle
Utah Schools for the Deaf
    and Blind
Utah State Board of Education
742 Harrison Boulevard
Ogden, UT 84404
801-629-4700 or 800-990-9328;
    TDD 801-629-4701
http://www.usdb.k12.ut.us

VIDPI News
Visually Impaired Data Processors
  International
Council of Citizens with
  Low Vision
5707 Brockton Drive
Suite 302
Indianapolis, IN 46220
317-254-1332 or 800-733-2258

VISTA Newsletter
Council of Citizens with
  Low Vision
5707 Brockton Drive
Suite 302
Indianapolis, IN 46220
317-254-1332 or 800-733-2258

Vendorscope
Council of Citizens with Low
  Vision

5707 Brockton Drive
Suite 302
Indianapolis, IN 46220
317-254-1332 or 800-733-2258

Visionary
Illinois Society for Prevention of
  Blindness
407 South Dearborn Street
Suite 1000
Chicago, IL 60605
312-922-8710 or 800-433-4772
http://eyehealthillinois.org

Washington Weekly Review
(AFB Washington Review)
American Foundation for
  the Blind
11 Penn Plaza, Suite 300
New York, NY 10001

212-502-7660 or 800-232-5463;
  TDD 212-502-7662
http://www.afb.org

Worksight
Mississippi State University
Rehabilitation Research and
  Training Center on Blindness
  and Low Vision
P.O. Box 6189
Mississippi State, MS 39762
601-325-2001 or 1-800-675-7782
www.blind.msstate.edu/irr

Alabama Radio Reading Service
  Network
650 11th Street South
Birmingham, AL 35294
205-934-6576 or 800-444-9246
http://www.wbhm.org

APPENDIX VIII
RADIO READING SERVICES

Arkansas Radio Reading for the
  Blind, Inc.
2600 West Markham
Little Rock, AR 72208
510-663-4540
http://pages.prodigy.com/blindnet

Central Indiana Radio Reading,
  Inc.
1401 North Meridian Street
Indianapolis, IN 46202
317-636-2020
http://www.wfyi.org

Central Ohio Radio Reading
  Service
2955 W. Broad Street
Columbus, Ohio 43204
614-274-7650
http://www.corrs.org

Central Savannah River Area
  Radio Reading Service Inc.
c/o WACG-FM, Augusta College
2500 Walton Way
Augusta, GA 39010
706-737-1661

Chicagoland Radio Information
  Service, Inc.
77 E. Randolph Pedestrian
  Walkway
Chicago, IL 60601
312-541-8400
http://www.mcs.net/~cmeans/cris
  .html

Connecticut Radio Information
  Services
589 Jordan Lane
Wethersfield, CT 06109
860-956-3579
http://www.cslib.org/cris

Detroit Radio Information
  Service
4600 Cass Avenue
Detroit, MI 48201
313-577-4146
http://www.wdetfm.org

Evergreen Radio Reading Service
  of the Washington Library
  for the Blind and Physically
  Handicapped
821 Lenora Street
Seattle, WA 98129
206-615-0400

Georgia Radio Reading Service
260 14th Street, NW
Atlanta, GA 30318
404-685-2820 or 877-937-3378
http://www.galinks.com/garrs

Houston Taping for the Blind
  Radio
3935 Essex Lane
Houston, TX 77027
713-622-2767

Iowa Radio Reading Information
  Service
100 E. Euclid Avenue
Des Moines, IA 50313
515-243-6833 or 877-404-4747

Idaho Radio Reading Service
P.O. Box 83720
Boise, ID 83720
208-334-3220

Illinois Radio Reader
59 East Armory
Champaign, IL 61820
217-333-6503
http://www.will.uiuc.edu

INSIGHT/WYMS
5225 West Vliet Street
Milwaukee, WI 53208
414-475-8488
http://www.wyms.org

In-Sight
43 Jefferson Boulevard
Warwick, RI 02888
401-941-3322

In Touch Networks
15 West 65th Street
New York, NY
212-769-6270 or 800-456-3166

KPBS-FM Radio Reading Service
San Diego State University
San Diego, CA 92182
619-594-8170
http://www.kpbs.org

KUT 90.5 FM
University of Texas at Austin
Communications Building B
Austin, TX 78712
512-471-4683
http://www.kut.org

Montana Radio Reading
  Service
126 East Broadway, #8
Missoula, MT 59802
406-721-1998 or 800-942-7323

North Eastern Indiana Radio
  Reading Service Inc.
920 Florence Avenue
Fort Wayne, IN 46808
219-422-8230

Northern Illinois Radio
  Information Service
Riverfront Museum Park

711 N. Main Street
Rockford, IL 61103
815-961-8000
http://www.northernpublicradio.
   org

Radio Information Center for
   the Blind
Division of Associated Services
   for the Blind
919 Walnut Street
Philadelphia, PA 19107
215-627-0700
http://www.asb.org

Radio Information Service
Wabash Valley College
2200 College Drive
Mt. Carmel, IL 62963
618-262-8641, ext. 253

Radio Reading Service
4235 Electric Road, SW
Suite 105
Roanoke, VA 24014
540-989-8900

Radio Information Service for
   Blind and Handicapped
9541 Church Circle Drive
Belleville, IL 62223
618-394-6221

Radio Information Service for
   Blind and Print Handicapped of
   West Central Illinois
Western Illinois University
504 Memorial Hall
Macomb, IL 61455
309-298-2403
http://www/wiu.edu/usus/miris/
   wiv

Radio Reading Network of
   Maryland
2901 Liberty Heights Avenue
Baltimore, MD 21215
410-333-5720 or 800-5605

Radio Reading Services of Great
   Cincinnati, Inc.
2045 Gilbert Avenue
Cincinnati, OH 45202
513-221-8558

Radio Talking Book Service, Inc.
7101 Newport Avenue
Suite 205
Omaha, NE 68152
402-572-3003 or 800-729-7826

Radio Vision
619 Route 17M
Middletown, NY 10940
845-343-1131 or 800-327-7343
http://www.rcls.org

Reading Radio Service
815 North Walnut
Hutchinson, KS 67501
316-662-6646

READ-OUT Radio Reading Services
P.O. Box 2400
Syracuse, NY 13220
315-453-2424
http://www.wcny.org

RISE
c/o WMHT-FM
P.O. Box 17
Schenectady, NY 12301
518-356-1700
http://www.wmht.org

Sight Seer
West Michigan Radio Reading
   Service
213 Sheldon Boulevard, SE
Grand Rapids, MI 49503
616-235-0020
http://www.thesightseer.org

South Carolina Educational Radio
   for the Blind
1430 Confederate Avenue
Columbia, SC 29201
803-898-8755 or 1-800-922-2222

Sun Sounds of KJZZ
3124 East Roosevelt Street
Phoenix, AZ 85008
602-231-0500
http://www.sunsounds.org

Talking Information Center
130 Enterprise Drive
P.O. Box 519
Marshfield, MA 02050
781-834-4400 or 1-800-696-9505
http://www.radioview.com

Trade Winds Radio Reading
   Service
5901 W. Seventh Street
Gary, IN 46406
219-949-4000 or 800-694-4242;
   TDD 219-944-3733
http://www.thetimesonline.com/
   org/tradewinds

UPDATE Radio Reading Service
Chautauqua Blind Association
510 W. Fifth Street
Jamestown, NY 14701
716-664-6660

Valley Voice Radio Reading Service for the Print Handicapped
WMRA-FM
James Madison University
Harrisonburg, VA 22807
703-568-3811
http://www.valleyvoice.org

Virginia Voice for the Print
   Handicapped
P.O. Box 15546
401 Azalea Avenue
Richmond, VA 23227
804-266-2477

Washington Ear Inc.
35 University Boulevard East
Silver Spring, MD 20901
301-681-6636
http://www.washear.org

WCBU Radio Information Service
1501 W. Bradley Avenue
Peoria, IL 61625
309-677-3585

WYPL-FM
1850 Peabody Avenue
Memphis, TN 38104
901-725-8833
http://www.memphis.lib.tn.us/
   wypl/wyptop.htm

Radio Reading Service GW
285 Dorset Street
Springfield, MA 01108
413-788-6981

Wichita Radio Reading Service
3317 East 17th Street

Wichita, KS 67208
316-987-6600

WKAR Radio Talking Book
283 Communication Arts and
   Sciences Building
East Lansing, MI 48824
517-353-9124; TDD 517-355-
   7508
http://www.wkar.org

WLRN-FM School Board of
   Dade County Florida
172 N.E. 15th Street
Miami, FL 33132
305-995-2218 or 1-800-273-
   6677
http://www.wlrn.org

WPLN Talking Library
700 Second Avenue

Nashville, TN 37210
615-862-5874

WRKC-Radio Home Visitor
Kings College
Wilkes-Barre, PA 18711
520-208-5811

WTSU Radio Reading Service
252 Montgomery Street
Suite 312
Montgomery, AL 36104
334-241-9574

WRBH 88.3 FM Reading Radio
3606 Magazine Street
New Orleans, LA 70115
504-899-1144

WUSF Radio Reading Service
University of South Florida WRB
   209

4202 E. Fowler Avenue
Tampa, FL 33620
813-974-8695 or 800-444-4193
http://www.wusf.usf.edu

York County Blind Center's Radio
   Reading Service
1380 Spahn Avenue
York, PA 17403
717-848-1690
http://www.forsight.org

APPENDIX IX
REHABILITATION SERVICES (BY STATE)

ALABAMA

Alabama Department of
  Rehabilitation Services
2129 East South Boulevard
Montgomery, AL 36116-2455
334-281-8780 or 1-800-441-7607
http://www.rehab.state.al.us

Workshop and Rehabilitation Services for the Blind and Disabled
2129 East South Boulevard
Montgomery, AL 36116-2455
334-281-8780 or 1-800441-7607
http://www.rehab.state.al.us

ALASKA

Alaska Center for the Blind
3903 Taft Drive
Anchorage, AK 99517-3069
907-248-7770 or 1-800-770-7517
http://www.alaskablind.com

ARIZONA

Arizona Center for the Blind and
  Visually Impaired
3100 East Roosevelt Street
Phoenix, AZ 85008
602-273-7411
http://www.acbvi.org

Tucson Association for the Blind
  and Visually Impaired
3767 East Grant Road
Tucson, AZ 85716
520-795-1331

ARKANSAS

Arkansas Department of Human
  Services: Division of Services for
  the Blind

522 Main Street
Suite 100
Little Rock, AR 72203-3237
501-682-5463 or 1-800-960-9270;
  TDD/TTY 501-682-0093
http://www.state.ar.us/dhs/dsb

CALIFORNIA

California Department of Rehabilitation: Services for the Blind
2000 Evergreen Street
Sacramento, CA 95815-3832
916-263-8953; TDD/
  TTY 530-345-3897
http://www.rehab.cahwnet.gov/

Society for the Blind
2750 24th Street
Sacramento, CA 95818
916-452-8271
http://www.societyfortheblind.org

COLORADO

Colorado Department of Human
  Services: Rehabilitation Services
2211 West Evans Street
Building B
Denver, CO 80230
720-884-1234
http://www.state.co.us

CONNECTICUT

Connecticut State Board of Education and Services for the Blind
184 Windsor Avenue
Windsor, CT 06095
860-602-4000 or 1-800-842-4510;
  TDD/TTY 860-602-4002
http://www.besb.state.ct.us

DELAWARE

Delaware Department of Health
  and Social Services: Division for
  the Visually Impaired
1901 North Dupont Highway
Biggs Building
New Castle, DE 19720
302-577-4730; TDD/
  TTY 302-577-4750
http://www.state.de.us/dhss/dvi/
  dvihome.htm

DISTRICT OF COLUMBIA

Columbia Lighthouse for the
  Blind
1120 20th Street, NW
Washington, DC 20036
202-454-6400 or (toll free)
  877-324-5252
http://www.clb.org

FLORIDA

Center for the Visually Impaired
1187 Dunn Avenue
Daytona Beach, FL 32114
904-253-8879 or 1-800-227-1284
http://www.cfiflorida.org

Florida Department of
  Education: Division of
  Blind Services
2551 Executive Center Circle
Tallahassee, FL 32399
850-488-1330 or 1-800-342-1828
http://www.state.fl.us/dbs

Independent Living for Adult
  Blind
c/o Florida Community College at
  Jacksonville

101 West State Street
Jacksonville, FL 32202
904-633-8220

GEORGIA

Georgia Department of Human
   Resources: Division of
   Rehabilitation Services
Two Peachtree Street, NW
Suite 35-412
Atlanta, GA 30303-3142
404-657-3000
http://www.vocrehabga.org

Living Independence for Everyone
17-21 East Travis Street
Savannah, GA 31406
912-920-2414 or 1-800-948-
   4824; TDD/TTY 912-920-2419

HAWAII

Hawaii Department of Human
   Services: Ho'opono Services
   for the Blind, Vocational
   Rehabilitation and Services
   for the Blind Division
1901 Bachelot Street
Honolulu, HI 96817
808-692-7716
http://www.rrhi.com/
   hooponoblindservices

IDAHO

Idaho Commission for the Blind
   and Visually Impaired
341 West Washington Street
Boise, ID 83720-0012
208-334-3220
http://www.icbvi.state.id.us

ILLINOIS

Illinois Department of Rehabilitation Services: Bureau of
   Blind Services
623 East Adams Street
Springfield, IL 62794-9429
217-785-3887 or 1-800-275-
   3677; TDD/TTY 630-495-2294
http://www.state.il.us/agency/
   dhs/bsnp.html

Chicago Lighthouse for People
   Who Are Blind or Visually
   Impaired
1850 West Roosevelt Road
Chicago, IL 60608
312-666-1331; TDD/
   TTY 312-666-8874
http://www.thechicagolighthouse.
   org

INDIANA

Indiana Family and Social
   Services Administration:
   Division of Disability, Aging
   and Rehabilitative Services
Indiana Government Center
402 West Washington Street
Room W-453
Indianapolis, IN 46204
317-232-7020 or 1-800-545-7763
http://www.state.in.us/fssa

Trade Winds Rehabilitation Center
5901 West Seventh Avenue
Gary, IN 46406-0308
219-949-4000 or 1-800-694-
   4242; TDD/TTY 219-944-3733
http://www.thetimesonline.com/
   org/tradewinds

IOWA

Iowa Department for the Blind
524 Fourth Street
Des Moines, IA 50309-2364
515-281-1333 or 1-800-362-
   2587; TDD/TTY 515-281-1355
http://www.blind.state.ia.us/

KANSAS

Kansas Department of Social and
   Rehabilitation Services:
   Division of Services for
   the Blind, Rehabilitation
   Center for the Blind
2516 SW Sixth Avenue
Topeka, KS 66606
785-296-3311
http://www.state.ks.us/public/srs

Vision Rehabilitation Center
6100 East Central Avenue
Suite 5

Wichita, KS 67208-4237
316-682-4646

KENTUCKY

Kentucky Department for the
   Blind
209 St. Clair Street
Frankfort, KY 40602
502-575-7315 or 1-800-334-6920
http://www.state.ky.us/agen-
   cies/wforce//dfblind/index.htm

Kentucky Department for the
   Blind: Independent Living Services, Charles McDowell Center
8412 Westport Road
Louisville, KY 40242
502-327-6010 or 1-800-346-
   2115
http://www.state.ky.us/agencies/
   wforce/dfblind/kdfbhome.htm

LOUISIANA

Louisiana Center for the Blind
101 South Trenton Street
Ruston, LA 71270
318-251-2891 or 800-234-4166
http://www.lcb-ruston.com

Louisiana Department of Social
   Services: Louisiana Rehabilitation Services
8225 Florida Boulevard
Baton Rouge, LA 70806
225-925-3594 or 800-737-2958
http://www.dss.state.la.us/offlrs/

MAINE

Maine Department of Labor:
   Bureau of Rehabilitation
   Services, Division for the Blind
   and Visually Impaired
3 Anthony Avenue
#150 State House Station
Augusta, ME 04333-0150
207-624-5959; TDD/
   TTY 207-624-5955

MARYLAND

Johns Hopkins School of Medicine: Wilmer Ophthalmological

Institute, Lions Vision Research and Rehabilitation Center
550 North Broadway
Sixth Floor
Baltimore, MD 21205
410-955-0580
http://www.wilmereyeinstitute.org

Maryland State Department of Education: Division of Rehabilitation Services
2301 Argonne Drive
Baltimore, MD 21218-1696
410-767-9100 or (toll-free)
    1-888-200-7117; TDD/
    TTY 410-554-9411
http://www.dors.state.md.us/

Services for the Visually Impaired
8720 Georgia Avenue
Suite 210
Silver Spring, MD 20910
301-589-0894

MASSACHUSETTS

Massachusetts Association for the Blind
200 Ivy Street
Brookline, MA 02446
617-738-5110 or 1-800-682-9200
URL: http://www.mablind.org

Massachusetts State Commission for the Blind
88 Kingston Street
Boston, MA 02111-2227
617-727-5550 or 1-800-392-6450
http://www.magnet.state.ma.us/mcb

MICHIGAN

Michigan Commission for the Blind Training Center
1541 Oakland Drive
Kalamazoo, MI 49008
616-337-3848
http://www.mfia.state.mi.us/mcb

Visual Rehabilitation and Research Center of Michigan
15401 East Jefferson Avenue
Grosse Pointe Park, MI 48230
313-824-2401

Visually Impaired Center
725 Mason Street
Flint, MI 48503
810-235-2544

MINNESOTA

Minnesota State Academy for the Blind
P.O. Box 68
Fairbault, MN 55021
507-333-4800 or 1-800-657-3634
http://www.msab.state.mn.us

Minnesota State Services for the Blind
2200 University Avenue West
Suite 240
St. Paul, MN 55114-1840
651-642-0500 or 1-800-652-9000
TDD/TTY 651-642-0506
http://www.mnworkforcecenter.org/ssb/

MISSISSIPPI

Addie McBryde Rehabilitation Center for the Blind
2550 Peachtree Street
Jackson, MS 39296-5314
601-364-2700 or 1-800-443-1000; TDD/TTY 601-853-5100

Mississippi Department of Rehabilitation Services: Office of Vocational Rehabilitation for the Blind
1281 Highway 51 North
Madison, MS 39110
601-853-5100 or 1-800-443-1000
http://www.mdrs.state.ms.us

MISSOURI

Missouri Rehabilitation Services for the Blind
3418 Knipp Drive
Jefferson City, MO 65109
573-751-4249 or 1-800-592-6004
http://www.dss.state.mo.us/dfs/rehab.htm

Rehabilitation Institute: Center for Blindness and Low Vision

2801 Wyandotte Street
Third Floor
Kansas City, MO 64108
816-753-6533

MONTANA

Montana Department of Public Health and Human Services: Developmental Disabilities Program/Vocational Rehabilitation/Blind and Low Vision Services
111 North Sanders
Room 307
Helena, MT 59604
406-444-2590 or (toll free)
    1-877-296-1197

NEBRASKA

Nebraska Commission for the Blind and Visually Impaired
4600 Valley Road, Suite 100
Lincoln, NE 68510-4844
402-471-8100 or (toll free) 877-809-2419; TDD/TTY 402-471-2891

NEW HAMPSHIRE

New Hampshire Division of Vocational Rehabilitation: Services for the Blind and Visually Impaired
78 Regional Drive
Building #2
Concord, NH 03301
603-271-3537 or 800-581-6881
http://216.64.49.52/vrweb/blind.html

NEW JERSEY

New Jersey Commission for the Blind and Visually Impaired
153 Halsey Street, 6th Floor
Newark, NJ 07101
973-648-3333

New Jersey Foundation for the Blind
230 Diamond Spring Road
Denville, NJ 07834
201-627-0055

NEW MEXICO

New Mexico Commission for the
  Blind
1120 Paseo de Peralta
PERA Building, Room 553
Santa Fe, NM 87504
505-827-4479 or (toll free) 1-
  888-513-7968
http://www.state.nm.us/cftb

NEW YORK

Helen Keller Worldwide
90 West Street
Second Floor
New York, NY 10006
212-766-5266 or 1-800-535-5374
http://www.hkworld.org

New York State Education
  Department: Office of Vocational and Educational Services
  for Individuals with Disabilities
One Commerce Plaza
Room 1606
Albany, NY 12234
518-474-2714 or 1-800-222-5627
http://web.nysed.gov/vesid

Resource Center for Independent
  Living
401-409 Columbia Street
Utica, NY 13503-0210
315-797-4642; TDD/TTY 315-
  797-5837
http://www.rcil.com

Westchester Independent Living
  Center
200 Hamilton Avenue
Second Floor
White Plains, NY 10601
914-682-3926; TDD/TTY 914-
  682-0926
http://www.wilc.org

NORTH CAROLINA

North Carolina Division of Services for the Blind
2601 Mail Service Center
309 Ashe Avenue
Raleigh, NC 27699-260

919-733-9822; TDD/TTY 919-
  733-9700
http://www.dhhs.state.nc.us/dsb/

NORTH DAKOTA

North Dakota Department of
  Human Services: Vocational
  Rehabilitation
600 South Second Street, Suite
  1B
Bismarck, ND 58504
701-328-8950 or 1-800-755-
  2745; TDD/TTY 701-328-8968

OHIO

Ohio Rehabilitation Services
  Commission: Bureau of Services for the Visually Impaired
400 East Campus View Boulevard
Columbus, OH 43235-4604
614-438-1255 or 1-800-282-
  4536; TTD/TTY 614-995-1161
http://www.state.oh.us/rsc

Ohio State University: College of
  Optometry, Vision Rehabilitation Service
338 West 10th Avenue
Columbus, OH 43210
614-292-1104
http://www.optometry.ohio-
  state.edu

OKLAHOMA

Oklahoma Department of Rehabilitation Services
3535 N.W. 58th Street, Suite 500
Oklahoma City, OK 73112
405-951-3400 or 1-800-845-8476
http://www.onenet.net/~drspi-
  owm

OREGON

Independent Living Resources
4506 S.E. Belmont, Suite 100
Portland, OR 97215-1658
503-232-7411; TDD/TTY 503-
  232-8408
http://www.ilr.org

Oregon Commission for the Blind
535 12th Avenue, SE
Portland, OR 97214
503-731-3221 or (toll-free) 1-
  888-202-5463; TDD/TTY 503-
  731-3224
http://www.cfb.state.or.us

PENNSYLVANIA

Associated Services for the Blind
919 Walnut Street
Philadelphia, PA 19107
215-627-0600
http://www.asb.org

Association for the Blind and
  Visually Impaired
614 North 13th Street
Allentown, PA 18102-2199
610-433-6018
http://www.abvi.org

Center for Vision Rehabilitation
Allegheny General Hospital
Suite 116
Ophthalmology Department
Pittsburgh, PA 15212
412-359-6300 or 1-800-637-3762

RHODE ISLAND

Rhode Island Department of
  Human Services: Services for
  the Blind and Visually Impaired
40 Fountain Street
Providence, RI 02903-1898
401-277-2382 or 1-800-752-
  8088
http://www.ors.state.ri.us

SOUTH CAROLINA

South Carolina Commission for
  the Blind
1430 Confederate Avenue
Columbia, SC 29201
803-898-8800 or 1-800-922-2222
http://www.sccb.state.sc.us

SOUTH DAKOTA

South Dakota Department of
  Human Services: Division of

Service to the Blind and
Visually Impaired
East Highway 34
500 East Capitol
Pierre, SD 57501-5070
605-773-5990 or 1-800-265-9684
http://www.state.sd.us/dhs/

TENNESSEE

Tennessee Rehabilitation Center
460 Ninth Avenue
Smyrna, TN 37167-2010
615-741-4921

Tennessee Services for the Blind
and Visually Impaired
400 Deaderick Street, 11th Floor
Nashville, TN 37248-6200
615-313-4914

TEXAS

Texas Commission for the Blind:
Criss Cole Rehabilitation Center
4800 North Lamar
Austin, TX 78756
512-377-0300 or 1-800-252-5204
http://www.tcb.state.tx.us/
criss_cole.asp

UTAH

Utah Industries for the Blind
P.O. Box 1258
Salt Lake City, UT 84110-1258
Local Telephone: (801) 485-3847

Utah State Division of Services for
the Blind and Visually Impaired

250 North 1950 West, Suite B
Salt Lake City, UT 84116-7902
801-323-4343 or 1-800-284-
1823; TDD/TTY 801-323-4395

VERMONT

Vermont Association for the Blind
and Visually Impaired
37 Elmwood Avenue
Burlington, VT 05401
802-863-1358 or 1-800-639-5861

VIRGINIA

Virginia Rehabilitation Center for
the Blind and Vision Impaired
401 Azalea Avenue
Richmond, VA 23227
804-371-3151

WASHINGTON

Washington State Department of
Services for the Blind
402 Legion Way, SE, Suite 100
Olympia, WA 98504-0933
360-586-1224 or 1-800-552-
7103; TDD/TTY 206-764-4051
http://www.wa.gov/dsb

WEST VIRGINIA

West Virginia Department of Education and the Arts: Division of
Rehabilitation Services, Information and Referral Services
for the Blind and Visually
Impaired

P.O. Box 50890
State Capitol Complex
Charleston, WV 25305-0890
304-766-4891 or 1-800-642-
3021; TDD/TTY 304-766-4970

WISCONSIN

Wisconsin Center for the Blind
and Visually Impaired
1700 West State Street
Janesville, WI 53546
608-758-6146 or 1-800-832-
9784; TDD/TTY 608-758-6127

Wisconsin Council of the Blind
354 West Main Street
Madison, WI 53703-3115
608-255-1166 or 1-800-783-5213
http://www.wcblind.org

Wisconsin Department of Health
and Family Services: Division of
Supportive Living, Bureau for
the Blind
1 West Wilson Street
Madison, WI 53707
608-266-3139
http://www.dhfs.state.wi.us/

WYOMING

Wyoming Division of Vocational
Rehabilitation
1100 Hershler Building
Cheyenne, WY 82002
307-777-7389
http://onestop.state.wy.us/
appview/ujn-home.asp

APPENDIX X
SCHOLARSHIPS FOR THE BLIND

American Council on Rural Special Education Scholarships
Kansas State University
2323 Anderson Avenue
Suite 226
Manhattan, KS 66501-2912
785-532-2737
http://www.kus.edu

American Council of the Blind Scholarships
1155 15th Street, NW
Suite 270
Washington, DC 20005
202-467-5081 or 800-424-8666

American Foundation for the Blind Scholarships
11 Penn Plaza
Suite 300
New York, NY 10001
212-502-7600 or 800-232-5463
http://www.afb.org

Amy Reiss Blind Student Scholarship
Fordham University Financial Aid Office
140 W. 62nd Street
Room 125
New York, NY 10023
http://www.acenet.edu

Association for Education and Rehabilitation of the Blind and Visually Impaired
Ferrell Scholarship Fund
4600 Duke Street
Suite 430
Alexandria, VA 22397
703-823-9690

Barbara Jackman Zuckert Scholarship

George Washington University
Disabled Support Services
Marvin Center
Suite 436
Washington, DC 20052
202-994-8250

Blinded Veterans Association Scholarships
Blinded Veterans Association
477 H Street, NW
Washington, DC 20001
202-371-8880

Christian Record Braille Foundation Scholarships
444 South 52nd Street
Lincoln, NE 68506
402-488-0981

Citizens Scholarship Foundation of America
Jenneth Cote
Citizens Scholarship Foundations of America
Box 112A
Londonderry Turnpike
RFD #7
Manchester, NH 13104
and
Ingrid LeMarie
New Hampshire Charitable Fund
One South Street
Concord, NH 03301
http://www.csfa.org

Council of Citizens with Low Vision International
1155 15th Street, NW
Suite 1004
Washington, DC 20005
800-733-2258
http://www.cclvi.org

Council of Citizens with Low Vision, Carl E. Foley Scholarship
Pennsylvania College of Optometry
1200 West Godfrey Street
Philadelphia, PA 19141
215-276-6268

Equal Opportunity Publications
445 Broad Hollow Road
Suite 425
Melville, NY 11747
631-421-9421
http://www.eop.com

The Foundation for Exceptional Children Scholarships
1920 Association Drive
Reston, VA 20190
703-264-3507

Foundation for Science and the Handicapped Scholarships
Chairperson of the Science Grant Committee
Division of Rehabilitation Education
154 Juliet Court
Clarenden Hills, IL 60514

George Peabody College, Vanderbilt University Department of Special Education
Nashville, TN 37203
615-322-2249

Itzhak Perlman Award
Denise Warner
Very Special Arts Education Office
Kennedy Center
Washington, DC 20566
202-662-8899

Jewish Braille Institute of America Inc. Scholarship
110 East 30th Street
New York, NY 10016
212-889-2525

Lighthouse International
Career Incentive and Achievement Awards
111 East 59th Street
New York, NY 10022
212-821-9428

National Federation of the Blind
Scholarship Committee
805 Fifth Avenue
Grinnell, LA 50112-1653
641-236-3369
http://www.nfb.org

The New Hampshire Charitable Foundation
37 Pleasant Street
Concord, NH 03301-4005
603-225-6641

Opportunities for the Blind Ind., Scholarships
P.O. Box 510
Leonardtown, MD 20650
800-884-1990
http://www.oppblind.com

Recording for the Blind Scholastic Achievement Awards
Public Relations Department
Recording for the Blind
20 Roszel Road
Princeton, NJ 08540
609-452-0606, ext. 246

Ronnie Milsap Foundation
600 Renaissance Center
Suite 1300
Detroit, MI 48243

Rotary Ambassadorial Scholarships
Rotary International
Scholarship Dept.
1560 Sherman Avenue
Evanston, IL 60601
847-866-3000
http://www.rotary.org

University of Kansas
Research and Training Center on Independent Living
BCR/4089 Dole
Lawrence, KS 66045
913-864-4095

Vinland National Center
P.O. Box 308
3675 Ihduhapi Road
Loretto, MN 55357
612-479-3555

Vermont Association for the Blind
Charles E. Leonard Memorial Scholarship Fund
P.O. Box 2000
Champlain Mill
Winooski, VT 05404

VSA (Very Special Arts)
1300 Connecticut Avenue, NW
Suite 700
Washington, DC 20036
800-933-8721

Western Michigan University
Department of Rehabilitation
Western Michigan University
Kalamazoo, MI 49008

APPENDIX XI
SPORTS AND RECREATION ORGANIZATIONS AND PUBLICATIONS

Access to Art: An Art Resource Directory for the Blind and Visually Impaired
American Foundation for the Blind
11 Penn Plaza
Suite 300
New York, NY 10001
212-502-7660 or 800-232-5463;
 TDD 212-502-7662
http://www.afb.org

American Alliance for Health, Physical Education, Recreation and Dance
1900 Association Drive
Reston, VA 22091
703-476-3481
http://www.aahperd.org

American Blind Bowling Association
411 Sheriff Street
Mercer, PA 16137
412-662-5748

American Blind Skiers, Inc.
2325 Wilshire Boulevard
Santa Monica, CA 90403
213-828-5514

American Camping Association
5000 State Road 67 North
Martinsville, IN 46151
765-342-8456
http://www.ACAcamps.org

American Horticulture Therapy Association
909 York Street
Denver, CO 80206

720-865-3616
http://www.ahta.org

American Red Cross
Program of Swimming for the Handicapped
431 18th Street, NW
Washington, DC 20006
800-797-8022
http://redcross.org

American Music Therapy Association
8455 Colesville Road, Suite 1000
Silver Spring, MD 20910
301-589-3300
http://www.namt.org

American Printing House for the Blind
1839 Frankfort Avenue
P.O. Box 6085
Louisville, KY 40206
502-895-2405 or 800-223-1839
http://www.aph.org

Association of Disabled American Golfers
P.O. Box 280649
Lakewood, CO 80228
303-922-5228
http://www.toski.com/golf/adag

Association of Handicapped Artists
5150 Broadway
Depew, NY 14043
716-683-9316

Association of Radio Reading Services

Sun Sound Reading Service
3124 East Roosevelt Street
Phoenix, AZ 85008
1-800-255-2777

Bemidji State University
Outdoor Program Center
Hobson Memorial Union
Bemidji, MN 56601
218-755-2999

Bibles and Other Scriptures in Special Media
National Library Service for the Blind and Physically Handicapped
Reference Circular
Library of Congress
Washington, DC 20542
212-287-5100

Bible Outdoor Leisure Development (BOLD)
533 East Main Street
Aspen, CO 81611
303-925-2086

Bradford Woods Outdoor Center
5040 State Road
67 North
Martinsville, IN 46151
765-342-8456

Braille Sports Foundation
4601 Excelsior Avenue South
St. Louis Park, MN 55416
612-920-9363

Breckenridge Outdoor Education Center
917 Airport Road

P.O. Box 697
Breckenridge, CO 80424
970-453-6422

Challenge Alaska
P.O. Box 110065
Anchorage, AK 99511
907-344-7399
http://www.challenge.ak.org

Choice Magazine
100 Riverview Center
Middletown, CT 06457
860-347-6933

Council for Disabled Sailors
American Sailing Association
60 Padanaram Road
Unit 16
Danbury, CT 06810

Courage Center
Department of Sports, Physical
    Education and Recreation
3915 Golden Valley Road
Golden Valley, MN 55422
763-520-0520
http://www.courage.org

Disabled Sports USA
41 Hungerford Drive
Suite 100
Rockville, MD 20850
301-217-0960
http://www.dsusa.org

Discovery Blind Sports Interna-
    tional
6811 Aitkem Drive
Oakland, CA 94611
510-399-0777

Evergreen Travel Service
4114 North Avenue, SW
#13
Lynnwood, WA 98036
800-435-2288

Independent Living Aids
200 Robbins Lane
Jericho, NY 11753
800-537-2118
http://www.independentliving.
    com

Information and Research Utiliza-
    tion Center

American Alliance for Health,
    Physical Education, Recreation
    and Dance
1900 Association Drive
Reston, VA 20191
800-213-7193
http://www.aahperd.org

Information Center for
    Individuals with Disabilities
P.O. Box 750119
Arlington Heights, MA 02475
781-860-0673
http://www.disability.net

International Bicycle Tours Inc.
12 Mid Place
Chappaqua, NY 10514
914-238-4576

Kirkwood Instruction for Blind
    Skiers
P.O. Box 138
Kirkwood, CA 95646

Louis Braille Foundation for
    Blind Musicians
112 East 19th Street
New York, NY 10003

*Matilda Ziegler Magazine for the
    Blind*
80 Eighth Avenue, Room 1304
New York, NY 10011
212-242-0263
http://zieglermag.org

National Arts and the Handi-
    capped Information Service
Arts and Special Constituency
    Project
National Endowment for the Arts
2401 E Street, NW
Washington, DC 20506

National Association for Sports
    for Cerebral Palsy
66 East 34th Street
New York, NY 10016
212-481-6359
http://www.uscpaa.org

National Beep Baseball
    Association
2231 W. First Avenue
Topeka, KS 66606

785-234-2156
http://www.nbaa.org

National Braille Association
3 Towline Circle
Rochester, NY 14623
716-427-8260
http://www.nationalbraille.org

National Camp Directory for the
    Blind and Visually Impaired
American Foundation for the
    Blind
11 Penn Plaza, Suite 300
New York, NY 10001
212-502-7660 or 800-232-5463;
    TDD 212-502-7662
http://www.afb.org

National Committee/Arts for the
    Handicapped
1300 Connecticut Avenue
Suite 700
Washington, DC 20036
202-628-2800 or 800-933-8721
http://vsarts.org

National Exhibits by Blind Artists
919 Walnut Street, First Floor
Philadelphia, PA 19107
1-800-222-1764

National Gardening Association
180 Flynn Avenue
Burlington, VT 05401
802-863-1308

National Handicapped Sports and
    Recreation Association
5932 Illinois Avenue
Orangevale, CA 95662
916-989-0402

National Therapeutic Recreation
    Society
22377 Belmont Ridge Road
Ashburn, VA 20148
703-858-0784
http://www.health.gov/nhic

North American Riding for the
    Handicapped Association
P.O. Box 33150
Denver, CO 80233
303-252-4610
http://www.harha.org

Outward Bound
945 Pennsylvania Street
Denver, CO 80203
800-243-8520
http://www.outwardbound.org

People-to-People Committee for
the Handicapped
1111 20th Street, NW, Suite 660
Washington, DC 20036
202-653-5007

Peter Burwash International Ltd.
2203 Timberloch Place, #126
The Woodlands, TX 77380
218-363-4707
http://www.pbi-tennis.com

President's Committee on
Employment of People with
Disabilities
1331 F Street, NW
Washington, DC 20004
202-376-6200
http://www.health.gov/nhic

Recording for the Blind Inc.
20 Roswell Road
Princeton, NJ 08540
609-452-0606
http://www.rfbdnj.org

Santa Monica Blind Skiers Inc.
2325 Wilshire Boulevard
Santa Monica, CA 90403

Science Products
Box A
Southeastern, PA 19399
1-800-888-7401

SIRE, Inc. (Self Improvement
Through Riding)
Rt. 2, Box 56
Hockley, TX 77447
281-356-7588

Skating for the Blind and Handicapped
1200 East and West Road
West Seneca, NY 14224
716-675-7222
http://www.sabahinc.org

Ski for Light
1400 Carole Lane
Green Bay, WI 54313
414-494-5572

SOAR
5404 NE Alameda Avenue
Portland, OR 97214

Society for the Advancement of
Travel for the Handicapped
374 Fifth Avenue, Suite 610
New York, NY 10016
212-447-7284
http://www.sath.org

Sports Illustrated
Available through the National
Library Service for the Blind
and Physically Handicapped
1291 Taylor Street, NW
Washington, DC 20542

Telesensory Systems
455 North Bernardo Avenue
P.O. Box 7455

Mountain View, CA 94043-5274
1-800-286-8484

Travel Industry and Disabled
Exchange (TIDE)
5435 Donna Avenue
Tarzana, CA 91356

Travel Information Center
Moss Rehabilitation Hospital
12th Street and Tabor Road
Philadelphia, PA 19141
215-329-5715

United States Blind Chess Association
30 Snell Street
Brockton, MA 02410

United States Blind Golfers Association
3094 Shamrock Street North
Tallhassee, FL 32308
850-893-4511
http://www.usbga.org

Vinland National Center
3675 Ihduhapi Road
P.O. Box 308
Loreetto, MN 55357
615-479-3555

West Chester University Outdoor
Resource Center
West Chester, PA 19380
215-436-1000

APPENDIX XII

DIAGRAM OF THE EYE

NOTE

The diagram of the eye that appears below will be useful in clarifying matters of anatomy and structure, and will be essential in understanding many of the entries throughout the book.

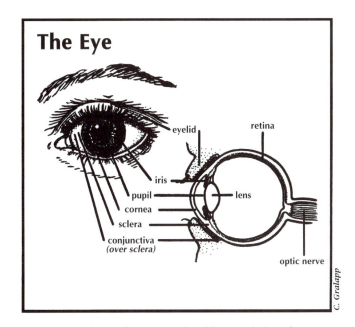

Cross section of the eye. Reprinted by permission of the American Academy of Ophthalmology.

BIBLIOGRAPHY

ABLEDATA. *Braille Telephone Device for the Deaf.* Newington, Conn.: ABLEDATA, 1989.

———. *Electronic Travel Aids Printout.* Newington, Conn.: ABLEDATA, 1989.

———. *Kurzweil Reader Printout.* Newington, Conn.: ABLEDATA, 1989.

———. *Speech Synthesizers Printout.* Newington, Conn.: ABLEDATA, 1989.

———. *Telebraille.* Newington, Conn.: ABLEDATA, 1989.

———. *Voice Output Module.* Newington, Conn.: ABLE-DATA, 1989.

Abel, Robert. *The Eye Care Revolution: Prevent and Reverse Common Vision Problems.* Clifton, N.J.: Kensington Publishing Corporation, 1999.

Alexandidis, E. *The Pupil.* New York: Springer-Verlag, 1985.

Alpert, Joseph S. *The Heart Attack Handbook.* Boston: Little, Brown, 1985.

American Academy of Ophthalmology. Medem. "Air Bags May Cause Serious Eye Injuries in Children." Available online. URL: http://www.medem.com/MedLB/article_detaillb.cfm?article_ID=ZZZ14RKP6BC.

———. "American Academy of Ophthalmology Says Newly Approved Drug, Visudyne, is Promising." Available online. URL: http://www.medem.com/MedLB/article_detaillb.cfm?article_ID=ZZZY6EF428C.

———. "Corneal Rings Safe and Effective for Correcting Nearsightedness, Two-Year Study Shows." Available online. URL: http://www.medem.com/MedLB/article_detaillb.cfm?article_ID=ZZZHDXJB8RC. Posted September 2001.

———. "Early Ophthalmic Examination Can Lead to Child Abuse Detection and Prevention." Available online. URL: http://www.medem.com/MedLB/article_detaillb.cfm?article_ID=ZZZASLAS2AC.

———. "90% of Sports-Related Eye Injuries Are Preventable, Eye M.D.s Say." Available online. URL: http://www.medem.com/MedLB/article_detaillb.cfm?article_ID=ZZZVYGPIJ7C. Posted on March 23, 2000.

American Foundation for the Blind. *A Different Way of Seeing.* New York: AFB, 1984.

———. *Aging and Vision.* New York: AFB, 1987.

———. *Career Choice for Blind and Visually Impaired Students: Career Planning and Placement Offices.* New York: AFB, 1987.

———. *Directory of Services for Blind and Visually Impaired Persons in the United States.* 23rd ed. New York: AFB, 1988.

———. *Facts about the American Foundation for the Blind.* New York: AFB, 1986.

———. *A Good Employee Is a Good Employee.* New York: AFB, 1987.

———. *Helen Keller,* New York: AFB, 1987.

———. *How Does a Blind Person Get Around?* New York: AFB, 1988.

———. *Is Your Child Blind?* New York: AFB, 1975.

———. *Louis Braille.* New York: AFB, 1987.

———. *Low Vision Questions and Answers: Definitions, Devices, Services.* New York: AFB, 1987.

———. *The M. C. Migel Memorial Library and Information Center.* New York: AFB, 1986.

———. *Parenting Preschoolers: Suggestions for Raising Young Blind and Visually Impaired Children.* New York: AFB, 1984.

———. *The Preschool Deaf-Blind Child: Suggestions for Parents.* New York: AFB, 1974.

———. *Touch the Baby.* New York: AFB, 1987.

———. *Understanding and Living with Glaucoma.* New York: AFB, 1984.

———. *Understanding Braille.* New York: AFB, 1970.

———. *Visually Impaired Professional Personnel.* New York: AFB, 1986.

———. *What Do You Do When You See A Blind Person?* New York: AFB, 1970.

———. *What To Do When You Meet A Deaf-Blind Person.* New York: AFB, 1985.

American Heart Association. *Recovering From a Stroke.* Dallas: AHA, 1986.

———. *1989 Stroke Facts.* Dallas: AHA, 1988.

———. *Stroke: Why Do They Behave that Way?* Dallas: AHA, 1974.

Anderson, Douglas R. *Testing the Field of Vision.* St. Louis: C. V. Mosby Company, 1982.

Anderson, Harry C. *An Experience: Students with Usher Syndrome and their Parents.* Baltimore: RP Foundation Fighting Blindness, 1977.

Anderson, Julia, "How Technology Brings Blind People into the Workplace." *Harvard Business Review* (March–April 1989): 36–39.

Annala, Linda. *Facing the Future with Usher's Syndrome.* Baltimore: RP Foundation Fighting Blindness, 1976.

Apolloni, Tony. "Effective Advocacy: How to Be a Winner." *Exceptional Parent* (February 1985): 14–19.

Architectural and Transportation Barriers Compliance Board. *Uniform Federal Accessibility Standards.* Washington, D.C.: ATBCB, 1984.

Arkenstone, Inc. *Arkenstone Reader with TrueScan.* Sunnyvale, Calif.: Arkenstone, 1989.

———. *Calera Recognition Systems.* Sunnyvale, Calif.: Arkenstone, 1989.

———. *What Is Arkenstone?* Sunnyvale, Calif.: Arkenstone, 1989.

Arthur, Julietta K. *Employment for the Handicapped.* New York: Abingdon Press, 1967.

Artic Technologies. *ARTIC CRYSTAL.* Troy, Mich.: AT, 1989.

———. *ARTIC D'LIGHT.* Troy, Mich.: AT, 1989.

———. *Artic ENCORE!* Troy, Mich.: AT, 1989.

———. *Artic Navigates the Channel.* Troy, Mich.: AT, 1989.

———. *Artic Turbo-Pedals.* Troy, Mich.: AT, 1989.

———. *Artic Vision.* Troy, Mich.: AT, 1989.

———. *SynPhonix.* Troy, Mich.: AT, 1989.

Bailey, Ian L. "The Aged Blind." *The Australian Journal of Optometry* (January 1975): 31–39.

Bankes, James L. Kennerley. *Clinical Ophthalmology.* New York: Churchill Livingstone, 1987.

Barnes, Broda O., and Lawrence Galton. *Hypothyroidism: The Unsuspected Illness.* New York: Thomas Y. Crowell Company, 1976.

Barraga, Natalie C. *Visual Handicaps and Learning.* Belmont, Calif.: Wadsworth Publishing Company Inc., 1976.

Bath, Patricia E. "Blindness Prevention Through the Programs of Community Ophthalmology in Developing Countries." In *Ophthalmology.* Vol. 2. Edited by K. Shimizu and J. Oosterhuis. Amsterdam: Excerpta Medica, 1979.

Begbie, G. Hugh. *Seeing and the Eye.* New York: Doubleday, 1973.

Berkeley Systems, Inc. *Corporate Background.* Berkeley, Calif.: BSI, 1989.

———. *inLARGE: The Software Magnifying Glass.* Berkeley, Calif.: BSI, 1989.

———. *inTOUCH: The Tactile Macintosh Screen.* Berkeley, Calif.: BSI, 1989.

———. *outSPOKEN: The Talking Macintosh Interface.* Berkeley, Calif.: BSI, 1989.

Berland, Theodore, and Richard A. Perritt, M.D. *Living With Your Eye Operation.* New York: St. Martin's Press, 1974.

Berlinski, Peter. "A Hidden Resource." *Worklife* (Fall 1988): 2.

Biklen, Douglas, and Robert Bogdan. "Media Portrayals of Disabled People: A Study in Stereotypes." *Interracial Books for Children Bulletin* 8, no. 6–7 (1977): 4–9.

"Bill of Rights for People with Disabilities." *Tips and Trends* 1, no. 6 (June–July 1989): 1.

BIT Corporation. *Winter 1989 Catalog, Edition #9.* Boston: BIT, 1989.

Bitter, James A. *Introduction to Rehabilitation.* St. Louis: C. V. Mosby Company, 1979.

Blacker, M. M., and D. R. Wekstein, eds. *Your Health After Sixty.* New York: E. P. Dutton, 1979.

Blau, Sheldon Paul, and Dodi Schultz. *Lupus: The Body Against Itself.* New York: Doubleday and Company, Inc., 1977.

Blinded Veterans Association. *BVA Fact Sheet.* Washington, D.C.: BVA, 1989.

———. *Alternatives for Blind or Visually Impaired Veterans.* Washington, D.C.: BVA, 1989.

Blodi, Frederick C. *Herpes Simplex Infections of the Eye.* New York: Churchill Livingstone, 1984.

Boardman, Louise S. *My Son Has Usher's Syndrome.* Baltimore: RP Foundation Fighting Blindness, 1985.

Bonfanti, Barbara H. "Effects of Training on Nonverbal and Verbal Behaviors of Congenitally Blind Adults." *Journal of Visual Impairment and Blindness* (January 1979): 1–9.

Bowe, Frank. *Jobs for Disabled People.* New York: Public Affairs Committee Inc., 1985.

———. "Recruiting Workers with Disabilities." *Worklife* (Summer 1989): 37–41.

Brady, Frank B. *A Singular View—The Art of Seeing With One Eye.* Annapolis, Md.: Frank B. Brady Publisher, 1985.

Braille Institute. *How to Help a Blind Person.* Los Angeles: BI, 1980.

———. *Track and Field Olympics.* Los Angeles: BI, 1989.

———. *When Glasses No Longer Help.* Los Angeles: BI, 1980.

Braille Sports Foundation. *Feeling Sports: February 1989.* Minneapolis: BSI, 1989.

———. *Feeling Sports: September–October 1989.* Minneapolis: BSI, 1989.

Braverman, Sydell. "The Psychological Roots of Attitudes Toward the Blind." *Attitudes Toward Blindness*. New York: American Foundation for the Blind, 1951.

Brock, Peter. *Love in the Lead*. New York: E. P. Dutton, 1954.

Brockhurst, Robert J. *Controversy in Ophthalmology*. Philadelphia: W. B. Saunders Company, 1977.

Brooks, Dennis L. *Don't Be Afraid of Cataracts*. Secaucus, N.J.: Arthur Henley, Lyle Stuart, 1978.

Brown, Bruce. "Supercharging Your Scanner." *PC Magazine* (March 28, 1989): 5.

Burde, Ronald M., Peter J. Savino and Jonathan D. Trobe. *Clinical Decisions in Neuro-Ophthalmology*. St. Louis: The C. V. Mosby Company, 1985.

Butler, Beverly. *Maggie By My Side*. New York: Dodd, Mead and Company, 1987.

Caird, F. I., and John Williamson, eds. *The Eye and It's Disorders in the Elderly*. Bristol: John Wright and Sons Ltd., 1986.

California State Health and Welfare Agency. *California State Plan for Rehabilitation Facilities Part I 1979–1984*. Sacramento, Calif.: CSHWA, 1984.

California State University, Northridge. *CSUN Assistive Technology Center*. Northridge, Calif.: CSUN, 1989.

———. Personal correspondence between Dr. Harry Murphy, Director of the Office of Disabled Student Services, and the writer. October 24, 1989.

Calne, R. Y. *The Oxford Companion to Medicine Volume II N–Z*. New York: Oxford University Press, 1986.

Carden, Robert G. "Vitamins for Healthier Eyes." *Let's LIVE* (September 1985): 10–11.

Carr, Ronald E., et al. *The Eye and Your Vision*. New York: National Association for Visually Handicapped, 1988.

Carroll Center for the Blind. *The Carroll Center for the Blind*. Newton, Mass.: CCB, 1989.

———. *Services for the Carroll Center for the Blind*. Newton, Mass.: CCB, 1989.

Carroll, Rev. Thomas J. "A Look at Aging." *The New Outlook* (April 1972): 97–103.

———. *Blindness*. Boston: Little, Brown and Company, 1961.

Cassel, Gary H., Michael D. Billig, and Harry G. Randall. *The Eye Book: A Complete Guide to Eye Disorders and Health*. Baltimore: Johns Hopkins University Press, 1998.

Cassie, Dhyan. *So Who's Perfect*. Scottdale, Pa.: Herald Press, 1984.

Cauwels, Janice M. *The Body Shop*. St. Louis: C. V. Mosby Company, 1986.

Cawood, Liz Tilton, ed. *WORDS: Work Oriented Rehabilitation Dictionary and Synonyms*. Seattle: Northwest Association of Rehabilitation Industries Inc., 1976.

The Center for the Partially Sighted. *Myths and Realities of Visual Impairment*. Santa Monica, Calif.: CPS, 1985.

———. *The Center for the Partially Sighted and You*. Santa Monica, Calif.: CPS, 1985.

———. *The CPS at a Glimpse*. Santa Monica, Calif.: CPS, 1987.

Chase, Allan. *The Truth About STD*. New York: William Morrow, 1983.

Chawla, Hector Bryson. *Essential Ophthalmology*. New York: Churchill Livingstone, 1981.

Chong, Curtis. "Speech Output for the IBM Personal Computer." *The Braille Monitor* (January 1986): 37–47.

Clark, Matt, Carl Robinson and Ingrid Wickelgren, "Interchangeable Parts." *Newsweek* (September 12, 1988): 61–63.

Clearinghouse on the Handicapped. *Programs for the Handicapped*. Washington, D.C.: CH, 1983.

———. *Pocket Guide to Federal Help for Individuals with Disabilities*. Washington, D.C.: CH, 1987.

Cohen, Jerome. "The Effects of Blindness on Children's Development." *Children* (January/February 1966): 23–27.

Computerized Books for the Blind. *Computerized Books for the Blind*. Missoula, Mont.: CBB, 1989.

Conte, Luca E. *Sheltered Employment Services and Programs*. Washington, D.C.: National Rehabilitation Information Center, 1983.

Cook, Paul F., Peter R. Dahl and Margaret Ann Gale. *Vocational Opportunities*. Salt Lake City, Utah: Olympus Publishing Company, 1978.

Cooley, Donald G. *After 40 Health and Medical Guide*. Des Moines, Iowa: Better Homes and Gardens Books, 1980.

Coombs, Jan. *Living With the Disabled: You Can Help*. New York: Sterling Publishing Co. Inc., 1984.

Corsaro, Maria, and Carole Korzeniowsky. *STD: A Commonsense Guide*. New York: St. Martin's Press, 1980.

Council for Exceptional Children. *Overview: 1988–89*. Reston, Va.: CEC, 1989.

County of Santa Clara: Social Services Agency. *Social Services Agency Guide*. San Jose, Calif.: SSA, 1989.

Cull, John G., and Richard E. Hardy. *Behavior Modification in Rehabilitation Settings*. Springfield, Ill.: Charles C. Thomas, 1974.

Cupak, K. "The Importance of Eye Camps in Underdeveloped Countries." In *Ophthalmology*. Vol. 2. Edited by K. Shimizu and J. Oosterhuis. Amsterdam: Excerpta Medica, 1979.

Curtis, Patricia. *Greff: The Story of a Guide Dog*. New York: E. P. Dutton, 1982.

Cutsworth, T. *The Blind in School and Society*. New York: American Foundation for the Blind Inc., 1951.

D'Amato, Robert, and Joan Snyder. *Macular Degeneration: The Latest Scientific Discoveries and Treatments for Preserving Your Sight*. New York: Walker & Company, 2000.

Davidoff, Jules B. *Differences in Visual Perception*. New York: Academic Press Inc., 1975.

Davidson, Margaret. *Louis Braille*. New York: Hastings House Publishers, 1971.

Department of Health and Human Services. *Section 504 of the Rehabilitation Act of 1973*. Washington, D.C.: DHHS, 1989.

Deur, Lynne. *Doers and Dreamers: Social Reformers of the Nineteenth Century*. Minneapolis: Lerner Publications Company, 1972.

DeVita, Vincent, et al., eds. *AIDS: Etiology, Diagnosis, Treatment, Prevention*. New York: J. B. Lippincott, 1985.

Dickman, Irving R. *What Can We Do About Limited Vision?* Public Affairs Pamphlet Number 491A, New York: Public Affairs Committee Inc., 1984.

Dickman, Irving R., and Sol Gordon. *Getting Help for a Disabled Child—Advice from Parents*. Public Affairs Pamphlet Number 615, New York: Public Affairs Committee Inc., 1983.

Dickey, Thomas W. "Meeting the Vocational Needs of the Older Blind Person." *The New Outlook* (May 1975): 218–225.

Dietl, Dick. "Operation Job Match Helping Fill the Worker Void." *Worklife* (January/February/March 1988): 10–11.

Discovery Blind Sports International. *Discovery Blind Sports International*. Kirkwood, Calif.: DBSI, 1989.

Dodds, Allan G., David D. Clark-Carter and C. Ian Howarth. "The Sonic Pathfinder: An Evaluation." *Journal of Visual Impairment and Blindness* (May 1984): 203–206.

Dudley, Rosemary, and Wade Rowland. *How to Find Relief from Migraine*. New York: Beaufort Books Inc., 1982.

Duke-Elder, Stewart, and Peter A. MacFaul. *System of Ophthalmology: Volume XIV: Injuries, Part 2 Non-Mechanical Injuries*. St. Louis: C. V. Mosby Company, 1972.

Dukeminier, Jesse. "Organ Donation: Legal Aspects." In *The Encyclopedia of Bioethics*, edited by Warren T. Reich. New York: Macmillan (1978): 1157–1159.

Duncan, John, ed., *Environmental Modifications for the Visually Impaired: A Handbook*. New York: American Foundation for the Blind, 1988.

Dyke, Peter J., Gunter Haase and Mark May. "Diagnosis and Care of Bell's Palsy." *Patient Care* (October 1988): 107–118.

Eden, John. *The Eye Book*. New York: Penguin Books, 1978.

Editors of Prevention Magazine. *Prevention's New Encyclopedia of Common Diseases*. Emmaus, Pa.: Rodale Press, 1984.

Eichel, Valerie J. "A Taxonomy for Mannerisms of Blind Children." *Journal of Visual Impairment and Blindness* (May 1979): 167–177.

Emiliani, P. L., ed. *Development of Electronic Aids for the Visually Impaired*. Boston: Dr. W. Junk Publishers, 1986.

Enabling Technologies Company. *The Marathon Brailler*. Stuart, Fla.: ETC, 1989.

———. *PED-30*. Stuart, Fla.: ETC, 1989.

———. *Romeo Braille Printer*. Stuart, Fla.: ETC, 1989.

———. *The TED-600*. Stuart, Fla.: ETC, 1989.

ERIC Clearinghouse on Handicapped and Gifted Children. *ERIC Digest: Selecting Software for Special Education Instruction*. Reston, Va.: ERIC, 1986.

———. *ERIC Digest: Visual Impairments*. Reston, Va.: ERIC, 1982.

———. *Research and Resources on Special Education: Abstract 13*. Reston, Va.: ERIC, 1987.

———. *Research and Resources on Special Education: Abstract 14*. Reston, Va.: ERIC, 1987.

———. *Research and Resources on Special Education: Abstract 19*. Reston, Va.: ERIC, 1988.

Esche, Jeanne, and Carol Griffin. *A Handbook for Parents of Deaf-Blind Children*. Lansing, Mich.: Michigan School for the Blind, 1980.

Esterman, Ben. *The Eye Book*. Arlington: Great Ocean Publishers, 1977.

Eye Bank Association of America. *Background Information on Eye Bank Association of America*. Washington, D.C.: EBAA, 1988.

———. *Questions Most Frequently Asked About Eye Donation and Corneal Transplantation*. Washington, D.C.: EBAA, 1988.

———. *A Summary of the Programs and Services of the Eye Bank Association of America*. Washington, D.C.: EBAA, 1988.

EyeCare Info.com. "Ocular Pharmacology." Available online. URL: http://www.eyecareinfo.com/professionals/ocular_pharmacology.shtml.

Faye, Eleanor, E. *Clinical Low Vision*. Boston: Little, Brown, 1984.

Featherstone, Helen. *A Difference in the Family*. New York: Basic Books Inc., 1980.

Feman, Stephen S., and Robert D. Reinicke, eds. *Handbook of Pediatric Ophthalmology*. New York: Grune & Stratton, 1978.

Ferguson, Dianne L. "Parent Advocacy Network." *Exceptional Parent* (March 1984): 41–45.

Ferrara, Peter J., ed. *Social Security*. Washington, D.C.: Cato Institute, 1985.

Finkelstein, Daniel. "Blindness and Disorders of the Eye." *The Braille Monitor* (December 1988): 578–579.

"First Lady's Thyroid to be Irradiated." *San Jose Mercury News,* 12 April 1989, pp. 2A.

Foley, Conn, and H. F. Pizer. *The Stroke Fact Book.* New York: Bantam Books, 1985.

Fonda, Gerald E. *Management of Low Vision.* New York: Thieme-Stratton Inc., 1981.

Foundation Fighting Blindness (the). "Clinical Trial Finds Antioxidants and Zinc Beneficial in Reducing Risk of Severe AMD." Available online. URL: http://www.blindness.org/html/science/wzinc.html.

———. "Foundation Hosts Important Stem Cell Meeting." Available online. URL: http://www.blindness.org/html/science/wstemcell.html. Posted November 2000.

———. "Gene Therapy Reverses Blindness in Dogs, Opens Possibility for Human Treatment Trials." Available online. URL: http://www.blindness.org/html/science/wdogcomments.html.

———. "Researchers Restore Vision in an Animal Model of Childhood Blindness." Available online. URL: http://www.blindness.org/html/science/rpe65rev.html.

———. "Usher Syndrome Gene Identified." Available online. URL: http://www.blindness.org/html/science/wusherwork.html.

Foundation for the Junior Blind. *Needs Assessment: California Services for Persons with Visual Impairments.* Los Angeles: FJB, 1987.

Fraiberg, S. *Insights from the Blind.* New York: Basic Books, 1977.

Frames, Robin. "Insight Into Eyesight." *MS Facts and Issues.* New York: National Multiple Sclerosis Society, 1985.

Freeman, Paul B. "Optical and Nonoptical Aids for Patients with Age-Related Macular Degeneration." *Sightsaving* 54, no. 1 (1985): 20–23.

Freese, Arthur S. *Cataracts and Their Treatment.* Public Affairs Pamphlet Number 545, New York: Public Affairs Pamphlets, 1977.

———. *The Bionic People Are Here.* New York: McGraw-Hill Book Company, 1979.

———. *The Miracle of Vision.* New York: Harper & Row, Publishers, 1977.

———. *Stroke: The New Hope and the New Help.* New York: Random House, 1980.

Freid, Jacob. "The Blind Senior Citizen's Needs." *The Braille Monitor* (March/April 1977): 110–112.

Froyd, Helen E. "Counseling Families of Severely Visually Handicapped Children." *The New Outlook* (June 1973): 251–257.

Gallin, John I., and Anthony S. Fauci, eds. *Acquired Immunodeficiency Syndrome (AIDS).* New York: Raven Press, 1985.

Galloway, N. R. *Common Eye Diseases and Their Management.* Berlin: Springer-Verlag, 1985.

Garrett, James F., and Edna S. Levine, eds. *Rehabilitation Practices with the Physically Disabled.* New York: Columbia University Press, 1973.

Geist, Chrisann Schiro, and William A. Calzaretta. *Placement Handbook for Counseling Disabled Persons.* Springfield, Ill.: Charles C. Thomas, 1982.

Gilbard, Jeffrey P. "Can My Eye Irritation Be Related to My Lupus?" *Lupus News* 8, no. 1 (1988): 2.

Gittinger Jr., John W. *Ophthalmology: A Clinical Introduction.* Boston: Little, Brown, 1984.

Gliedman, John, and William Roth. *The Unexpected Minority.* New York: Harcourt, Brace, Jovanovich, 1980.

Goldberg, Maxwell H., and John R. Swinton. *Blindness Research: The Expanding Frontiers.* University Park: Pennsylvania State University Press, 1969.

Goldenson, Robert M., ed. *Disability and Rehabilitation Handbook.* New York: McGraw-Hill Book Company, 1978.

Graedon, Joe, and Teresa Graedon. *The Graedon's People's Pharmacy For Older Adults.* New York: Bantam Books, 1988.

———. *The People's Pharmacy.* New York: St. Martin's Press, 1985.

Green, Charles. "Disabled Rights Bill Endorsed." *San Jose Mercury News.* 8 September 1989, pp. 1A.

Grover, John W. *VD: The ABC's.* Englewood Cliffs, N.J.: Prentice-Hall, 1971.

Guide Dog Foundation for the Blind Inc. *Guide Dog Foundation for the Blind Inc. Puppy Program.* Smithtown, New York: GDFB, 1989.

———. *Guide Dog Foundation for the Blind Inc. Training Program.* Smithtown, N.Y.: GDFB, 1989.

———. The Guideway. Smithtown, N.Y.: GDFB, 1989.

Guide Dogs for the Blind Inc. *Legislation Pertaining to Dog Guides in the United States (1970).* San Rafael, Calif.: GDB, 1970.

———. *Fact Sheet.* San Rafael, Calif.: GDB, 1987.

Guiding Eyes for the Blind Inc. *Guiding Eyes for the Blind.* Yorktown Heights, N.Y.: GEB, 1987.

———. *Guiding Eyes for the Blind: The Pursuit of Independence.* Yorktown Heights, N.Y.: GEB, 1987.

Hadley School for the Blind. *Student Course Catalog 1988–1989.* Winnetka, Ill.: HSB, 1988.

Hagen, Dolores. *Microcomputer Resource Book for Special Education.* Reston, Va.: Reston Publishing Company Inc., 1984.

Hamilton, Helen Klusek, ed. *Professional Guide to Diseases, Second Edition.* Springhouse, Pa.: Springhouse Corporation, 1987.

Hamilton, Richard. *The Herpes Book.* Los Angeles: J. P. Tarcher Inc., 1980.

Harper, Forine Watson. "Gestures of the Blind." *Education of the Visually Handicapped* (Spring 1978): 14–20.

Haskins, James. *Who Are the Handicapped?* New York: Doubleday, 1978.

Havener, William H. *Ocular Pharmacology.* St. Louis: C. V. Mosby Company, 1970.

———. *Synopsis of Ophthalmology: The Ophthalmoscopy Book.* St. Louis: C. V. Mosby Company, 1984.

Keller, Helen. *Midstream.* Westport, Conn.: Greenpress Publishers, 1929.

Helen Keller International. *Facts About Helen Keller International.* New York: HKI, 1988.

———. Personal correspondence between Victoria Sheffield and the writer. August 14, 1989.

Helen Keller National Center for Deaf-Blind Youths and Adults. *Helen Keller National Center for Deaf-Blind Youths and Adults.* Sands Point, N.Y.: HKNC, 1988.

———. *Guidelines for Helping Deaf-Blind Persons.* Sands Point, N.Y.: HKNC, 1988.

Henkind, Paul, Martin Mayers, and Arthur Berger, eds. *Physicians' Desk Reference for Ophthalmology.* Oradell, N.J.: Medical Economics Company Inc., 1987.

Henter-Joyce Inc. *The Experts in Access Technology.* St. Petersburg, Fla.: HJI, 1989.

———. *Forum-Mate.* St. Petersburg, Fla.: HJI, 1989.

———. *JAWS.* St. Petersburg, Fla.: HJI, 1989.

Heppe, Cherie. *Of Dog Guides and White Canes.* Baltimore: National Federation of the Blind, 1986.

Herman, Scott C., ed. *Transportation Research Record 934,* Washington, D.C.: Transportation Research Board, National Research Council, 1983.

Hayes, Anthony D. "The Sonic Pathfinder: A New Electronic Travel Aid." *Journal of Visual Impairment and Blindness* (May 1984): 200–202.

Holleb, Arthur I., ed. *American Cancer Society Cancer Book.* New York: Doubleday and Company Inc., 1986.

Hoshmand, Lisa T. "Blindisms: Some Observations and Propositions." *Education of the Visually Handicapped* (May 1975): 56–59.

Howard, Ian P. *Human Visual Orientation.* New York: John Wiley, 1982.

Howe Press of Perkins School for the Blind. *Newsletter Summer 1987.* Watertown, Mass.: HP, 1987.

———. *Newsletter Summer 1988.* Watertown, Mass.: HP, 1988.

———. *Newsletter Winter 1987.* Watertown, Mass.: HP, 1987.

HumanWare, Inc. *Braille-n-Print.* Loomis, Calif.: HWI, 1989.

———. *ClearView.* Loomis, Calif.: HWI, 1989.

———. *Index Advanced.* Loomis, Calif.: HWI, 1989.

———. *Index Classic.* Loomis, Calif.: HWI, 1989.

———. *Index Domino.* Loomis, Calif.: HWI, 1989.

———. *KeyBraille.* Loomis, Calif.: HWI, 1989.

———. *KeyNote PC.* Loomis, Calif.: HWI, 1989.

———. *Mountbatten Brailler.* Loomis, Calif.: HWI, 1989.

———. *Mowat Sensor.* Loomis, Calif.: HWI, 1989.

———. *Sonicguide.* Loomis, Calif.: HWI, 1989.

———. *Speakwriter 2000.* Loomis, Calif.: HWI, 1989.

———. *Viewpoint.* Loomis, Calif.: HWI, 1989.

IBM Corporation. *Resource Guide for Persons with Vision Impairments.* Atlanta: IBM, 1989.

———. *Technology for Persons with Disabilities.* Atlanta: IBM, 1989.

Independent Living Aids Inc. *Can-Do Products.* Plainview, N.Y.: ILA, 1989.

———. *Portable Electronic Magnifying Viewers for People on the Go.* Plainview, N.Y.: ILA, 1989.

International Association of Lions Clubs. *Glaucoma.* Oak Brook, Ill.: IALC, 1987.

International Conference on the Education of the Deaf. *Deaf-blind Children and Their Education.* Rotterdam: University Press, 1971.

Jackson, Tom, and Paul Krantz. "Removing Everyday Barriers." *Better Homes and Gardens* (September 1988): 37–41.

Jacobbi, Marianne. "Battling Lyme Disease." *Family Circle Magazine* (July 25, 1989): 17–20.

James, John S. "CMV Retinitis—Ganciclovir, Foscarnet, and Other Treatments: Background, History, and Emerging Controversy." *AIDS Treatment News,* no. 71 (December 1988): 1–7.

Jampol, Lee M. "Lasers—Past, Present, and Future." *Sight-saving* 53, no. 4 (1984–85): 10–11.

Jenkins, William M., et al. *Rehabilitation of the Severely Disabled.* Dubuque, Iowa: Kendall/Hunt Publishing Company, 1976.

Jernigan, Kenneth. *Blindness: Is the Public Against Us?* Baltimore: National Federation of the Blind, 1975.

———. *Blindness: Of Visions and Vultures.* Baltimore: National Federation of the Blind, 1976.

———. *Blindness, Simplicity, Complexity, and the Public Mind.* Baltimore: National Federation of the Blind, 1982.

———. *Blindness: The Coming of the Third Generation.* Baltimore: National Federation of the Blind, 1986.

———. *Blindness: The Pattern of Freedom.* Baltimore: National Federation of the Blind, 1985.

———. *Disability and Visibility: Uncle Tom, Blind Tom, and Tiny Tim.* Baltimore: National Federation of the Blind, 1970.

———. "Facts You Should Know Concerning Disability Insurance." *The Braille Monitor* (June 1989): 362–364.

———. *Focus on the Education of Blind Children.* New York: National Federation of the Blind, 1988.

Job Accommodation Network. JAN. Morgantown, W. Va.: JAN, 1989.

———. *JAN Update.* Morgantown, W. Va.: JAN, 1989.

———. *Job Accommodation Network: Typical Questions.* Morgantown, W. Va.: JAN, 1989.

———. *Job Accommodation Network: A System that Works for the Employer.* Morgantown, W. Va.: JAN, 1989.

———. *Job Accommodation Network: A System that Works for the Job-Ready Person with a Disability.* Morgantown, W. Va.: JAN, 1989.

———. *Job Accommodation Network: A System that Works for the Rehabilitation Professional.* Morgantown, W. Va.: JAN, 1989.

Joffee, E. "Role of Electronic Travel Aids: Field Applications of the Russell Pathsounder." *Journal of Visual Impairment and Blindness* (October 1987): 389–390.

John-Hall, Annette. "Blindness Can't Stop These Athletes." *San Jose Mercury News,* 14 July 1989, pp. 1D.

Johnson, Eric W. *V.D.* New York: J.B. Lippincott Company, 1978.

Johnson, Kurt L. *Incentives and Disincentives in the Vocational Rehabilitation Process.* Washington D.C.: National Rehabilitation Information Center, 1983.

Johnson, Patty T. *Helen Keller: Girl From Alabama.* Huntsville, Ala.: Strode Publishers, 1980.

Jose, Randall T. *Understanding Low Vision.* New York: American Foundation for the Blind, 1983.

Kaplan, Elizabeth W., ed., *Transportation Research Record 1098.* Washington D.C.: Transportation Research Board, National Research Council, 1986.

Katz, Alfred H., and Knute Martin. *A Handbook of Services for the Handicapped.* Westport, Conn.: Greenwood Press, 1982.

Katz, Susan. *Empowering the Disabled.* HealthNet Reference Library. Columbus, Ohio: CompuServe, 1987.

Keith, C. Gregory. *Genetics and Ophthalmology.* London: Churchill Livingstone, 1978.

Keller, Helen. "My Dreams." *Century Magazine* 77, no. 1 (1908): 69–74.

———. *The World I Live In.* New York: Century Company, 1908.

Kelman, Charles D. *Cataracts: What You Must Know About Them.* New York: Crown Publishers Inc., 1982.

———. *Through My Eyes.* New York: Crown Publishers, 1985.

Kelley, Jerry D., ed. *Recreation Programming for Visually Impaired Children and Youth.* New York: American Foundation for the Blind, 1981.

Kendrick, Deborah. *Jobs to be Proud of: Profiles of Workers Who are Blind or Visually Impaired.* New York: American Foundation for the Blind Press, 1993.

Kestenbaum, Alfred. *Applied Anatomy of the Eye.* New York: Grune and Stratton, 1963.

Kimmins, Charles W. *Children's Dreams.* London: George Allen & Unwin Ltd., 1937.

Kirchner, Corinne, and Ziva Simon. "Blind and Visually Handicapped College Students—Part I: Estimated Numbers." *Journal of Visual Impairment and Blindness* (February 1984): 78–81.

Kirtley, Donald. *The Psychology of Blindness.* Chicago: Nelson-Hall, 1975.

Kirtley, Donald, and Katherine Cannistraci. "Dreams of the Visually Handicapped: Toward a Normative Approach." *AFB Research Bulletin #27* (April 1974): 111–133.

Kirtley, Donald, and Kenneth Sabo. "Aggression in the Dreams of Blind Women." *Journal of Visual Impairment and Blindness.* 77, no. 6 (June 1983): 269–270.

———. "Symbolism in the Dreams of the Blind." *International Journal of Rehabilitation Research.* 2, no. 2 (1979): 225–232.

Knight, John J. "Mannerisms in the Congenitally Blind Child." *The New Outlook* (November 1972): 297–301.

Koby, Melvin M. *The "Eyes" Have It—The Eyes and Lupus.* San Jose, Calif.: Bay Area Lupus Foundation, 1981.

Koek, Karin E., Susan B. Martin, and Annette Novallo, eds. "American Association of the Deaf-Blind." *Encyclopedia of Associations,* 23rd ed. Detroit: Gale Research Inc., 1989.

Koestler, Frances A. *The Unseen Minority.* New York: David McKay Company Inc., 1976.

Kornzweig, Abraham L. "Progress in the Prevention of Blindness Among the Aged." *The New Outlook* (September 1971): 210–213.

Kozin, Franklin. *General Clinical Overview of Lupus.* San Jose, Calif.: Bay Area Lupus Foundation, 1986.

Krames Communications. *A Guide to Eye Safety.* Daly City: Kans., 1987.

Kraus, Lewis E. "Disability and Work." *Worklife* (Fall 1989): 37–39.

Kreisler, Nancy, and Jack Kreisler. *Catalog of Aids for the Disabled.* New York: McGraw-Hill, 1982.

Kubler-Ross, Elisabeth. *On Death and Dying.* New York: MacMillan Publishing Co. Inc., 1969.

Kugelmass, J. Alvin. *Louis Braille.* New York: Julian Messner, 1951.

Kuklin, Susan. *Mine for a Year.* New York: Coward-McCann Inc., 1984.

Kwitko, Marvin L., and Frank J. Weinstock. *Geriatric Ophthalmology.* New York: Grune & Stratton Inc., 1985.

Lance, James W. *Migraine and Other Headaches.* New York: Scribner's, 1986.

Langston, Deborah P. *Living With Herpes.* New York: Doubleday, 1983.

Lash, Joseph P. *Helen and Teacher.* New York: Dell, 1980.

Lassiter, Robert A., et al., eds. *Vocational Evaluation, Work Adjustment, and Independent Living for Severely Disabled People.* Springfield, Ill.: Charles C. Thomas, 1983.

Lauer, Harvey, and Leonard Mowinski. *Computer Aids for the Visually Impaired.* HealthNet Reference Library. Columbus, Ohio: Compuserve, 1989.

———. *Recommending Computers for the Visually Impaired: A Moving Target or a Losing War?* HealthNet Library. Columbus, Ohio: CompuServe, 1989.

Lavin, John H. *Stroke: From Crisis to Victory.* New York: Franklin Watts, 1985.

Lee, Yvonne, "Lyon Makes Text Bigger Now Without Add-In Card." *InfoWorld* (July 10, 1989): 24.

Leflar, Robert B., and Helen Lillie. *Cataracts.* Washington, D.C.: Public Citizen's Health Research Group, 1981.

"Legal Services Corporation." *The Guide to American Law.* Vol. 7. Washington, D.C.: Legal Services Corporation (1984): 132–133.

Lehrer, Steven. *Alternative Treatments for Cancer.* Chicago: Nelson-Hall, 1979.

Leontief, Wassily, "The New Technology: How Did We Get Here, Where Are We Going?" *The Future of Work for Disabled People: Employment and the New Technology.* New York: American Foundation for the Blind, 1986.

Leslie, G. Robert, ed. *Supportive Personnel in Rehabilitation Centers: Current Practices and Future Needs.* Pittsburg: Association of Rehabilitation Centers Inc., 1967.

Lesnoff-Caravaglia, Gavi, eds. *Aging and the Human Condition.* New York: Human Services Press Inc., 1982.

Lindenberg, Richard, Frank B. Walsh, and Joel G. Sacks. *Neuropathology of Vision.* Philadelphia: Lea and Febiger, 1973.

Lions Clubs International. Fact Sheet. Oak Brook, Ill.: LCI, 1989.

Lions Clubs History. Oak Brook, Ill.: LCI, 1989.

Lions International Helen Keller Day. Oak Brook, Ill.: LCI, 1987.

Lions Dog Guide Schools. Oak Brook, Ill.: LCI, 1988.

Llyod, Judy H. "Use of Telescopic Aids for Vocational Purposes." *Journal of Visual Impairment and Blindness* (May 1984): 216–220.

Lowenfeld, Berthold. "The Social Impact of Blindness upon the Individual." *New Outlook for the Blind* 58, no. 4 (April 1964): 273–277.

Luckiesh, M. *Visual Illusions.* New York: Dover Publications Inc., 1965.

Lukoff, Irving, et al. *Attitudes Toward Blind Persons.* New York: American Foundation for the Blind, 1972.

Lunt, Suzanne. *A Handbook for the Disabled.* New York: Scribner's, 1982.

Lyme Borreliosis Foundation, Inc. *Lyme Disease: A Serious Health Threat.* Tolland, Conn.: LBF, 1989.

Lyon Computer Discourse Limited. *Lyon Large Print Program.* North Vancouver, B.C.: LCD, 1989.

Lyon, John. Personal Correspondence. November 9, 1989.

MacDonald, A. B. "Lyme Disease: A Neuro-ophthalmologic View." *Journal of Clinical Neuro-ophthalmology* 7, no. 4 (1987): 10.

Mainstream Inc. *Putting Disabled People in Your Place: Focus on Blind and Vision-Impaired Individuals.* Washington, D.C.: MI, 1985.

Malcolm, Andrew H. "Is There Too Little Order in the Transplant Business?" *The New York Times,* 13 April 1986.

Malikin, David, and Herbert Rusalem, eds. *Vocational Rehabilitation of the Disabled: An Overview.* New York: University Press, 1969.

Malone, Mary. *Annie Sullivan.* New York: G. P. Putnam's Sons, 1971.

Maloney, William F., Lincoln Grindle and Donald E. Pearcy. *Consumer Guide to Modern Cataract Surgery.* Fallbrook, Calif.: Lasenda Publishers, 1986.

Mangold, Sally. Personal Interview. San Francisco, Calif.: July 13, 1989.

Mann, Richard C. *Diagnosis: Cerebral Palsy.* Oklahoma City: United Cerebral Palsy of Oklahoma, 1986.

Manninen, Diane L., and Roger Evans. "Public Attitudes and Behavior Regarding Organ Donation." *Journal of American Medical Association* 253, no. 21 (June 7, 1985): 3111–3115.

Martin, Paul. "Medicine's New Superstar: The Atom." *The Lion* (February 1989): 14–16.

Massengill, R. K. *Supersight: The Lens Implant Miracle.* Boston: Health Institute Press, 1986.

Maumenee, Irene H. "Discoveries in Genetic Eye Disease." *Sightsaving* 53, no. 4 (1984–85): 14–15.

Maurer, Marc. *Preparation and the Critical Nudge.* Baltimore: National Federation of the Blind, 1988.

May, Michael, and Ronald Salviolo. *Blind Alpine Skiing and Racing.* Kirkwood, Calif.: Kirkwood Instruction of Blind Skiers, 1986.

McGarry, Barbara D. "Legislative Advocacy for the Blind in America: The Historical Involvement of Consumers and Professionals." In *Yearbook of the AERBVI 1983.* Alexandria, Va.: The Association for Education and Rehabilitation of the Blind and Visually Impaired (1983): 31–39.

McGlen, Brian. Pfizer International. Telephone interview. May 5, 1989.

McInnes, J. M., and J. A. Treffry. *Deaf-Blind Infants and Children.* Toronto: University of Toronto Press, 1982.

Meehan, Michaelann. RP Foundation. Telephone interview. May 11, 1989.

Meighan, Thomas. *An Investigation of the Self Concept of Blind and Visually Handicapped Adolescents.* New York: American Foundation for the Blind, 1971.

Mendelsohn, Steven B. *Financing Adaptive Technology.* New York: Smiling Interface, 1987.

Menitove, Jay E., and Jerry Kolins, eds. *AIDS.* Arlington: American Association of Blood Banks, 1986.

Meredith, Travis A. *The Eye: Disease, Diagnosis, Treatment.* Bowie, Md.: Robert J. Brady Company, 1975.

Miller, Barbara S., and William H. Miller. "Extinguishing 'Blindisms': A Paradigm for Intervention." *Education of the Visually Handicapped* (Spring 1976): 7–14.

Miller, David. *Ophthalmology: The Essentials.* Boston: Houghton Mifflin Professional Publishing, 1979.

Miller, Stephen J. H. *Parson's Diseases of the Eye.* New York: Churchill Livingstone, 1978.

Mitchell, Joyce Slayton. *See Me More Clearly.* New York: Harcourt, Brace, Jovanovich, 1980.

Moore, Thomas, Eye Bank Association of America. Telephone interview. March 6, 1989.

Morain, Claudia. "First Lady Slimmer, But Illness Isn't Worth It." *San Jose Mercury News,* 1 April 1989, pp. 3C.

Morris, Ian. "Technology and Disabled People: A Global View." *The Future of Work for Disabled People: Employment and the New Technology.* New York: American Foundation for the Blind, 1986.

Moses, Howard. "Americans with Disabilities Act—1989: Extending Civil Rights Protection." *NARIC Quarterly* 2, no. 2 (Summer 1989): 1–13.

Mueller, Conrad G., and Mae Rudolph. *Light and Vision.* New York: Time-Life Books, 1972.

Mullen, Peggy Boucher. *Consumer Guide to Prescription Drugs.* Lincolnwood, Ill.: Publications, International, 1987.

Munna, Raymond. *As I See It: Radial Keratotomy Before, During, and After Surgery.* Metairie, La.: Granite Publishers, 1985.

Murphy, Jo Anne. *How Does a Blind Person Get Around?* New York: American Foundation for the Blind, 1988.

Myers, Lawrence. *Living with MS.* Healthnet Library. Columbus, Ohio: CompuServe, 1988.

Murray, Thomas H. "The Gift of Life Must Always Remain a Gift." *Discover* (March 1986): 90–92.

Nash, David T. *Coronary! Prediction and Prevention.* New York: Scribner's, 1978.

National Alliance for Eye and Vision Research. "The Demographics of Eye and Vision Disorders." Available online. URL: http://www.eyeresearch.org/naevr/demographics.html.

———. "Age-Related Macular Degeneration: Questions and Answers." Available online. URL: http://www.eyeresearch.org/naevr/amd_qa.html.

———. "Age-Related Macular Degeneration: Facts and Figures." Available online. URL: http://www.eyeresearch.org/naevr/amd_ff.html.

National Association for Parents of the Visually Impaired. *Awareness: First Quarter.* Camden, N.Y.: NAPVI, 1989.

National Association for Visually Handicapped. *Classification of Impaired Vision.* New York: NAVH, 1973.

———. *Every Low Vision Patient Should Know* . . New York: NAVH, 1985.

———. *Fact Sheet.* New York: NAVH, 1985.

———. *Family Guide.* New York: NAVH, 1980.

———. *Guide to Visual Aids and Illumination.* New York: NAVH, 1986.

———. *The Heartbreak of Being "A Little Bit Blind!"* New York: NAVH, 1982.

———. *Problems of the Partially Seeing.* New York: NAVH, 1985.

National Braille Association. *National Braille Association.* HealthNet Reference Library. Columbus, Ohio: Compuserve 1989.

National Eye Institute (The). "Glaucoma Awareness Month Emphasizes Treatments that Reduce Side Effects, Help Save Vision." Available online. URL: http://www.nei.nih.gov/news/121300.htm. Posted December 13, 2001.

———. "New Eye Disease Treatment May Improve Patients' Quality of Life." Available online. URL: http://www.nei.nih.gov/news/6_21_99.htm. Posted June 21, 1999.

———. "Help Now Available for People with Low Vision. New Program Targets 1 in 20 Americans." Available online. URL: http://www.nei.nih.gov/news/1099.htm. Posted October 19, 1999.

———. "Blacks, Whites Benefit from Different Surgical Glaucoma Treatments." Available online. URL: http://www.nei.nih.gov/news/pr798.htm. Posted July 6, 1998.

———. "Antiviral Drug Sharply Reduces Return of Herpes of the Eye." Available online. URL: http://www.nei.nih.gov/news/hedsII.htm. Posted July 29, 1998.

———. "Life With Low Vision: A Report on Qualitative Research Among People With Low Vision and Their Caregivers." Available online. URL: http://www.nei.nih.gov/nehep/execsum.htm. Posted June 1997.

———. "New Treatment for Eye Disease Reduces Need for Strong Drugs." Available online. URL: http://www.nei.nih.gov/news/newtreatment.htm. Posted May 27, 1997.

National Eye Research Foundation. *The National Eye Research Foundation.* Northbrook, Ill.: NERF, 1988.

National Federation of the Blind. *Do You Know a Blind Person?* New York: NFB, 1988.

———. *What Is the National Federation of the Blind?* New York: NFB, 1988.

National Industries for the Blind. *National Industries for the Blind.* Wayne, N.J.: NFB, 1989.

National Information Center for Handicapped Children and Youth. *General Information about Handicaps and People with Handicaps.* Washington, D.C.: NICHCY, 1982.

National Institute on Disability and Rehabilitation Research. *Data on Disability from the National Health Interview Survey, 1983–85.* Washington, D.C.: NIDRR, 1988.

———. *Disability Statistics Bulletin, No. 1, Spring 1988.* Washington, D.C.: NIDRR, 1988.

National Institute of Handicapped Research. *Rehab Brief: Disabled Americans: Self Perceptions.* Washington, D.C.: NIHR, 1987.

———. *Rehab Brief: Sports for Disabled Individuals.* Washington, D.C.: NIHR, 1981.

———. *Rehab Brief: Works Disincentives.* Washington, D.C.: NIHR, 1980.

———. *Rehab Brief: Sensory Aids for Visually Impaired Clients.* Washington, D.C.: NIHR, 1987.

National Multiple Sclerosis Society. *What is Multiple Sclerosis?* New York: NMSS, 1987.

National Rehabilitation Association. *Technology and Employment of Persons with Disabilities.* Alexandria, Va.: NRA, 1989.

National Rehabilitation Information Center. *Consumerism and Advocacy in Vocational Rehabilitation.* Silver Spring, Md.: NARIC, 1983.

———. *NARIC Guide to Disability and Rehabilitation Periodicals.* Silver Spring, Md.: NARIC, 1989.

———. *REHABDATA.* Silver Spring, Md.: NARIC, 1989.

National Society to Prevent Blindness. *AMD.* New York: NSPB, 1985.

———. *Annual Report.* New York: NSPB, 1988.

———. *Cataract.* New York: NSPB, 1986.

———. *Diabetic Retinopathy.* New York: NSPB, 1986.

———. *Facts and Figures: Adult Eye Problems.* New York: NSPB, 1980.

———. *Glaucoma . . . Sneak Thief of Sight.* New York: NSPB, 1985.

———. *The Sight Saving People.* New York: NSPB, 1987.

———. *1987 Sports and Recreational Eye Injuries.* New York: NSPB, 1987.

———. *Vision Problems in the U.S.: Facts and Figures.* New York: NSPB, 1980.

Neal, Helen. *Low Vision.* New York: Simon & Shuster, 1987.

Nelson, Eugene C., and Ellen Roberts, Jeannette Simmons and William A. Tisdale, *Medical and Health Guide for People Over Fifty.* Glenview, Ill.: Scott, Foresman and Company, 1986.

"New Cell-transplant Operation May Eventually Be Able to Treat Blindness." *San Jose Mercury News,* 9 September 1989, pp. 19A.

Newell, Frank W. *Ophthalmology: Principles and Concepts.* St. Louis: C. V. Mosby Company, 1982.

Newington Children's Hospital. *ABLEDATA.* Newington, Conn.: NCH, 1989.

———. *ABLEDATA Printout.* Newington, Conn.: NCH, 1989.

New York State Office of Advocate for the Disabled. *What Makes Disabled People Disabled?* Albany, N.Y.: NYOAD, 1982.

Noir Medical Technologies. *Noir: A Chemical Sunglass.* South Lyon, Mich.: NMT, 1985.

Northern California Society to Prevent Blindness. *Coping with Sight Loss in Northern California.* San Francisco: NCSPB, 1989.

O'Brien, Robert, and Morris Chafetz. *The Encyclopedia of Alcoholism.* New York: Facts On File Publications, 1982.

O'Bryant, Tom. "Facts About Hiring People with Disabilities." *Worklife* (Fall 1988): 8–10.

Oi, Walter Y., and William F. Gallagher. "Attitudes Toward Employment, Technology and Independence: Introductory Remarks." *The Future of Work for Disabled People: Employment and the New Technology.* New York: American Foundation for the Blind, 1986.

Opteq Vision Systems. *Opteq II Typing System.* Brookfield, Wisc.: OVS, 1989.

———. *Opteq IV.* Brookfield, Wisc.: OVS, 1989.

———. *Opteq V.* Brookfield, Wisc.: OVS, 1989.

———. *Opteq VFF.* Brookfield, Wisc.: OVS, 1989.

———. *Opteq Vision Systems.* Brookfield, Wisc.: OVS, 1989.

Orlansky, Michael D. *Mainstreaming the Visually Impaired Child.* Camden, N.Y.: National Association for Parents of the Visually Impaired Inc., 1989.

Ottoson, David, and Semir Zeki. *Central and Peripheral Mechanisms of Color Vision.* London: Macmillan Press Ltd., 1985.

Owen, Mary Jane. "Hammers, Saws and Obligations: The Control of Specialized Tools in a Competitive Marketplace." *Worklife* (Spring 1989): 30–32.

Pagon, Roberta A. "Retinitis Pigmentosa." *Survey of Ophthalmology* 33, no. 3 (November–December 1988): 137–153.

"Parental Leave on Line." *NAPVI Awareness* (Third Quarter 1987): 5.

Parr, John Cuthbert. *Introduction to Ophthalmology.* New York: Oxford University Press, 1978.

Perkins School for the Blind. *1987 Annual Report.* Watertown, Mass.: PSB, 1987.

———. *Perkins' Programs.* Watertown, Mass.: PSB, 1988.

Perry, Lewis C. "Howe, S.G." *McGraw-Hill Encyclopedia of World Biography* 5 (1973): 378–379.

Pfaffenberger, Clarence J., et al. *Guide Dogs for the Blind: Their Selection, Development, and Training.* New York: Elsevier Scientific Publishing Company, 1976.

Phillips, Calbert I. *Basic Clinical Ophthalmology.* London: Pitman Publishers Limited, 1984.

Pimentel, Albert. *Handling the Upper Secondary and College Usher's* Syndrome Student. Baltimore: RP Foundation Fighting Blindness, 1976.

Pinckney, Cathey and Edward R. *The Patient's Guide to Medical Tests.* New York: Facts On File Publications, 1982.

President's Committee on Employment of People With Disabilities. *Annual Work Plan 1989.* Washington, D.C.: PCEPD, 1989.

———. *Disabled Adults in America.* Washington, D.C.: PCEPD, 1985.

———. *People with Disabilities in Our Nation's Job Training Partnership Act Programs.* Washington, D.C.: PCEPD, 1987.

———. *Ready, Willing, and Available.* Washington, D.C.: PCEPD, 1989.

———. *This is the President's Committee.* Washington, D.C.: PCEPD, 1988.

Price, Ira Marc, and Linda Comac. Coping with Macular Degeneration: *A Guide for Patients and Families to Understand and Living With Degenerative Vision Disorder.* New York: Putnam, 2000.

Pritikin, Roland I. "Eyeglasses." *Groliers Academic American On-Line Encyclopedia.* Columbus, Ohio: Grolier Electronic Publishing, 1988.

Raised Dot Computing Inc. *Raised Dot Computing.* Madison, Wisc.: RDC, 1989.

Read, Leah Fowler. "An Examination of the Social Skills of Blind Kindergarten Children." *Education of the Visually Handicapped* (Winter 1989): 142–155.

Recording for the Blind. *Recording for the Blind: A Service to People.* Princeton, N.J.: RB, 1986.

———. *Recording for the Blind: How the Service Works.* Princeton, N.J.: RB, 1986.

———. *What is Recording for the Blind?* Princeton, N.J.: RB, 1986.

Retinitis Pigmentosa Foundation Fighting Blindness. *Answers to Your Questions About Retinitis Pigmentosa.* Baltimore: RPFFB, 1983.

———. *Answers to Your Questions About Usher's Syndrome.* Baltimore: RPFFB, 1988.

———. *Backgrounder: Usher's Syndrome.* Baltimore: RPFFB, 1988.

———. *Explore the Bright Side of Darkness.* Baltimore: RPFFB, 1988.

———. *Night Vision Aid Fact Sheet.* Baltimore: RPFFB, 1987.

———. Personal correspondence between Michaelann R. Meehan. Information and Referral Coordinator, and the winter. 6 July 1989.

Reynolds, James D. *Amblyopia.* HealthNet Reference Library. Columbus, Ohio: CompuServe, 1989.

———. *Cataracts.* HealthNet Reference Library. Columbus, Ohio: CompuServe, 1989.

———. *Cataract Surgery.* HealthNet Reference Library. Columbus, Ohio: CompuServe, 1989.

———. *Color Blindness.* HealthNet Reference Library. Columbus, Ohio: CompuServe, 1989.

———. *Corneal Transplant.* HealthNet Reference Library. Columbus, Ohio: CompuServe, 1989.

———. *Diabetic Retinopathy.* HealthNet Reference Library. Columbus, Ohio: CompuServe, 1989.

———. *Eye Care Professionals.* HealthNet Reference Library. Columbus, Ohio: CompuServe, 1989.

———. *Glaucoma.* HealthNet Reference Library. Columbus, Ohio: CompuServe, 1989.

———. *Glaucoma Surgery.* HealthNet Reference Library. Columbus, Ohio: CompuServe, 1989.

———. *Hypertensive Retinopathy.* HealthNet Reference Library. Columbus, Ohio: CompuServe, 1989.

———. *Lasers in Ophthalmology.* HealthNet Reference Library. Columbus, Ohio: CompuServe, 1989.

———. *Miscellaneous Neurological Disorders.* HealthNet Reference Library. Columbus, Ohio: CompuServe, 1989.

———. *Nasolacrimal System.* HealthNet Reference Library. Columbus, Ohio: CompuServe, 1989.

———. *Ocular Herpes.* HealthNet Reference Library. Columbus, Ohio: CompuServe, 1989.

———. *Ocular Trauma (Eye Injury).* HealthNet Reference Library. Columbus, Ohio: CompuServe, 1989.

———. *Orbital Cellulitis.* HealthNet Reference Library. Columbus, Ohio: CompuServe, 1989.

———. *Radial Keratotomy.* HealthNet Reference Library. Columbus, Ohio: CompuServe, 1989.

———. *Refractive Errors.* HealthNet Reference Library. Columbus, Ohio: CompuServe, 1989.

———. *Retinal Detachment.* HealthNet Reference Library. Columbus, Ohio: CompuServe, 1989.

———. *Retinal Detachment Surgery.* HealthNet Reference Library. Columbus, Ohio: CompuServe, 1989.

———. *Retinitis Pigmentosa.*HealthNet Reference Library. Columbus, Ohio: CompuServe, 1989.

———. *Strabismus.* HealthNet Reference Library. Columbus, Ohio: CompuServe, 1989.

———. *Strabismus Surgery.* HealthNet Reference Library. Columbus, Ohio: CompuServe, 1989.

———. *Uveitis.* HealthNet Reference Library. Columbus, Ohio: CompuServe, 1989.

Rhode, Stephen J., and Stephen P. Ginsberg, eds. *Ophthalmic Technology.* New York: Raven Press, 1987.

Rice, Mary. *Medications In Lupus Therapy.* San Jose, Calif.: Bay Area Lupus Foundation, 1983.

Rivlin, Barbara Pogul. "Recent Study Compares Employment Trends." *NARIC Quarterly* 2, no. 2 (Fall 1989): 1, 8–10.

Roehrig, Arthur. *Living with Usher's Syndrome.* Baltimore: RP Foundation Fighting Blindness, 1985.

Roth, Wendy Carol. "Let Us Work!" *Parade Magazine,* 17 September 1989, p. 16.

Rudrud, Eric H., et al. *Proactive Vocational Habilitation.* Baltimore: Paul H. Brookes Publishing Company, 1984.

Sabo, Kenneth, and Donald Kirtley. "Objects and Activities in the Dreams of the Blind." *International Journal of Rehabilitation Research* 5, no. 2 (1982): 241–242.

Sachsenweger, Rudolf. *The Illustrated Handbook of Ophthalmology.* London: Wright PSG, 1984.

San Francisco Lighthouse for the Blind. *At Ease!* San Francisco: SFLB, 1982.

Saper, Joel R., and Kenneth R. Magee. *Freedom from Headaches.* New York: Simon & Shuster, 1981.

Sargent, Jean Vieth. *An Easier Way.* New York: Walker & Company, 1981.

Sarno, John E., and Martha Taylor Sarno. *Stroke: A Guide for Patients and Their Families.* New York: McGraw-Hill Book Company, 1969.

Scadden, Lawrence. "The Changing Workplace: View from a Disabled Technologist." *The Future of Work for Disabled People: Employment and the New Technology.* New York: American Foundation for the Blind, 1986.

Scholl, Geraldine T. *Foundations of Education for Blind and Visually Handicapped Children and Youth.* New York: American Foundation for the Blind Inc., 1986.

Schweitzer, N. M. J., ed. *Ophthalmology.* Amsterdam: Excerpta Medica, 1982.

Scoblionkov, Deborah. "Blindness Isn't a Handicap—It's a Nuisance." *McCall's* (October 1989): 49–52.

Scott, Eileen P. *Your Visually Impaired Student.* Baltimore: University Park Press, 1982.

Scott, Neil. Personal interview. Northridge, Calif.: March 10, 1989.

Seeing Eye Inc. A Digest of Legislation Relating to Travel with Dog Guides in the United States and Canada. Morristown, N.J.: SEI, 1988.

———. *Can a Seeing Eye Dog Help You or Someone You Know?* Morristown, N.J.: SEI, 1989.

———. *Q and A: Facts About the Seeing Eye.* Morristown, N.J.: SEI, 1980.

———. *The Seeing Eye.* Morristown, N.J.: SEI, 1980.

———. *The Seeing Eye Has a Scientific Breeding Station.* Morristown, N.J.: SEI, 1989.

———. *The Seeing Eye, How It Started.* Morristown, N.J.: SEI, 1989.

Seeing Technologies Inc. *The SEETEC Systems.* Minneapolis: STI, 1989.

Sensory Aids Foundation. *Annual Program Report, 1988.* Palo Alto, Calif.: SAF, 1988.

———. *Doing the Job is Easy. The Hard Part is Getting It!* Palo Alto, Calif.: SAF, 1989.

———. *SAF Fact Sheet.* Palo Alto, Calif.: SAF, 1989.

Shafto, Marjorie, and Gerald L. Hunt. *Every Woman's Guide to the Body at 40.* New York: Perigee Books, 1987.

Sherman, Spencer E. *A Consumer's Guide to Contact Lenses.* New York: The Dial Press, 1982.

Shields, M. Bruce. "Major Advances in Glaucoma Therapy." *Sightsaving* 53, no. 4 (1984–85): 6–11.

Shimizu, Koichi, and Jendo A. Oosterhuis. *Ophthalmology.* Vol. 1. Amsterdam: Excerpta Medica, 1979.

Sholton, David B. *The Dry Eye Syndrome.* San Jose, Calif.: Bay Area Lupus Foundation, 1981.

"Shopping Bag." *NAPVI Awareness* (First Quarter 1989): 2–7.

Shulman, Julius. *Cataracts.* New York: Simon & Shuster, New York 1984.

———. *No More Glasses.* New York: Simon & Shuster, 1987.

Sickle Cell Anemia Research and Education, Inc. *Facts About Sickle Cell Anemia.* Oakland, Calif.: SCARE, 1977.

Silverman, Harold M., and Gilbert I. Simon. *The Pill Book.* New York: Bantam Books, 1979.

Skurzynski, Gloria. *Bionic Parts for People.* New York: Four Winds Press, 1978.

Smith, Eleanor. *Earning Power.* HealthNet Reference Library. Columbus, CompuServe, 1989.

Smith, Elizabeth Simpson. *A Guide Dog Goes to School.* New York: William Morrow, 1987.

Smith-Kettlewell Eye Research Institute. *The Smith-Kettlewell Eye Research Institute.* San Francisco: SKERI, 1989.

———. *The Smith-Kettlewell Rehabilitation Engineering Center: Annual Report of Progress.* San Francisco: SKERI, 1987.

———. *The Smith-Kettlewell Rehabilitation Engineering Center: Annual Report of Progress.* San Francisco: SKERI, 1988.

Sobel, David S., and Tom Ferguson. *The People's Book of Medical Tests.* New York: Summit Books, 1985.

Sommer, A. *Field Guide to the Detection and Control of Xerophthalmia.* Geneva: World Health Organization, 1982.

Sperber, Al. *Out of Sight.* Boston: Little, Brown and Company, 1976.

Staff of Ready Reference Press. *Directory of Information Resources for the Handicapped.* Santa Monica, Calif.: Ready Reference Press, 1980.

Staff of Peninsula Center for the Blind. *The First Steps.* Palo Alto, Calif.: Peninsula Center for the Blind, 1980.

Stark, Walter J. *Cataracts: A Guide for Patients.* Wall Township, N.J.: H I N, Inc., 1997.

State of California Department of Rehabilitation. *Business Enterprise Training Program.* Sacramento, Calif.: CDR, 1983.

———. *Regulations: Business Enterprise Program for the Blind.* Sacramento, Calif.: CDR, 1983.

Stephens, John W. *Understanding Diabetes.* Beaverton, Oreg.: The Touchstone Press, 1987.

Summers, Laureen. "Reimbursing Adaptive Technology." *NARIC Quarterly* 2, no. 4 (Winter 1989): 1, 7–11, 17.

Swail, J., and E. L. Bryenton. "Sensory 6: An Electronic Travel Aid for Blind Persons." *Journal of Visual Impairment and Blindness* (May 1987): 217–219.

Tait, Perla. "Play and the Intellectual Development of Blind Children." *The New Outlook* (December 1972): 361–369.

Talal, Norman, and Dan Lechay. *Are You Aware of Lupus?* San Jose, Calif.: Bay Area Lupus Foundation, 1989.

Talking Computers Inc. *NEWSBITS.* Falls Church, Va.: TCI, 1989.

———. *NEWSBITS Auditory Magazine: February 1989.* Falls Church, Va.: TCI, 1989.

———. *NEWSBITS Auditory Magazine: June 1989.* Falls Church, Va.: TCI, 1989.

———. *News From Talking Computers, Inc.* Falls Church, Va.: TCI, 1989.

———. *Talk-To-Me Tutorials.* Falls Church, Va.: TCI, 1989.

Taylor, Robert B. *Feeling Alive After 65.* New York: Arlington House Publishers, 1973.

Telephone Pioneers of America. *Pioneering: The Service Connection.* New York: TPA, 1986.

Telesensory Systems, Inc. *Focus on Technology.* Mountain View, Calif.: TSI, 1989.

———. *LapVert.* Mountain View, Calif.: TSI, 1989.

———. *Navigator.* Mountain View, Calif.: TSI, 1989.

———. *Optacon II.* Mountain View, Calif.: TSI, 1989.

———. *See What You've Been Missing.* Mountain View, Calif.: TSI, 1989.

———. *Voyager.* Mountain View, Calif.: TSI, 1989.

Thackray, John. "The High Cost of Workplace Eye Trauma." *Sightsaving* 51, no. 1 (1982): 19–22.

Thijssen, J. M., and A. M. Verbeek, eds. *Ultrasonography in Ophthalmology.* Boston: Dr. W. Junk Publishers, 1981.

Transceptor Technologies, Inc. *Introducing the Personal Companion.* Ann Arbor, Mich.: TTI, 1989.

Transcript of Phil Donahue Show. *"What They Did for Love."* 13 February 1989, Mutimedia Entertainment, New York.

Trevor-Roper, P. D. and P. V. Curran. *The Eye and Its Disorders.* Oxford, U.K.: Blackwell Scientific Publications, 1984.

Turriff, Tod W. National Society to Prevent Blindness. Telephone interview. 16 November 1989.

"UCLA Finds Gene Tied to Blindness in Mice." *San Jose Mercury News,* 15 December 1989, pp. 17A.

United Cerebral Palsy Association. *Cerebral Palsy—Facts and Figures.* New York: UCPA, 1986.

———. *What Is Cerebral Palsy.* New York: UCPA, 1978.

United States Association for Blind Athletes. *SportsScoop: July and August 1989.* Colorado Springs, Colo.: USABA, 1989.

———. *Sports Summaries: Alpine Skiing.* Colorado Springs, Colo.: USABA, 1989.

———. *Sports Summaries: Goal Ball.* Colorado Springs, Colo.: USABA, 1989.

———. *Sports Summaries: Gymnastics.* Colorado Springs, Colo.: USABA, 1989.

———. *Sports Summaries: Judo.* Colorado Springs, Colo.: USABA, 1989.

———. *Sports Summaries: Nordic Skiing.* Colorado Springs, Colo.: USABA, 1989.

———. *Sports Summaries: Powerlifting.* Colorado Springs, Colo.: USABA, 1989.

———. *Sports Summaries: Speed Skating.* Colorado Springs, Colo.: USABA, 1989.

———. *Sports Summaries: Swimming.* Colorado Springs, Colo.: USABA, 1989.

———. *Sports Summaries: Tandem Cycling.* Colorado Springs, Colo.: USABA, 1989.

———. *Sports Summaries: Track and Field.* Colorado Springs, Colo.: USABA, 1989.

———. *Sports Summaries: Wrestling.* Colorado Springs, Colo.: USABA, 1989.

———. *United States Association for Blind Athletes.* Colorado Springs, Colo.: USABA, 1989.

University of Maryland Medicine. "Refractive Errors." Available online. URL: http://www.umm.edu/eye-care/visprobs.htm.

———. "Age-Related Macular Degeneration (AMD)." Available online. URL: http://www.umm.edu/eye-care/macular.htm.

U.S. Bureau of the Census. *Disability, Functional Limitation, and Health Insurance Coverage: 1984/85.* Washington, D.C.: USBC, 1986.

U.S. Department of Health and Human Services. *Diabetic Retinopathy.* NIH Publication No. 85–2171. Washington, D.C.: Government Printing Office, 1987.

———. *Vision Research: A National Plan, 1983–1987 Volume Two/Part One.* NIH Publication No. 83–2471. Washington, D.C.: Government Printing Office, 1987.

———. *Vision Research: A National Plan, 1983–1987 Volume Two/Part Two*. NIH Publication No. 83–2472. Washington, D.C.: Government Printing Office, 1987.

———. *Vision Research: A National Plan, 1983–1987 Volume Two/Part Four*. NIH Publication No. 83–2472. Washington, D.C.: Government Printing Office, 1987.

———. *Vision Research: A National Plan, 1983–1987 Volume Two/Part Five*. NIH Publication No. 83–2475. Washington, D.C.: Government Printing Office, 1987.

U.S. Department of Labor. *Interviewing Guides for Specific Disabilities*. Washington, D.C.: DOL, 1977.

U.S. Postal Service. *Mailing Free Matter for Blind and Visually Handicapped Persons*. Washington, D.C.: USPS, 1985.

Vander, James F., and Janice A. Gault. *Ophthalmology Secrets*. Philadelphia: Hanley & Belfus, Inc., 1998.

Vaughn, Daniel, and Taylor Asbury. *General Ophthalmology*. Los Altos, Calif.: Lange Medical Publications, 1977.

Vaughn, Lewis, ed. *The Complete Book of Vitamins and Minerals for Health*. Emmaus, Pa.: Rodale Press, 1988.

Vernon, McCay, Joann A. Boughman and Linda Annala. *Considerations in Diagnosing Usher's Syndrome: RP and Hearing Loss*. Baltimore: RP Foundation Fighting Blindness, 1982.

Veterans Administration. *Federal Benefits for Veterans and Dependents*. Washington, D.C.: VA, 1988.

Vision Place (The). "Treating Glaucoma with Eye Drops." Available online. URL: http://www.thevisionplace.com/VisionPlaceIII/discover/treatglcdrops.htm.

———. "Laser Treatment for Glaucoma." Available online. URL: http://www.thevisionplace.com/VisionPlaceIII/discover/treatglclaser.htm.

Wall, M., and D. R. May. "Threshold Amsler Grid Testing in Maulopathies." *Ophthalmology* (September 1987): 1126–33.

Walsh, Sara R., and Robert Holzberg, eds. *Understanding and Educating the Deaf-Blind/Severely and Profoundly Handicapped*. Springfield, Ill.: Charles C. Thomas Publisher, 1981.

Ware, Mary A., and Lois O. Schwab. "Child Rearing by Blind Parents." *The New Outlook* (June 1971): 169–174.

Waring, A. O. "Results of the Prospective Evaluation of Radial Keratotomy (PERK) Study on Year After Surgery." *Ophthalmology* 92, no. 2 (February 1985): 177–198.

Warren, David H. *Blindness and Early Childhood Development*. New York: American Foundation for the Blind, 1977.

———. "Blindness and Early Development: Issues in Research Methodology." *The New Outlook* (February 1976): 53–60.

Weale, R. A. *Focus on Vision*. Cambridge, Mass.: Harvard University Press, 1982.

Weinberg, Nancy, and Rosina Santana. "Comic Books: Champions of the Disabled Stereotype." *Rehabilitation Literature* 39, nos. 11–12 (November–December 1978): 327–331.

Weiner, Florence. *No Apologies*. New York: St. Martin's Press, 1986.

Weisgerber, Robert A., et al., eds. *Training the Handicapped for Productive Employment*. Rockville, Md.: Aspen Publications, 1980.

Western Blind Rehabilitation Center. *WBRC Clinical Summary*. Palo Alto, Calif.: WBRC, 1987.

———. *Western Blind Rehabilitation Center*. Palo Alto, Calif.: WBRC, 1987.

Wilensky, Jacob T., and John E. Read, eds. *Primary Ophthalmology*. New York: Grune and Stratton Inc., 1984.

World Health Organization. *Available Data On Blindness (Update 1987)*. New York: WHO, 1987.

———. *Control of Vitamin A Deficiency and Xerophthalmia*. Geneva: WHO, 1982.

———. *Guidelines for Programmes for the Prevention of Blindness*. Geneva: WHO, 1979.

———. *The Use of Residual Vision by Visually Disabled Persons*. Copenhagen: WHO, 1981.

Woods, Virgil L. *Update in Lupus Research*. San Jose, Calif.: Bay Area Lupus Foundation, 1984.

Woodworth, Robert S., and Harold Schlosberg. *Experimental Psychology*. New York: Henry Holt and Company, 1958.

Worden, Helen W. "Aging and Blindness." *The New Outlook* (December 1976): 433–437.

Yanoff, Myron. "Magnetic Views of the Eye and Brain." *Sightsaving* 53, no. 4 (1984–85): 16–17.

Yudkin, John. *The Penguin Encyclopedia of Nutrition*. New York: Viking Press, 1985.

Ziegler, Martha. "Strength in Numbers: The National Network of Parent Coalitions." *Exceptional Parent* (June 1983): 57–58.

Zimmerman, Phillip. "HealthWatch: Nutritional Approaches to Degenerative Eye Diseases." *Townsend Letter for Doctors* (February/March 1988): 2.

Zinn, Walter J., and Herbert Solomon. *The Complete Guide to Eye Care, Eyeglasses, and Contact Lens*. Hollywood, Fla.: Frederick Fell Publishers Inc., 1986.

INDEX

Boldface page numbers indicate major treatment of a subject.

A

abacus **1**
ABLEDATA **1**
Abraham, David 116
accelerated speech 3
Access-Able Travel Source **1**
accessibility **1–2**
Access World 12
accommodation **2**
Act to Promote the Education of the Blind **2**
acyclovir **2**, 52
ADA. *See* Americans With Disabilities Act (ADA)
adaptation, aging and 6
adaptive aids **2–5**
   aging and 7
Administration for Children, Youth and Families 93
Administration on Developmental Disabilities 93
adrenergic agents 70
adventitiously blind, defined 29
advocacy **5**
AFB. *See* American Foundation for the Blind (AFB)
AFDC. *See* Aid to Families with Dependent Children (AFDC)
Age-Related Maculopathy (ARM) 6–7, 19–20
   central vision and 39
   laser treatment 135
   progression of 145–146
aging **5–7**
AIDS 7

Aid to Families with Dependent Children (AFDC) **7–8**, 95, 97
air bags **8**
Air Carrier Access Act 235
albinism **8**, 46
alcohol amblyopia **8–9**
Alice in Wonderland syndrome 153
Alliance for Eye and Vision Research 9, 159
Alva Access Group 9
amaurosis 9
amblyopia 8, **9–10**, 46, 183, 218
   anisometropia and 15
   central vision and 39
American Academy of Ophthalmology **10–11**, 86, 210
American Association of Instructors of the Blind (AAIB) 74
American Association of the Deaf-Blind (AADB) **11**
American Association of Workers for the Blind (AAWB) 21
American Braille Press 129
American Cancer Society 35
American Council of Blind Lions 139
American Council of the Blind (ACB) **11–12**
American Foundation for Overseas Blind 129
American Foundation for the Blind (AFB) **12**, 175, 194
   education and 74
   employment and 78, 79
American National Standards Institute (ANSI) 1–2, **13**
American Printing House for the Blind (APH) 2, **12–13**, 225

Americans With Disabilities Act (ADA) **13–14**, 165, 235
American Thermoform Corporation (ATC) **13**
ametropia **14**
Amsler, Marc 14
Amsler grid **14**, 146
Amtrak Improvement Act of 1973 193, 235
anesthetic drugs 69–70
aneurysm **14–15**
angioid streaks 200
aniridia **15**, 46
anisocoria **15**
anisometropia **15**
ANSI. *See* American National Standards Institute (ANSI)
anterior chamber **15**, 26, 85
antibiotics **16**
antifungal drugs 69
anti-inflammatory drugs 69
antiprotozoal drugs 69
antiviral drops 87
antiviral drugs 2, **16**, 51, 69
aphakia **16**
appetite suppressants **16–17**
aqueous fluid 15, **17**, 54, 81, 85
ARA-A **17**
Architectural and Transportation Barriers compliance Board 1
Architectural Barriers Act of 1968 **17**, 93, 165
arcus senilis 6, **17–18**
argon laser **18**, 135
Arianne Beheer B.V. 116
ARM. *See* Age-Related Maculopathy (ARM)
arterial occlusion **18–19**, 200